Office-Based Maxillofacial Surgical Procedures

Elie M. Ferneini • Michael T. Goupil
Editors

Office-Based Maxillofacial Surgical Procedures

A Step-by-step Approach

Springer

Editors
Elie M. Ferneini
Greater Waterbury OMS
Beau Visage Med Spa
Cheshire, CT
USA

Division of Oral and Maxillofacial Surgery
University of Connecticut School of Dental Medicine
Farmington, CT
USA

Michael T. Goupil
Division of Oral and Maxillofacial Surgery
University of Connecticut School of Dental Medicine
Farmington, CT
USA

ISBN 978-3-030-22370-0 ISBN 978-3-030-22371-7 (eBook)
https://doi.org/10.1007/978-3-030-22371-7

This Springer imprint is published by the registered company Springer Nature Switzerland AG
The registered company address is: Gewerbestrasse 11, 6330 Cham, Switzerland

Foreword

This book provides the reader a guide to the procedures that may be undertaken in a contemporary oral and maxillofacial surgery office setting. This work by Drs. Ferneini and Goupil is of excellent quality and could definitely be utilized as a curriculum model for office-based oral and maxillofacial surgical procedures. In general, it is divided into three broad sections when it comes to office-based procedures: perioperative techniques, dentoalveolar procedures, and maxillofacial cosmetic procedures.

Section one deals with perioperative techniques including general medical and facial assessment, laboratory studies, sedation techniques, and informed consent. It includes thorough discussions of both general and basic perioperative topics of interest to a wide range of surgeons, residents, and students. Section two focuses on dentoalveolar procedures in a step-by-step and well-illustrated fashion. It includes comprehensive explanations of procedures including biopsies, frenectomies, management of fistulas, and a couple of nice chapters on the removal of impacted teeth, as well as the coronectomy of third molars. The detail is excellent, and the references are consistently up-to-date. Section three explores the realm of aesthetic surgery of the maxillofacial region. The reader is provided an easy-to-follow, stepwise explanation of the more commonly performed cosmetic procedures including scar revision surgery, fillers, and nerve conduction blockers, as well as more advanced procedures such as blepharoplasty, genioplasty, and neck lifting.

This book is quite attractive because of its completeness and contemporary nature in an easy-to-read format. Drs. Ferneini and Goupil have been able to recruit a good mixture of both seasoned and younger contributors. They are to be commended for including the work of younger talents and giving them this exposure going forward. The multidisciplinary nature of the contributions will be attractive to many surgical specialties that manage disorders in and about the head and neck region.

I commend both Drs. Ferneini and Goupil for providing this ambitious and concise treatise which, I believe, will appeal to a wide readership at multiple levels.

Shreveport, LA, USA

G. E. Ghali

Contents

Contributors

Mohammad Banki Artistic Contours, Warwick, RI, USA

Daniel Beauvais Department of Oral and Maxillofacial Surgery, School of Dental Medicine, University of Connecticut, Farmington, CT, USA

Eric R. Bernstein University of Connecticut School of Dental Medicine, Farmington, CT, USA

Gregory Biron University of Pittsburgh Medical Center, Pittsburgh, PA, USA

Mina Boulos Thomas Jefferson University Hospital, Philadelphia, PA, USA

A. Michael Brown Division of Periodontology, University of Connecticut School of Dental Medicine, Farmington, CT, USA

Vernon Burke High Desert Oral and Facial Surgery, El Paso, TX, USA

Charles L. Castiglione Hartford Hospital, Connecticut Children's Medical Center, Hartford, CT, USA

Joy Xun Chen New York Presbyterian Hospital, Columbia University Medical Center, New York, NY, USA

Justin Clemow Case Western Reserve School of Dental Medicine, Metrohealth Medical Center, Cleveland, OH, USA

Kristopher Cooper University of Pittsburgh School of Dental Medicine and University of Pittsburgh Medical Center, Pittsburgh, PA, USA

L. Angelo Cuzalina OSU Medical School/Surgical Residency Program, Tulsa, OK, USA

Jonny Feldman Division of Orthodontics, UConn School of Dental Medicine, Farmington, CT, USA

Elie M. Ferneini Beau Visage Med Spa, Greater Waterbury OMS, Cheshire, CT, USA

Division of Oral and Maxillofacial Surgery, University of Connecticut, Farmington, CT, USA

Matthew J. Goldschmidt The Cosmetic Surgery Center, Independence, OH, USA

Michael T. Goupil University of Connecticut School of Dental Medicine, Farmington, CT, USA

Stephan Goupil Emerson Family Medicine at Emerson Hospital, Concord, MA, USA

Steven Halepas Department of Oral and Maxillofacial Surgery, New York Presbyterian Hospital, Columbia University Medical Center, New York, NY, USA

Christopher Haxhi UCLA Oral and Maxillofacial Surgery Department, Los Angeles, CA, USA

Douglas Johnson University of Florida Shands Jacksonville, Jacksonville, FL, USA

Neel S. Joshi Department of Surgery, University of Connecticut School of Medicine, Farmington, CT, USA

James E. Kennedy Division of Periodontology, University of Connecticut School of Dental Medicine, Farmington, CT, USA

Alia Koch New York Presbyterian Hospital, Columbia University Medical Center, New York, NY, USA

Regina Landesberg Oral/Maxillofacial Surgery, Simsbury, CT, USA

Frank de Latour William Beaumont Army Medical Center, Ft Bliss, TX, USA

Christy Lottinger University of Connecticut Oral and Maxillofacial Surgery, Farmington, CT, USA

Killian MacCarthy OMS Associates, South Portland, ME, USA

Tarryn MacCarthy Mbrace Orthodontic, Falmouth, ME, USA

Damon McIntire Warren Alpert Medical School of Brown University, Providence, RI, USA

Julie McNeish University of Connecticut Oral and Maxillofacial Surgery, Farmington, CT, USA

Nicholas A. Nagaki University of Connecticut Oral and Maxillofacial Surgery, Farmington, CT, USA

Frank C. Nichols Division of Periodontology, University of Connecticut School of Dental Medicine, Farmington, CT, USA

Christine Niekrash Frank H Netter MD School of Medicine, Quinnipiac University, Hamden, CT, USA

Benjamin Noblitt University of Cincinnati Oral and Maxillofacial Surgery, Cincinnati, OH, USA

Erik J. Nuveen Cosmetic Surgery Affiliates, Oklahoma City, OK, USA

Department of Oral and Maxillofacial Surgery, The University of Oklahoma, Oklahoma City, OK, USA

Frank Paletta Warren Alpert Medical School of Brown University, Providence, RI, USA

Joseph A. Perrone Yale New Haven Hospital, New Haven, CT, USA

Eric Ress UConn School of Dental Medicine, Farmington, CT, USA

Craig H. Rhyne United States Air Force, Alamo Heights, TX, USA

Amir Tadros Division of Oral and Maxillofacial Surgery, School of Dental Medicine, University of Connecticut, Farmington, CT, USA

Tyler J. Thomas Indiana Restorative Dentistry, Carmel, IN, USA

Clarence L. Trummel Division of Periodontology, University of Connecticut School of Dental Medicine, Farmington, CT, USA

Zulara N. Wahla Department of Surgery, University of Connecticut School of Medicine, Farmington, CT, USA

Part I

Perioperative Techniques

1 Medical Assessment

Joseph A. Perrone

The treatment of patients is becoming more and more complex every day. It is not practical to simply learn a procedure and expect that it will be successful in every patient. Rather, one must consider modifications based on each patient's specific history. New advances and technologies are continually transforming medicine and dentistry into fields that are more specialized and complex than ever. Patients are now expecting more individualized treatments as well. As new conditions continue to be discovered, new medications developed, and new treatment modalities invented, the environment in which oral surgeons practice can seem overwhelming. However, as trained medical professionals, there is an established protocol to assessing every individual patient, no matter how complex things may seem. Medicine has developed a systematic way to recognize and categorize the risks with which any individual may present. It becomes the surgeon's job, when treating patients, to become aware of each individual's potential risks, and then provide a patient-specific and comprehensive treatment plan. It all starts with an appropriate medical assessment.

Patient Registration Forms

In this digital world, it is often possible to start the medical assessment of a patient before they ever enter the office. This is done with patient registration forms that incorporate both demographic information and a medical history questionnaire. This should be done in a simple, easy-to-read format that is comprehensive but not overly cumbersome. There are several recommended forms available by organizations such as the ADA. Figure 1.1 shows an example of a patient registration form. This can be emailed, faxed, mailed in paper form, or even picked up in person by

J. A. Perrone (✉)
Yale New Haven Hospital, New Haven, CT, USA
e-mail: jperrone@ctomfs.com

E. M. Ferneini, M. T. Goupil (eds.), *Office-Based Maxillofacial Surgical Procedures*, https://doi.org/10.1007/978-3-030-22371-7_1

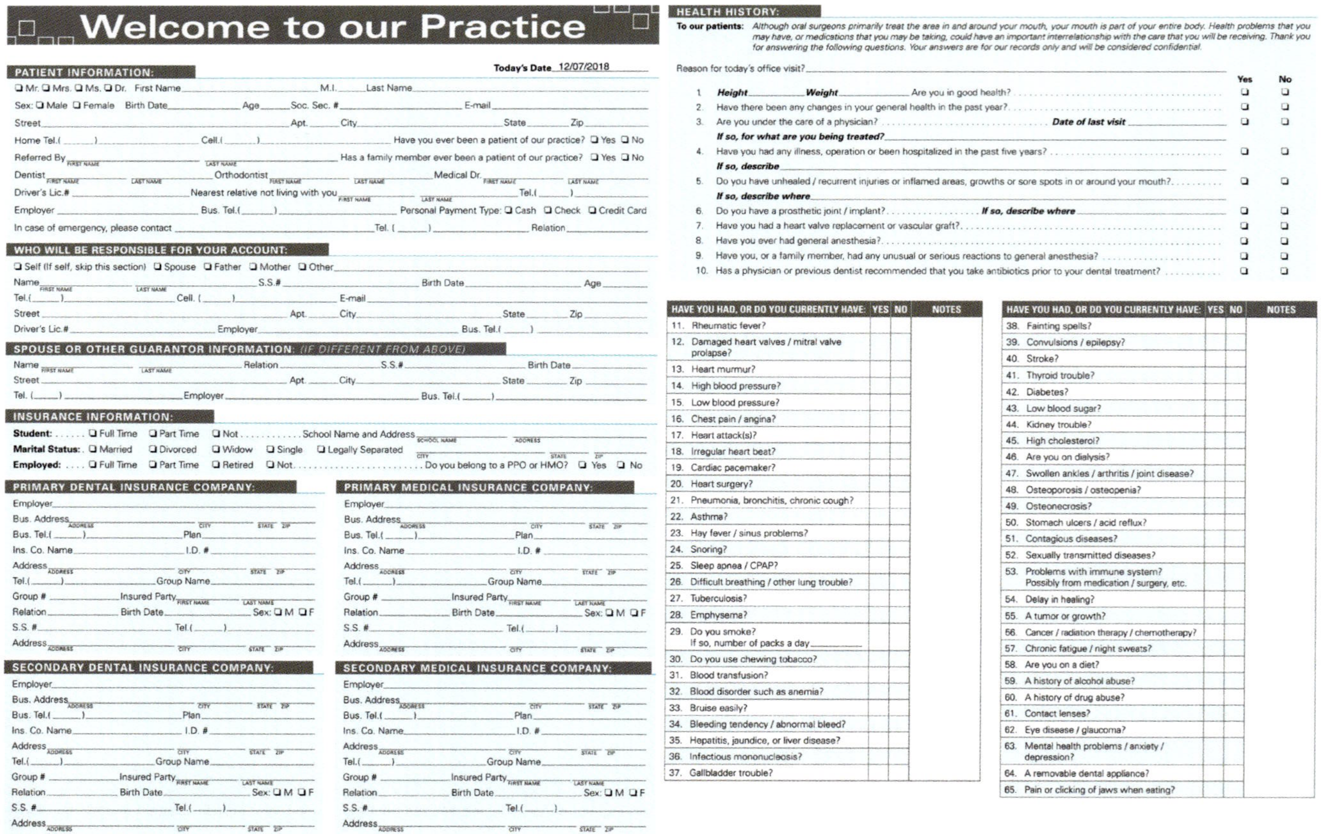

Welcome to our Practice

PATIENT INFORMATION: Today's Date 12/07/2018

❑ Mr. ❑ Mrs. ❑ Ms. ❑ Dr. First Name ___ M.I. ___ Last Name ___
Sex: ❑ Male ❑ Female Birth Date ___ Age ___ Soc. Sec. # ___ E-mail ___
Street ___ Apt. ___ City ___ State ___ Zip ___
Home Tel.( ) ___ Cell.( ) ___ Have you ever been a patient of our practice? ❑ Yes ❑ No
Referred By ___ (FIRST NAME / LAST NAME) Has a family member ever been a patient of our practice? ❑ Yes ❑ No
Dentist ___ (FIRST NAME / LAST NAME) Orthodontist ___ (FIRST NAME / LAST NAME) Medical Dr. ___ (FIRST NAME / LAST NAME)
Driver's Lic.# ___ Nearest relative not living with you ___ (FIRST NAME / LAST NAME) Tel.( ) ___
Employer ___ Bus. Tel.( ) ___ Personal Payment Type: ❑ Cash ❑ Check ❑ Credit Card
In case of emergency, please contact ___ Tel. ( ) ___ Relation ___

WHO WILL BE RESPONSIBLE FOR YOUR ACCOUNT:

❑ Self (If self, skip this section) ❑ Spouse ❑ Father ❑ Mother ❑ Other ___
Name ___ (FIRST NAME / LAST NAME) S.S.# ___ Birth Date ___ Age ___
Tel.( ) ___ Cell. ( ) ___ E-mail ___
Street ___ Apt. ___ City ___ State ___ Zip ___
Driver's Lic.# ___ Employer ___ Bus. Tel.( ) ___

SPOUSE OR OTHER GUARANTOR INFORMATION: *(IF DIFFERENT FROM ABOVE)*

Name ___ (FIRST NAME / LAST NAME) Relation ___ S.S.# ___ Birth Date ___
Street ___ Apt. ___ City ___ State ___ Zip ___
Tel. ( ) ___ Employer ___ Bus. Tel.( ) ___

INSURANCE INFORMATION:

Student: ...... ❑ Full Time ❑ Part Time ❑ Not .... School Name and Address ___ (SCHOOL NAME / ADDRESS / CITY / STATE / ZIP)
Marital Status: . ❑ Married ❑ Divorced ❑ Widow ❑ Single ❑ Legally Separated
Employed: .... ❑ Full Time ❑ Part Time ❑ Retired ❑ Not........................ Do you belong to a PPO or HMO? ❑ Yes ❑ No

PRIMARY DENTAL INSURANCE COMPANY:

Employer ___
Bus. Address ___ (ADDRESS / CITY / STATE / ZIP)
Bus. Tel.( ) ___ Plan ___
Ins. Co. Name ___ I.D. # ___
Address ___ (ADDRESS / CITY / STATE / ZIP)
Tel.( ) ___ Group Name ___
Group # ___ Insured Party ___ (FIRST NAME / LAST NAME)
Relation ___ Birth Date ___ Sex: ❑ M ❑ F
S.S. # ___ Tel.( ) ___
Address ___ (ADDRESS / CITY / STATE / ZIP)

PRIMARY MEDICAL INSURANCE COMPANY:

Employer ___
Bus. Address ___ (ADDRESS / CITY / STATE / ZIP)
Bus. Tel.( ) ___ Plan ___
Ins. Co. Name ___ I.D. # ___
Address ___ (ADDRESS / CITY / STATE / ZIP)
Tel.( ) ___ Group Name ___
Group # ___ Insured Party ___ (FIRST NAME / LAST NAME)
Relation ___ Birth Date ___ Sex: ❑ M ❑ F
S.S. # ___ Tel.( ) ___
Address ___ (ADDRESS / CITY / STATE / ZIP)

SECONDARY DENTAL INSURANCE COMPANY:

Employer ___
Bus. Address ___ (ADDRESS / CITY / STATE / ZIP)
Bus. Tel.( ) ___ Plan ___
Ins. Co. Name ___ I.D. # ___
Address ___ (ADDRESS / CITY / STATE / ZIP)
Tel.( ) ___ Group Name ___
Group # ___ Insured Party ___ (FIRST NAME / LAST NAME)
Relation ___ Birth Date ___ Sex: ❑ M ❑ F
S.S. # ___ Tel.( ) ___
Address ___ (ADDRESS / CITY / STATE / ZIP)

SECONDARY MEDICAL INSURANCE COMPANY:

Employer ___
Bus. Address ___ (ADDRESS / CITY / STATE / ZIP)
Bus. Tel.( ) ___ Plan ___
Ins. Co. Name ___ I.D. # ___
Address ___ (ADDRESS / CITY / STATE / ZIP)
Tel.( ) ___ Group Name ___
Group # ___ Insured Party ___ (FIRST NAME / LAST NAME)
Relation ___ Birth Date ___ Sex: ❑ M ❑ F
S.S. # ___ Tel.( ) ___
Address ___ (ADDRESS / CITY / STATE / ZIP)

HEALTH HISTORY:

To our patients: *Although oral surgeons primarily treat the area in and around your mouth, your mouth is part of your entire body. Health problems that you may have, or medications that you may be taking, could have an important interrelationship with the care that you will be receiving. Thank you for answering the following questions. Your answers are for our records only and will be considered confidential.*

Reason for today's office visit? ___

	Yes	No
1. ***Height*** ___ ***Weight*** ___ Are you in good health?	❑	❑
2. Have there been any changes in your general health in the past year?	❑	❑
3. Are you under the care of a physician? ***Date of last visit*** ___	❑	❑
If so, for what are you being treated? ___		
4. Have you had any illness, operation or been hospitalized in the past five years?	❑	❑
If so, describe ___		
5. Do you have unhealed / recurrent injuries or inflamed areas, growths or sore spots in or around your mouth?	❑	❑
If so, describe where ___		
6. Do you have a prosthetic joint / implant? ***If so, describe where*** ___	❑	❑
7. Have you had a heart valve replacement or vascular graft?	❑	❑
8. Have you ever had general anesthesia?	❑	❑
9. Have you, or a family member, had any unusual or serious reactions to general anesthesia?	❑	❑
10. Has a physician or previous dentist recommended that you take antibiotics prior to your dental treatment?	❑	❑

HAVE YOU HAD, OR DO YOU CURRENTLY HAVE:	YES	NO	NOTES
11. Rheumatic fever?			
12. Damaged heart valves / mitral valve prolapse?			
13. Heart murmur?			
14. High blood pressure?			
15. Low blood pressure?			
16. Chest pain / angina?			
17. Heart attack(s)?			
18. Irregular heart beat?			
19. Cardiac pacemaker?			
20. Heart surgery?			
21. Pneumonia, bronchitis, chronic cough?			
22. Asthma?			
23. Hay fever / sinus problems?			
24. Snoring?			
25. Sleep apnea / CPAP?			
26. Difficult breathing / other lung trouble?			
27. Tuberculosis?			
28. Emphysema?			
29. Do you smoke? If so, number of packs a day ___			
30. Do you use chewing tobacco?			
31. Blood transfusion?			
32. Blood disorder such as anemia?			
33. Bruise easily?			
34. Bleeding tendency / abnormal bleed?			
35. Hepatitis, jaundice, or liver disease?			
36. Infectious mononucleosis?			
37. Gallbladder trouble?			

HAVE YOU HAD, OR DO YOU CURRENTLY HAVE:	YES	NO	NOTES
38. Fainting spells?			
39. Convulsions / epilepsy?			
40. Stroke?			
41. Thyroid trouble?			
42. Diabetes?			
43. Low blood sugar?			
44. Kidney trouble?			
45. High cholesterol?			
46. Are you on dialysis?			
47. Swollen ankles / arthritis / joint disease?			
48. Osteoporosis / osteopenia?			
49. Osteonecrosis?			
50. Stomach ulcers / acid reflux?			
51. Contagious diseases?			
52. Sexually transmitted diseases?			
53. Problems with immune system? Possibly from medication / surgery, etc.			
54. Delay in healing?			
55. A tumor or growth?			
56. Cancer / radiation therapy / chemotherapy?			
57. Chronic fatigue / night sweats?			
58. Are you on a diet?			
59. A history of alcohol abuse?			
60. A history of drug abuse?			
61. Contact lenses?			
62. Eye disease / glaucoma?			
63. Mental health problems / anxiety / depression?			
64. A removable dental appliance?			
65. Pain or clicking of jaws when eating?			

Fig. 1.1 Patient intake form that can be filled out online prior to the appointment (Copyright PBHS, Inc.)

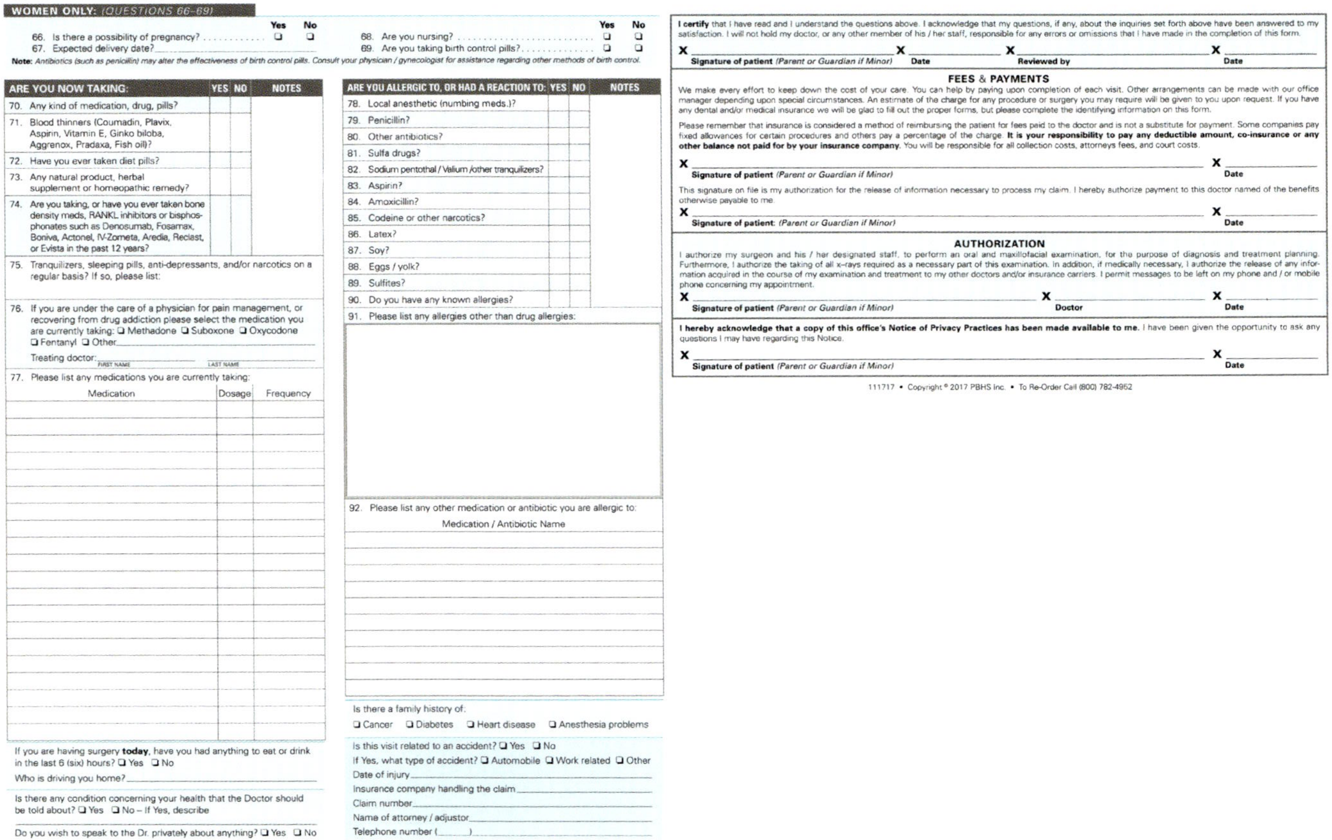

WOMEN ONLY: *(QUESTIONS 66–69)*

	Yes	No
66. Is there a possibility of pregnancy?	❑	❑
67. Expected delivery date? ______		
68. Are you nursing?	❑	❑
69. Are you taking birth control pills?	❑	❑

Note: *Antibiotics (such as penicillin) may alter the effectiveness of birth control pills. Consult your physician / gynecologist for assistance regarding other methods of birth control.*

ARE YOU NOW TAKING:	YES	NO	NOTES
70. Any kind of medication, drug, pills?			
71. Blood thinners (Coumadin, Plavix, Aspirin, Vitamin E, Ginko biloba, Aggrenox, Pradaxa, Fish oil)?			
72. Have you ever taken diet pills?			
73. Any natural product, herbal supplement or homeopathic remedy?			
74. Are you taking, or have you ever taken bone density meds, RANKL inhibitors or bisphosphonates such as Denosumab, Fosamax, Boniva, Actonel, IV-Zometa, Aredia, Reclast, or Evista in the past 12 years?			

75. Tranquilizers, sleeping pills, anti-depressants, and/or narcotics on a regular basis? If so, please list:

76. If you are under the care of a physician for pain management, or recovering from drug addiction please select the medication you are currently taking: ❑ Methadone ❑ Suboxone ❑ Oxycodone ❑ Fentanyl ❑ Other ______

Treating doctor: ______ (FIRST NAME) ______ (LAST NAME)

77. Please list any medications you are currently taking:

Medication	Dosage	Frequency

If you are having surgery **today**, have you had anything to eat or drink in the last 6 (six) hours? ❑ Yes ❑ No

Who is driving you home? ______

Is there any condition concerning your health that the Doctor should be told about? ❑ Yes ❑ No – If Yes, describe ______

Do you wish to speak to the Dr. privately about anything? ❑ Yes ❑ No

ARE YOU ALLERGIC TO, OR HAD A REACTION TO:	YES	NO	NOTES
78. Local anesthetic (numbing meds.)?			
79. Penicillin?			
80. Other antibiotics?			
81. Sulfa drugs?			
82. Sodium pentothal / Valium /other tranquilizers?			
83. Aspirin?			
84. Amoxicillin?			
85. Codeine or other narcotics?			
86. Latex?			
87. Soy?			
88. Eggs / yolk?			
89. Sulfites?			
90. Do you have any known allergies?			

91. Please list any allergies other than drug allergies:

92. Please list any other medication or antibiotic you are allergic to:

Medication / Antibiotic Name

Is there a family history of:
❑ Cancer ❑ Diabetes ❑ Heart disease ❑ Anesthesia problems

Is this visit related to an accident? ❑ Yes ❑ No
If Yes, what type of accident? ❑ Automobile ❑ Work related ❑ Other
Date of injury ______
Insurance company handling the claim ______
Claim number ______
Name of attorney / adjustor ______
Telephone number (____) ______

I certify that I have read and I understand the questions above. I acknowledge that my questions, if any, about the inquiries set forth above have been answered to my satisfaction. I will not hold my doctor, or any other member of his / her staff, responsible for any errors or omissions that I have made in the completion of this form.

X ______ **Signature of patient** *(Parent or Guardian if Minor)* X ______ **Date** X ______ **Reviewed by** X ______ **Date**

FEES & PAYMENTS

We make every effort to keep down the cost of your care. You can help by paying upon completion of each visit. Other arrangements can be made with our office manager depending upon special circumstances. An estimate of the charge for any procedure or surgery you may require will be given to you upon request. If you have any dental and/or medical insurance we will be glad to fill out the proper forms, but please complete the identifying information on this form.

Please remember that insurance is considered a method of reimbursing the patient for fees paid to the doctor and is not a substitute for payment. Some companies pay fixed allowances for certain procedures and others pay a percentage of the charge. **It is your responsibility to pay any deductible amount, co-insurance or any other balance not paid for by your insurance company.** You will be responsible for all collection costs, attorneys fees, and court costs.

X ______ **Signature of patient** *(Parent or Guardian if Minor)* X ______ **Date**

This signature on file is my authorization for the release of information necessary to process my claim. I hereby authorize payment to this doctor named of the benefits otherwise payable to me.

X ______ **Signature of patient:** *(Parent or Guardian if Minor)* X ______ **Date**

AUTHORIZATION

I authorize my surgeon and his / her designated staff, to perform an oral and maxillofacial examination, for the purpose of diagnosis and treatment planning. Furthermore, I authorize the taking of all x–rays required as a necessary part of this examination. In addition, if medically necessary, I authorize the release of any information acquired in the course of my examination and treatment to my other doctors and/or insurance carriers. I permit messages to be left on my phone and / or mobile phone concerning my appointment.

X ______ **Signature of patient** *(Parent or Guardian if Minor)* X ______ **Doctor** X ______ **Date**

I hereby acknowledge that a copy of this office's Notice of Privacy Practices has been made available to me. I have been given the opportunity to ask any questions I may have regarding this Notice.

X ______ **Signature of patient** *(Parent or Guardian if Minor)* X ______ **Date**

Fig. 1.1 (continued)

the patient ahead of time. Ideally, this information is available to the oral surgeon for review prior to the patient's appointment.

Demographic information obtained on these forms typically includes the patient's name, age, sex, occupation, email, phone number, and home address among other things. This information is valuable for providing the office with a means of communication with the patient. It also is able to provide some insight into the patient's level of healthcare literacy and investment in their care. Forms that are filled out incompletely or haphazardly should be a clue that perhaps the patient is not invested in their care or doesn't understand the importance of the requested information. It could be a clue about the patient's level of education and/or literacy. It is important to remember that these forms are typically being completed by people who do not have a significant background in medicine and/or dentistry. That makes it the surgeon's job to extract the information that is pertinent to the care that he or she will be providing.

The second portion of the form is the medical history, which will have a list of common conditions that may impact the patient's dental or surgical treatment. These will act as prompts to remind the patient of things they may not otherwise recall while filling out the form. There should also be a section that allows for the patient to enter free text information if they so desire. Sometimes a patient's issue does not seem to fit in any one box or category, and often that information may be left out if there is not an area for the patient to include any other important information. There will also be a section for the patient to fill out the list of their medications, and an area for allergies, also with prompts and a write-in or free-text area.

Once this information is collected, it is the job of the surgeon to review everything, and to make sure that the information contained in the different sections of the form are consistent with each other. A common occurrence is for patients to fill out the form with few or even no health conditions listed, yet they provide a list of six or seven medications. This is a clue that the patient may not have fully understood the purpose of the form, or perhaps they may not understand their own medical history. This should prompt the clinician to address the inconsistencies in the form to obtain a complete and accurate picture of the patient's medical status.

History and Physical

One of the most important jobs of any clinician upon meeting a patient for the first time is to obtain an accurate history. Often times a thorough and detailed history will provide the clinician with the majority of the information they need, with the physical exam, labs, and radiographs acting as confirmatory information to what the clinician already knows. There is a standard format for medical history taking (Table 1.1). Practicing and following this pattern each and every time will ensure that no information is skipped or missed. It also allows for effective and efficient communication among providers. When multiple clinicians all utilize the same format for transfer of information, each person is able to anticipate what is about to be discussed, so they are prepared to hear and digest the implications of the

Table 1.1 History and physical exam

Chief complaint
History of present illness
Past medical history
Surgical history
Family history
Social history
Medications
Allergies
Review of systems
Physical examination
Laboratory data and imaging

Table 1.2 Chief complaint

"What is the main reason you have come to see me today?"
Addresses the patient's #1 concern

information being conveyed. The medical history always starts with the patient's chief complaint (CC), then progresses to a history of present illness (HPI), past medical history (PMH), surgical history (SxH), family history (FH), social history (SH), a list of medications, and allergies. This is then followed by a review of systems (ROS), which is a way for the provider to screen for potential undiagnosed issues that may be of importance for the patient's upcoming care.

Chief Complaint

It is critical to always start with the patient's chief complaint. The chief complaint is the single most important reason that the patient is seeking care (Table 1.2). It is important to have the patient specify, in their own words, what is the main purpose of their visit to the office. This reason is twofold. First, it gives the provider an opportunity to understand what is most important to the patient. Secondly, it forces the patient to think about and express clearly in words the reason that they have come to your office. Once the chief complaint has been established, there may be other concerns that the patient would like to have addressed as well. However, they are unlikely to be satisfied if the chief complaint is not specifically addressed. Addressing the chief complaint gives the patient the feeling that the clinician is listening to their concerns and cares about helping them with what they are most concerned about. If the surgeon doesn't ask, he or she will never truly know what the patient hopes to get out of the appointment.

History of Present Illness

The chief complaint is always followed up by a series of questions by the provider to elucidate the history of present illness (Table 1.3). If the patient's chief complaint is pain in a tooth, the doctor will need to find out more specific information.

Table 1.3 Common HPI questions

When did this start?
What were you doing when it started?
How long has it lasted?
Do the symptoms fluctuate?
What makes it worse? Better?
Where exactly are you experiencing these symptoms?
How intense is it?
What have you done so far to deal with it?
Have you been treated for this already, and if so, what has been done?

Table 1.4 Common medical conditions that may need attention

Cardiac	Coronary Artery Disease, Heart Valve Disease, Congestive Heart Failure, Arrhythmias
Pulmonary	Asthma, COPD, Obesity
Renal	Chronic Kidney Disease, Dialysis
Hepatic	Hepatitis, Cirrhosis, Fatty Liver
Hematological	von Willebrand Disease, Hemophilias, Antiphospholipid Antibody Syndrome
Autoimmune	Lupus, Grave's Disease, Hashimoto's Thyroiditis
Endocrine	Diabetes Mellitus, Thyroid Disease, Adrenal Insufficiency
Neurological	Seizures, Stroke, Dementia
Musculoskeletal	Total joint replacement, spinal conditions, osteoporosis
Cancer	Head and neck, Non-Head and neck
Drug Abuse	Opiates, Cocaine, Marijuana, Methamphetamines
Pregnancy	

Follow-up questions would include things like "When did the pain start? What were you doing when it started? How bad is the pain? When is it at its worst? Does anything make it better? Does anything make it worse? What is the character of the pain? Where is the pain? Does it radiate anywhere? What does it feel like? Have you had any swelling?" All of this information will allow the doctor to begin to formulate a picture of what is going on and start to create a list of potential diagnoses. It is also important to understand what treatments the patient may have already had. "Have you seen any other doctors? Did they start you on antibiotics? Did they do any procedures for you?" Knowing all of this information will give the surgeon the full picture of where the patient has been, what has been done, where they need to be, and what options are left.

Past Medical History

Once there is a satisfactory understanding of the patient's current problem, the surgeon needs to review the patient's past medical history. Generally, for the oral surgeon, it is acceptable to briefly review things that are not likely to have a major impact on treatment, but more time should be spent on conditions that may have significant consequences (Table 1.4). These would include cardiac, pulmonary, liver, renal, and hematologic diseases among others. At this point it is advisable to also review the patient's medication list again to make sure that the PMH includes all the conditions that the patient is being medicated for, and none that they should be medicated for, but aren't. This is a way for the surgeon to double check the patient's memory and the forms that have been filled out. It is not unusual for patients to omit significant medical conditions because they are being effectively treated with medication. One such example is the patient who fails to disclose his congestive heart failure because it is effectively controlled by medication. An absence of cardiac issues in the PMH but several cardiac medications in the med list should immediately prompt the surgeon to ask about the reason the patient is on cardiac medication. The clinician can then explore the history of the condition, and how it has led to the need for medical management. In today's world, patients are living longer and are commonly seeking out elective care at advanced ages. Many of these elderly patients are being managed for multiple medical conditions, and new drugs are coming out seemingly every day. It is important to be well versed in the medications that are commonly prescribed and how they work. This is becoming more difficult, but fortunately there are a wide variety of tools for practitioners to use to find out critical information about medications.

Surgical History

The next section of the history is the patient's surgical history. Just like the PMH, surgical history can be brief or very extensive. Even if the surgical history seems unrelated or irrelevant, there is always valuable information that can be obtained. Most surgical procedures have several things in common (Table 1.5). These include anesthesia, bleeding, pain, and recovery time. Exploring a patient's prior experience with surgery can give the surgeon many clues about potential risks that may be experienced in an upcoming surgery. If planning for an IV anesthetic, it would be foolish to ignore previous IV anesthetic experiences. If a patient experienced significant nausea and vomiting following a colonoscopy, perhaps the surgeon should consider antiemetic medications in conjunction with the upcoming anesthetic. If a patient had postoperative bleeding following foot surgery, perhaps the surgeon should obtain preoperative labs and plan to have local hemostatic materials available for surgery. Prior uncontrolled pain after a surgery should lead to a discussion about the ineffective means of controlling that pain. The surgeon and the patient should have a different preoperative plan for postoperative pain control. If patients have previously had poor or prolonged healing, perhaps nutritional deficiencies

Table 1.5 Things to ask about past surgical experiences

Were there any anesthetic complications?
Were there any surgical complications?
Did you have excessive postoperative bleeding?
Did you have a postoperative infection?
How was your pain control following surgery?
Did you have any unusual delay in healing?

exist that should be rectified prior to surgery. It is easy to see that in preparing for an oral surgical procedure, an otherwise unrelated surgery could provide clues to how the patient will respond to the proposed treatment.

Family History

Family history is typically the next area to explore. Many times, it is helpful to have family members present at the consultation to help with gathering this information. Particularly in younger patients, who may not have a significant PMH of their own, family history can provide some important clues for the oral surgeon. While it is not necessary to figure out every condition that every relative was ever diagnosed with, it is important to focus on things that could seriously impact the patient's health or could present considerable risk for a planned surgery. Things such as sudden death as a result of hypertrophic obstructive cardiomyopathy or severe anesthetic complications such as malignant hyperthermia may be cause for postponing surgery until it can be verified that these things are not applicable to your patient. If they are applicable, modification of the treatment plan may be necessary, and often times this will include coordination with additional providers.

Social History

The last section of history taking is the social history. Many providers are hesitant to ask about this because it may be uncomfortable or seem impolite. In the doctor's office, there is no judgement about a patient's risky behaviors. It is inappropriate to avoid asking questions that may have implications for the patient's care simply because it is uncomfortable. Typically, the things to explore in this section include drug use, alcohol use, smoking, sexual activity, and other risky behavior such as occupational or recreational hazards. Of all the history questions that doctors typically ask, these questions are the ones most likely to be answered untruthfully on purpose. Patient's may not understand the importance of these questions and think that they are unrelated to their care. That will make them less likely to report the truth. They may have fear of getting in trouble with the law if the behavior is illegal. They may be embarrassed about their behavior, making it difficult to share with someone whom they have only just met. More importantly, they may want to keep this information secret from a friend or family member who is also present in the room. It is critical for these questions to be asked in a nonthreatening setting, absent of any other family members or friends, and with assurances of confidentiality.

Review of Systems

Once all of the patient's known history is reviewed with pertinent information recorded, the surgeon should proceed to the review of systems. While it may seem repetitive at first glance, the review of systems is not simply a second round of the

PMH. The ROS is a series of questions to attempt to determine if the patient may have a medical condition that they have not yet had diagnosed. An example of this would asking, "Do you get dehydrated and find yourself having to urinate an excessive number of times per day?" instead of asking, "Do you have diabetes?" This allows the surgeon to investigate any suspicious part of the health history that does not seem to be accounted for. It is yet another way to gather important information that may affect the outcome of a procedure, but it also is a service to the patient to potentially get them medical treatment they didn't even know they needed.

Physical Exam

The next step of the initial patient interview is to proceed with the physical exam (Table 1.6). In the dental office, the majority of the exam will focus on the head and neck, paying particular attention to the mouth and the dentition. It is not necessary to have the patient remove clothing (with the exception perhaps of glasses, hats, gloves, scarves, and winter coats). As with history taking, it is important to have an established, systematic approach to examining a patient. By following the same routine every time, the surgeon can ensure that he or she does not neglect a portion of the physical exam.

Vital Signs

It seems obvious that vital signs are a vital portion of your examination. Vital signs should be taken on every patient. Vital signs include heart rate, blood pressure, respiratory rate, and temperature (Table 1.7). Most practitioners have staff that should be comfortable in obtaining a patient's vital signs. This can be accomplished

Table 1.6 Physical examination

Vital Signs	
General Appearance	
Head and Neck Examination	
H	Head (scalp, forehead)
E	Eyes
E	Ears
N	Nose
T	Throat/teeth (includes intraoral examination)
Neck	
Cardiopulmonary	
Any additional relevant systems	

Table 1.7 Vital signs

Heart rate
Blood pressure
Respiratory rate
Temperature

manually, via automated systems, or a combination of both. This information is typically available for the clinician to review prior to entering the room. It can give significant clues to the patient's overall well-being and ability to tolerate a procedure. Some of the most common abnormalities in vital signs encountered in the oral surgeon's office are hypertension and tachycardia. This can often be attributed to dental anxiety, but many times it is because patients haven't been taking their prescribed medications or they have not seen a physician in a long time. Another abnormality that may be encountered is an otherwise asymptomatic patient with a resting heart rate in the 30 s or 40 s. Recognizing an abnormality such as this and a referral to a cardiologist could potentially save someone's life, and at the very least would significant decrease the risk of that patient having an acute cardiac event while in the office.

General Appearance

After assessing the patient's vital signs, typically the next assessment will be the patient's general appearance (Table 1.8). This is done simply through observation. With practice and experience, there is a lot of information that one can gather simply through careful observation of the patient. These include, but are not limited to: Does the patient appear their stated age? Do they appear healthy with normal energy? Do they appear well developed? Do they appear malnourished? Does their color seem normal, or do they look pale, blue, or red? Is their breathing easy and relaxed? Are they sitting comfortably or are they anxiously looking around the room and squirming in the chair? Are they appropriately dressed? Do they appear clean? Do they appear disheveled? Do they interact appropriately with you, and make eye contact when speaking? This assessment can be done in a matter of seconds, and it is impressive how much information one can gather simply by carefully observing the patient and their body language. This is not typically done as a distinct portion of the exam, since staring at a patient in silence is likely to make them uncomfortable, but it is done subtly and discretely while the surgeon introduces himself and obtains the medical history.

Head and Neck Examination

After obtaining the medical history and going through the review of systems most clinicians will proceed to their hands-on physical examination. There are many different ways to do this. Some might argue one way is better than another,

Table 1.8 General appearance

Clean and wearing appropriate clothing?
Well developed or malnourished?
Good color? Energy?
Breathing normally with a normal rate?
Eye contact?
Normal and appropriate posture?

Table 1.9 Highlights of head and neck exam

Head	Visualize and palpate hair, scalp, and forehead, facial nerve exam
Eyes	Check gross vision, extraocular movements, pupillary light response, Look at color of sclera, shape of pupils
Ears	Assess gross hearing bilateral, look at external ear, look at canal and tympanic membrane with otoscope
Nose	Look for deviation, palpate bridge for mobility, assess nares are patent, use speculum to visualize inside the nose and rule out septal hematoma
Teeth (mouth)	Look for swelling, palpable along maxilla, mandible, and TMJ, measure MIO, check occlusion, look at all mucosal surfaces, look at teeth, palpation/percussion of teeth, probing depths, caries, fractured teeth, and periodontal defects
Neck	Visual inspection, palpation for cervical lymph nodes, palpation of thyroid, identify cricothyroid membrane, assess mobility

but generally speaking, as long as the examination is thorough and complete, any method will work as long as it is performed consistently. Consistency is the key to accomplishing a complete detailed examination every time. One method that seems to work well for many surgeons is to progress through the exam "Outside to inside, and top to bottom." Another technique is to specifically describe findings in the categories HEENT. This stands for Head (scalp, forehead), Eyes, Ears, Nose, and Teeth (or Throat) to emphasize doing an intraoral examination as well (Table 1.9). Depending on the patient's presentation and chief complaint, this exam can be tailored to focus on the problem at hand. It may not be necessary to do a comprehensive facial trauma examination when someone presents with dental pain from a carious tooth. However, it is useful to follow the same pattern in more or less detail depending on the circumstances. A comprehensive examination is important to learn and practice early in one's career. After you become comfortable with a comprehensive examination, you can quickly assess portions of the exam that are unlikely to be involved and focus more time on the pertinent areas of interest. A basic head and neck trauma evaluation is described below, and can be simplified as necessary for each particular patient. One final tip which is often overlooked in a trauma examination is to first thoroughly clean the patient of dirt, debris, and blood which could cover or hide injuries from the examiner.

Starting on the outside, in top-to-bottom fashion, first look at the scalp or hair. Notice any irregularities in the hair or in the skin of the scalp itself. Look for lacerations or signs of bleeding, bruising, or swelling. Then start to move down. Examine the forehead looking at the skin, contours, muscle animation and wrinkles. Do the muscles animate symmetrically? Assess facial nerve function. Are there any contour defects or indentations?

Progressing downwards, next is the eye exam. Look at the position of the eyebrows and lids, taking note of any asymmetry. Palpate the superior and inferior orbital rims looking for step-offs or irregularities. Check for enophthalmos or exophthalmos. Look for pupils that are round and of equal size. Check pupillary light response to ensure that both pupils constrict equally when a light is shined in either eye. Assess extraocular movements by taking the patient through the full range of eye movements. Look for any discoloration of the sclera. Assess vision grossly in each eye with an eye chart. In the event of traumatic injuries, it would often be wise to have an even more detailed eye exam completed by an ophthalmologist which would likely include a dilated exam with measurements of intraocular pressures among other tests.

Moving further down the face, next check the nose. Visual inspection should be first, looking for asymmetry or any deviation of the nasal bridge or tip. Palpate the bridge of the nose feeling for mobility or crepitus. Look for lacerations. Obstruct each nostril with a finger and evaluate the patient's ability to breathe through each side. Is there any epistaxis? Use a nasal speculum and light source to adequately visualize inside the nose to look for mucosal tears or other sources of bleeding. Importantly, look for a septal hematoma, which if untreated could result in a permanent nasal defect.

Then move posteriorly from the nose towards the ears. Look at the malar eminence while palpating along the cheek bones paying attention to asymmetries, swelling, bruising, lacerations, and bony irregularities. Continue to the ears. Test a patient's gross hearing in each ear. Look for lacerations both externally and within the canal. Use an otoscope to evaluate the tympanic membrane and internal canal. The ear is another place where untreated hematomas can lead to permanent deformities. Pay special attention to injuries that have resulted in edema of the soft tissue of the ear or collection of blood below the skin.

Lastly, we come to the lower face. This part is often divided into an extraoral examination and intraoral examination. Extraorally, look at the skin and lips for lacerations, bruising, asymmetry, or other gross abnormalities. Palpate both jaws, paying particular attention to the inferior border of the lower jaw. Assess the temporomandibular joints through palpation and have the patient function by opening and closing, as well as attempting excursive movements. Palpate the neck and submandibular regions looking for lymphadenopathy and palpating the thyroid. Have the patient open and record MIO. Then move to the intraoral exam. Again, this can be done in different ways, but it is advisable to have a consistent pattern so that each aspect of the oral cavity is examined. Look at all of the mucosal surfaces throughout the mouth including the lips, tongue, floor of mouth, buccal mucosa, gingiva, pharynx, and hard and soft palate. Palpate and attempt to move the upper and lower jaws looking for mobility of the entire jaw or any segments of the jaws. Are there any steps in the dentition or any gingival tears? Have the patient close and assess the occlusion. Is it stable and reproducible? Then check each of the teeth individually by looking at all of the surfaces, and palpating each one assessing for mobility and tenderness. Look for caries, fractures, and periodontal disease. Often times, periodontal probing will be of significant diagnostic value as well. This portion of the exam can also contain important information for patients who present with infections. Palpate the involved areas to assess swelling and where the boundaries of the infection are. A good understanding of anatomic landmarks and fascial spaces will be important in assessing a patient's acute risk in those situations.

Neck

Infections can often become dangerous, particularly if they spread into the neck. A thorough evaluation of the neck is both helpful and important in these situations. First the surgeon should visually inspect the neck looking for any asymmetry, edema, masses, or irregularities. The neck should then carefully be palpated, feeling for cervical lymphadenopathy, enlargement or nodules of the thyroid gland, masses, or irregularities. Palpate the cricoid cartilage and identify the area of the cricothyroid membrane. Feel along the anterior borders of the sternocleidomastoids bilaterally. Check the patient's extension and flexion of the neck, and measure the thyromental distance, particularly in candidates for office-based anesthesia.

Cardiovascular and Pulmonary Exam

As dental providers, it is not necessary to complete an entire head-to-toe physical examination. This is the role of the patient's primary care provider. However, valuable information can be gained by a quick examination of the organ systems that are most critical to safe treatment of patients. The cardiac and pulmonary systems are without a doubt the systems that can result in the most dramatic and devastating consequences. For that reason, palpation of the patient's pulse, and auscultation of the heart and lungs is advised, particularly in patients with a history of heart or lung disease, and in those patients planning to undergo anesthesia.

Additional Tests

After completing a patient's medical history, ROS, and physical examination, it is time to consider any additional testing that could be helpful to this patient's assessment. Within the dental office, the most common additional tests that are done include radiographic imaging (Table 1.10). Depending on the patient's presentation,

Table 1.10 Imaging studies

Bite wings	Typically not helpful for oral surgery
Periapical	Must display entire tooth of interest and some surrounding tissue
Panorex	Should be able to visualize entire maxilla and mandible, including TMJ, maxillary sinuses, entire dentition. Excellent screening tool
CBCT	Visualizes hard tissue in excellent detail but is subject to scatter from metal, helpful for visualizing details of the TMJ, individual teeth, pathology, 3D jaw relationships, and 3D planning for implants, orthognathic surgery, or reconstructive surgery with precise measurements
Medical CT	Similar advantages of CBCT but visualizes soft tissue in better detail, higher radiation dosage, usually needs a referral to a radiology center (not done in office)
MRI	Not routinely used for oral surgery. Best modality for imaging the articular disc in the TMJ, certain types of soft tissue lesions

Table 1.11 Useful outpatient lab tests

Complete blood count with differential (CBC w/diff)	Information regarding anemia, platelet counts, and immune cells
Coagulation panel (Coags)	Includes PT, PTT, INR. Evaluation of bleeding risk
Basic metabolic panel (BMP)	Information regarding patient's glucose, electrolyte balance, and information about kidney function
Hemoglobin A1c (HbA1c)	Indication of long-term glucose control in diabetics
Liver function tests (LFTs)	Provide indication regarding liver function, liver damage, and inflammation
Albumin and prealbumin	Indication of nutritional status

and the areas of concern, this may simply be a periapical radiograph, a Panorex, or even a CBCT. Typically, any more detailed imaging, such as MRIs and PET scans would be ordered to be done at a radiology center.

Laboratory tests will also be valuable in assessing a patient's medical fitness for surgery (Table 1.11). Often times, patients will have recent lab tests available which will provide the surgeon with the information required. If not, the necessary tests can be ordered, or a discussion with the patient's primary care physician (PCP) may be helpful to determine if there are additional lab tests the PCP feels that the patient may need. Suggestions for lab tests will be mentioned during the discussions of specific medical considerations later in this chapter.

Medical Consultation

As medical professionals in an ever more complex and specialized world, it is not practical to think that any one provider can know everything about everything. There will be times when the patient's medical condition is very complex and the procedure could put them at significant risk for adverse outcomes. There are also times when the patient, or family member providing the medical information, is uninformed or has low healthcare literacy. In this circumstance, the patient may or may not have significant risk factors. It is inappropriate to assume that because the patient doesn't know their own medical history, that they are not at risk of bad outcomes. In either of these circumstances, it may be wise to contact one of the patient's physicians to discuss the proposed treatment and potential risks. As a member of the medical community, the number one priority is providing the best and safest care for each patient. This will often require the collaboration of multiple providers (Table 1.12). A common misconception is that the patient's MD can provide medical consultation in the form of "Clearance" to do the procedure. This is a completely inappropriate request and/or response for a medical consultation. Even if the patient's medical doctor "clears them" for office-based anesthesia, this does not absolve the surgeon administering the anesthesia from responsibility should the patient suffer a complication, nor is it in any way a guarantee that the patient and procedure will be free from complications.

To believe either of those things is naive and irresponsible. Rather, a medical consultation should be a collaboration between two or more parties. The patients

Table 1.12 Medical consultation

Consultation is appropriate when a patient is unable to provide a detailed or accurate medical history, or when a patient has a significant medical history with modifiable risk factors
Be specific about the proposed oral surgery when talking to the patient's physician. Describe the procedure in moderate detail. Without this information, the physician may not understand the nature of the proposed surgery and may not be able to give appropriate recommendations
Ask for ways to optimize the patient's medical condition to minimize risks for surgery. Identify those risk factors with the consulting physician
Do NOT ask for "medical clearance." Another physician cannot "clear" you to perform surgery. Surgery will always have risks, particularly in a medically compromised patient. Instead, consider yourself "cleared" when you identify and mitigate modifiable risk factors
If the risks are not modifiable and remain moderate or high, it is advisable to discuss the necessity and timing of the procedure with the patient's physician. Perhaps oral surgery can be deferred until the patient is in a lower risk state. This is most commonly encountered with patients who are undergoing chemotherapy, or who are awaiting chemotherapy, organ transplantation or cardiac surgery
Do not be afraid to speak directly to the patient's physician, on the phone or in person. Sometimes fax communication and email can leave gaps in the information being conveyed. Document phone calls in the patient's chart promptly

that typically require medical consultations are never free of risk, nor are the procedures. Therefore, it is important for both parties to understand what the risks are, and how to best mitigate them. The idea of the medical consultation is to identify the known risks and to reduce them to the lowest level possible. To have the patient still undergo the procedure, there will always be some risk of adverse events, but if every reasonable step to prevent those events is taken, only then will each patient be getting the care they deserve.

Therefore, a medical consultation should typically contain two things. First is a request for specific information. This is most commonly necessary because of the lack of specific medical knowledge of the patient who is providing the surgeon with the history. Many people will know if they had heart surgery, but they may not know if they had stents placed or if these were bare metal stents or drug eluting stents. A consultation with the patient's MD can provide this specific information. The next part of the consultation should be to ask if the patient is medically optimized for surgery, and if not, what steps need to be taken prior to surgery to optimize that patient. This is an area that requires specific communication as well. Many errors can be made if the surgeon is not specific to the medical provider about what the proposed treatment entails. Many medical doctors may not realize what is involved in preparing a dentate patient with large tori and exostoses for dentures. If they think you are only taking out a couple teeth, they may have a very different recommendation than if you describe to them the process of removing multiple teeth, having open mucosal sockets, removing large amounts of bone with incisions across the entire arch, etc. It is important to be specific about what the procedure will entail, so the patient's medical doctor may provide his or her best recommendations for optimizing the patient's medical conditions.

Common Medical Conditions Encountered Requiring Further Investigation

As previously mentioned, the world of medicine is becoming more complex every day. Adults are living longer, with more medical problems than ever. There are new drugs being developed every day, and patients are increasingly on multiple drugs. For this reason, there are many medical conditions that are encountered in the dental office, and it is important to have at least a cursory understanding of these conditions before starting invasive treatment.

Cardiac

Heart disease is still the number one cause of death in America as reported by the CDC's National Vital Statistics System. Cardiac disease is both extremely common, and potentially catastrophic. For these reasons, it is critical to be aware of a patient's cardiac health prior to undergoing elective surgery (Table 1.13).

Coronary Artery Disease/Ischemic Heart Disease

Coronary artery disease/ischemic heart disease is the most commonly encountered cardiac condition that dental providers will face. The patients will have a range of presentations, including angina, remote myocardial infarction, and recent myocardial infarction with or without conduction abnormalities. These conditions can also lead to heart failure.

Angina pectoris is the term used to describe a syndrome of chest pain or heaviness as a direct result of ischemia to the cardiac muscle. Patients may also describe difficulty breathing, left arm pain, left jaw pain, or other less specific symptoms. There are basically two factors at play that contribute to angina. This results from either an increase in myocardial oxygen demand (resulting from increased heart rate, contractility, and/or afterload) or a decrease in the delivery of oxygen to the myocardium. Decreased oxygen supply is most often the result of narrowing of the coronary arteries which supply the myocardium, or spasm of those same vessels. This ischemia is reversible so that if perfusion and oxygen supply is restored, and myocardial oxygen demand is decreased, no permanent damage results. Angina can be classified as either stable or unstable. Stable angina is characterized by no recent changes in symptoms, predictable onset of symptoms, and predictable resolution of symptoms. If a patient relays that for the last 5 years, every time they mow the

Table 1.13 Commonly encountered cardiac conditions

Coronary artery disease
Congestive heart failure
Valvular heart disease
Conduction abnormalities
Congenital heart disease

lawn they get angina, and then one tab of nitroglycerin and a 5 min rest alleviates the condition, they have stable angina. However, if a patient states that they used to recover from a 5 min rest, but over the last month they have been unable to catch their breath after three rounds of nitroglycerin and 20 min of rest, they would be classified as having unstable angina. Angina at rest is also considered unstable. This is significantly more concerning and would warrant delaying elective surgery and a medical consultation to evaluate and optimize the patient's cardiac condition prior to surgery. When ischemia to the heart muscle results in irreversible damage to the myocardium and cell death, a myocardial infarction results. This is typically an acute event, with symptoms similar to angina that are not responsive to alteration of myocardial oxygen supply and demand. Rather than just narrowing of the arteries and increased O_2 demand, MI is often the result of a ruptured plaque and subsequent thrombus occluding the coronary arteries. MIs are variable in severity depending on the size and specific location of the ischemic event, but still are associated with significant morbidity and mortality. A small infarct involving tissue critical to the conduction system of the heart can induce arrhythmias requiring pacemaker or defibrillator implantation. Often times the surviving tissue can be excitable and is also capable of inducing arrhythmias. Contractility will likely be impaired and the efficiency of the heart will be reduced. All of these post-MI changes decrease a patient's cardiac reserve and can put patients at risk for an acute event while under the stress of an oral surgery procedure. Consultation with the patient's cardiologist is advised, and often times it may be appropriate to delay elective surgery for 3–6 months following an MI. In order to limit risks, attention should be given to minimize the stresses to the cardiovascular system. The two things that are most likely to stress the patient's cardiovascular system are anxiety and pain. The provider should have a discussion at the time of consultation with the patient to establish a plan that will help to relieve the patient's anxiety (Table 1.14). This will be an individualized plan depending on what the patient is most anxious about. Things like relaxing music, keeping instruments out of sight, talking to the patient as you are about to do things to avoid surprises, and minimizing wait times in the waiting room will all help to keep patients calm. Performing these procedures early in the morning, perhaps first case of the day, can significantly decrease the amount of time a patient has to sit and build up anxiety. In some circumstances, anxiolytics may be appropriate. As mentioned, it is also paramount to keep pain to a minimum. Topical anesthetic is recommended prior to injection of local anesthetic (LA), and local anesthesia should be profound. Give adequate time for LA to take effect. Regarding LA, some providers would argue that LA with epinephrine should be avoided in these patients. The argument is that epinephrine is dangerous to the compromised cardiovascular system because it is a potent vasoconstrictor, increases afterload, and increases heart rate. This combination of effects can directly cause increased myocardial oxygen demand and decreased perfusion to the myocardium. However, one cannot deny that the experience of having dental surgery will result in the release of endogenous epinephrine as a result of anxiety, or even more so if there is any pain during the procedure. Therefore, other providers advocate for the limited use of epinephrine. The advantages of having a more profound anesthesia

Table 1.14 Anxiety reduction techniques

Have a consultation and establish a rapport with the patient in a nonthreatening situation. Get to know each other a little bit before surgery
Plan for early morning appointments so the patient will not have to be sitting around nervously waiting all morning
Avoid situations where they hear or see other patients in various stages of surgery. Have postoperative patients leave through a separate exit
Do not allow the patient to wait for a long time in the waiting room or in the operatory. Keep them continually occupied until the surgery begins
Have calming music playing
Avoid loud or abrupt noises
Provide frequent verbal reassurance that everything is going well and as planned
Do not allow the patient to see the instruments or syringes
Encourage the patient to bring a support person who will be in the waiting room during the procedure
Avoid surprises. Always talk to the patient and warn them if there will be noises or other frightening things
Minimize pain. Ensure that you have profound local anesthesia prior to starting the procedure
Consider pharmacologic anxiolytics such as nitrous oxide or benzodiazepines where practical. It may be appropriate to consider preoperative anxiolytics in certain patients
After surgery, make sure the patient knows they are not on their own. Provide the patient with contact information in case they have a question or an emergency
A postoperative phone call to the patient will go a long way to give them the reassurance that someone is keeping an eye on them

Table 1.15 Management of patients with coronary artery disease

Anxiety reduction techniques
Take preoperative vitals and monitor vitals during surgery
Supplemental O_2
Consider N_2O or other anxiolytics
Keep procedures short
Adequate pain control, both during and after surgery
Limit epinephrine or avoid it all together
Consider preoperative dose of nitroglycerin

with a longer duration of action should help to limit the amount of endogenous epinephrine released both during and after the procedure. Most surgeons limit the amount of epinephrine administered to these patients to two dental carpules with 1:100,000 epinephrine solution, which equates to just under 0.04 mg.

Additional management strategies (Table 1.15) should include preoperative and intraoperative assessment of the patient's vitals. Supplemental oxygen should be considered because it may help to slightly increase myocardial oxygen supply as oxygen demand increases. Nitrous oxide can be considered as it will provide both anxiolysis and supplemental oxygen to the patient. The patient should be kept coherent, however, so that the provider can frequently touch base with the patient about how they are feeling. If a patient routinely takes nitroglycerin for angina, it may be helpful to have them take a dose preoperatively. As with any intervention, discussion with the patient's cardiologist ahead of time will help with deciding which techniques will be most helpful in minimizing the patient's cardiac risk.

Conduction Abnormalities

As mentioned above, conduction abnormalities can result from prior MI, or they can be due to other genetic or acquired factors. The most commonly seen conduction abnormality in the dental office is atrial fibrillation. Atrial fibrillation in and of itself does not typically cause significant concern for office-based dental surgery, but there are certain issues that may present a problem. Atrial fibrillation is most commonly managed with anticoagulation and heart rate control. Anticoagulation is used to prevent a thrombus from forming within the atria of the heart, which could then lead to an embolic event causing a stroke, pulmonary embolism, mesenteric ischemia, etc. This has implications in dental surgery, because one of the most common postoperative complications with oral surgery is prolonged bleeding. It is important to know the medications the patient is on, and decide with the cardiologist if they need to be modified. Coumadin levels can be easily checked with an INR the morning of surgery. Other newer medications such as direct thrombin inhibitors are becoming more widely used, and may not have direct lab tests available to indicate the patient's level of anticoagulation. Knowledge of the medication's half-life will help to determine how long the patient should hold the medication preoperatively. Consideration also has to be given to the amount of bleeding expected after a surgery. This information should be conveyed to the cardiologist as well. For minor procedures such as a single tooth extraction, the risk of bleeding may be small enough that stopping an anticoagulant may be unnecessary, and may actually be more harmful than helpful because of the increased risk of a thromboembolic event.

The second concern with atrial fibrillation is an event with rapid ventricular response (RVR). Typically, patients are managed with rate control, allowing the rhythm to be irregular but keeping the heart rate under 100 bpm. In certain circumstances, such as dehydration or sympathetic activation, atrial fibrillation can result in a rapid ventricular rate often well over 100 bpm. Patients are frequently symptomatic if this occurs with palpitations, chest pain, dizziness, and shortness of breath. Symptomatic atrial fibrillation with RVR is a medical emergency that should be treated without delay by activation of the 911 response system. Beta-blockers and calcium channel blockers are most commonly used as first-line therapy in the treatment of atrial fibrillation with RVR.

Other conduction abnormalities are often encountered as well. Some other common conditions are Wolff-Parkinson-White Syndrome (WPW), left bundle branch block, and varying degrees of heart block. All of these conditions increase the risk of developing dangerous arrhythmias during noncardiac surgery. If properly treated (such as WPW with an ablation of the abnormal electrical pathway), cardiac risk may be similar to a patient with no cardiac history. Other times, risks may be increased. This information and plans to minimize cardiac risk can and should be discussed with the patient's cardiologist or PCP.

Valvular Disease

Valvular heart disease can also cause concern for patients planning to undergo noncardiac surgery. The most commonly affected valves are the mitral valve and the aortic valve, although any valve can be affected. Certain conditions such as mild asymptomatic mitral valve regurgitation or mitral valve prolapse is usually not going to require any preoperative modifications, where as severe aortic stenosis can have fatal consequences, particularly in association with general anesthesia. Valvular disease can also lead to heart failure. Either stenosis (which causes resistance to the forward flow of blood) or regurgitation (which results in only a small portion of blood being pumped out of the heart moving in the forward direction) will cause decreased efficiency of forward flow of blood and cause the heart to work harder. This can cause changes over time that lead to decompensation and eventual heart failure. It is always important to find out what stage of compensation or decompensation the patient is in prior to undergoing elective surgery.

Valvular heart disease is also a potential risk for general anesthesia. A heart with impedance to forward flow of blood will inherently be less tolerant of the hemodynamic changes induced by general anesthesia. Aortic stenosis has been specifically implicated in increased morbidity and mortality in noncardiac surgery. Any patient with valvular heart disease considering general anesthesia warrants a consultation with a cardiologist and often would be better cared for by an anesthesiologist in the hospital setting.

Heart Failure

Heart failure is the inability of the heart to effectively pump blood to the rest of the body. This results in decreased oxygen delivery to the tissues of the body. Symptoms include fatigue, shortness of breath, and poor exercise tolerance among other things (Table 1.16). This can lead to dysfunction in other critical organ systems as well. Often, the severity of a patient's heart failure can be assessed by an evaluation of their metabolic equivalents (METS) that they can tolerate. One MET is defined as the oxygen consumption of a 70 kg 40-year-old male at rest [1]. Typically, if a patient can tolerate 4 METs or greater, they should have adequate functional reserve to tolerate the stress of a minor or moderate risk surgical procedure. A patient who cannot walk a city block or up a single flight of stairs has very little functional reserve, and will not likely tolerate the stresses of surgery.

Table 1.16 Signs/symptoms of heart failure

Fatigue
Shortness of breath
Poor exercise tolerance
Frequent dry cough
Difficulty breathing when lying flat
Swelling of the lower extremities/peripheral edema

Table 1.17 4 METs or greater

Can you climb a flight of stairs?
Can you run a short distance?
Can you do heavy housework, such as scrubbing floors, washing windows, moving furniture, or painting?
Can you tolerate gardening?
Can you participate in golf, bowling, tennis, or dancing?
Can you mow the lawn with a push mower, or shovel snow?
Can you participate in swimming, basketball, or skiing?

Table 1.17 shows a list of questions that approximate 4 METs [1]. The surgeon should also be aware of the fluctuations that can accompany heart failure. A patient who seems to be doing well at the consultation could easily return for surgery with decreased exercise tolerance, SOB, and peripheral edema. It is important to assess the patient at each visit to ensure that they will be able to tolerate the planned procedure.

Congenital Heart Defects

The oral surgeon will also tend to come across congenital heart defects from time to time. Many children are now having these defects surgically repaired at a young age. As always, it is important to get a detailed history of the condition, and assess the patient for their functional status. Consultation with the cardiologist can provide crucial information regarding the patient's cardiac risk. Having an understanding of the physiological and hemodynamic changes of the heart will help to anticipate potential complications and prepare the surgeon to deal with them should they arise.

AHA Guidelines

Dental work or other procedures involving the GI tract have the potential to introduce bacteria into the blood stream. This is not usually a major issue, as the immune system is capable of handling transient bacteremia. However, there is a certain population at risk for developing infective endocarditis from transient bacteremia. Large groups of patients historically were given prophylactic antibiotics before dental treatment. However, in 2007, the AHA released guidelines significantly reducing the subset of patients recommended to receive prophylactic antibiotics. This was updated in 2017, reinforcing the recommendations from 2007. At this time, only patients with a prosthetic heart valve, prosthetic material used for valve repair, prior infective endocarditis, a cardiac transplant with regurgitation due to a structurally abnormal valve, unrepaired cyanotic congenital heart disease, or repaired congenital heart disease with residual shunting

Table 1.18 AHA guidelines for antibiotic prophylaxis

Prosthetic cardiac valve
Previous infective endocarditis
Cardiac valvulopathy in a cardiac transplant recipient
Congential heart disease:
Defect completely repaired within the previous 6 months with prosthetic material
Repaired congenital heart disease with residual defects at the site or adjacent to the site of a prosthetic patch or device
Unrepaired cyanotic congenital heart disease, including palliative shunts and conduits

Table 1.19 Oral antibiotic prophylaxis regimens

Antibiotic	Adult dose	Child dose
Amoxicillin	2 g	50 mg/kg
Cephalexin (Keflex)	2 g	50 mg/kg
Clindamycin	600 mg	20 mg/kg
Azithromycin	500 mg	15 mg/kg

at the site of a prosthetic patch or device are recommended to take prophylactic antibiotics [2]. A table of the AHA guidelines is presented in Table 1.18. A list of recommended antibiotic regimens is provided in Table 1.19.

Pulmonary

Pulmonary disease will also play a significant role in the practice of the oral and maxillofacial surgeon. The most common pulmonary disorders seen in the office include asthma and COPD.

Asthma

Asthma is a condition where the small airways in the lungs become inflamed and constricted in response to some type of precipitating factor. These factors vary from person to person and include things like exercise, cold air, upper respiratory infections, chemicals, and even anxiety. The constriction of the small airways then results in wheezing and shortness of breath. The provider should question the patient about precipitating factors so they can be avoided. The severity of the condition can be assessed by asking about which controller medications they take, how often they use their rescue inhaler, and how frequently they have had to go to the ER or had a hospital admission for asthma. Once the severity of the patient's asthma is assessed, there are certain things that should be done to minimize risk (Table 1.20). These include the avoidance, as best as possible, of precipitating factors. Again, techniques to limit anxiety may be very valuable here. The provider should also consider a prophylactic preoperative dose of the rescue inhaler. Prevention of an acute event is much safer than the treatment of an attack. Once the procedure has begun, it would be wise to have the patient's inhaler out on the counter where it is

Table 1.20 Considerations for patients with asthma

Identify and avoid triggers
Use anxiety reduction techniques
Defer elective surgery if patient is not well controlled
Auscultate for breath sounds listening for wheezing prior to surgery
Have patient's bronchodilator rescue inhaler out and in plain sight ready to be used
Consider preoperative dose of inhaler
If patient is undergoing an anesthetic, have spacer and equipment necessary to administer an inhaler to a sedated patient with a facemask
Have epinephrine available
Avoid NSAIDs postoperatively

Table 1.21 Management of a patient with COPD

Avoid elective surgery during an acute exacerbation
Anxiety Reduction Techniques
Avoid respiratory depressants such as sedatives and narcotics
If patient is managed with supplemental O_2, continue supplemental O_2
Cautious use of supplemental O_2 in patients not managed with supplemental O_2. Consider medical consultation to discuss with the physician
If managed on steroids, discuss with physician if there is a need for a stress dose
Avoid supine position
Have rescue inhaler out on the counter where it is easily visible and readily accessible
May need to take breaks on longer procedures to allow patients a chance to manage secretions

visible and easily accessible. Postoperatively, the use of NSAIDs should be avoided, as NSAIDs increase the production of leukotrienes which will only serve to increase the reactivity of the airway and likelihood of an asthma attack.

Chronic Obstructive Pulmonary Disease (COPD)

As the name implies, COPD is a chronic obstructive lung disease. This is most often the result of smoking, but can be the result of some less common genetic conditions or environmental exposures as well. The pathogenesis of COPD involves the destruction of alveoli and the loss of the elastic recoil that is necessary to maintain patent airways upon expiration. Damage to the upper airways also occurs and patients typically produce thick mucus secretions from inflammation of the bronchi and upper airways. This combination of abnormalities results in collapse of the small airways upon exhalation, air trapping within the lung, and hyper-expansion of the chest. This can make it exhausting to breath a normal tidal volume, and can make it nearly impossible to compensate for activity by increasing the size of the breath (the lung is already close to total lung capacity). Increasing the rate of small breathes does very little to increase a patient's exercise tolerance. Therefore, patients with COPD often have high work of breathing, chronic cough with thick mucus secretions, and very poor exercise tolerance.

The dental management of a patient with COPD (Table 1.21) would first and foremost be the postponement of elective surgery in a patient with an acute exacerbation. Allow that patient to be appropriately treated and optimized from a pulmonary standpoint prior to undergoing surgery. Secondly, any medications that decrease the respiratory drive, such as sedatives and narcotics, should be avoided. For patients maintained on corticosteroid therapy, steroid therapy should be continued perioperatively, and consultation with the patient's physician is advisable to discuss if there is a need for an additional stress dose of steroid. Lastly, the use of supplemental O_2 has been debated. Traditionally, many surgeons would avoid the use of supplemental oxygen with the fear that it would suppress the patient's respiratory drive. The theory is that patients become accustomed to hypercapnia and therefore rely on hypoxia for their respiratory drive. There was concern that providing supplemental oxygen would decrease their respiratory drive. This theory has recently been called into question and some providers claim that supplemental O_2 is unlikely to have a significant effect on respiratory rate and drive. However, until further evidence is available on this topic, the most appropriate thing to do would be to discuss it with the patient's pulmonologist or PCP preoperatively.

Renal

The kidneys are critical organs that are directly related to the regulation of the cardiovascular system. By understanding the role of the kidney, it is easy to see how renal dysfunction could cause cardiac complications, which can lead to disastrous complications. Understanding a patient's renal status and function is critical to providing safe and effective care.

Acute Renal Failure

Acute renal failure is the term used when the kidneys are acutely damaged and are unable to effectively filter the blood and produce urine. Patients with acute renal failure will be very sick and most often hospitalized. There is very little reason to attempt elective office-based oral surgery in a patient with acute renal failure.

Chronic Kidney Disease

Chronic kidney disease (CKD) is the more common entity that dental providers will experience in the outpatient setting. Chronic kidney disease exists as a continuum, with different stages of disease, ultimately ending with Stage V CKD which requires hemodialysis to survive. Early stages of kidney disease are classified based on the patient's calculated glomerular filtration rate, which is based on the patient's clearance of creatinine from their bloodstream. Therefore, even without having a glomerular filtration rate calculated, a blood creatinine level can give a practitioner a reasonable indication of the renal function in most patients. Patients who are on dialysis, on the other hand, will not have stable labs as they will vary depending

Table 1.22 Management of patients on hemodialysis

Schedule surgery for the day after hemodialysis so the patient is at their optimal fluid and electrolyte status
Avoid surgery on the day of hemodialysis due to administration of heparin
Preoperative CBC and Coags
Avoid taking BP on arm with AV fistula and do not use fistula for venous access
Consult patient's physician regarding possible use of prophylactic antibiotics
Anxiety reduction techniques
Monitor vitals throughout surgery
Discuss dosage of any drugs eliminated or metabolized by the kidneys with patient's physician
Pay particular attention to bleeding and use local hemostatic measures where appropriate

upon when they were drawn in relation to the dialysis. Hemodialysis most often involves the creation of a high flow arterio-venous fistula, which can then be used as an access point for dialysis. In order to avoid blood clotting in the dialysis tubing, patients are usually heparinized for this procedure.

Therefore, a patient who undergoes dialysis should be scheduled for elective oral surgery the day following a dialysis treatment (Table 1.22). This allows the heparin used during dialysis to be completely out of the system. It also allows the patient to be at their optimal state regarding fluid balance and accumulation of waste products in the blood stream. Patients with renal disease also need to be carefully dosed with medications. Many medications can be nephrotoxic, such as NSAIDs. These medications should be avoided when possible, although they may be acceptable if a patient has no renal function and is already on dialysis. Other medications besides NSAIDs also rely on renal excretion or metabolism. Dosing of these medications will need to be adjusted in order to avoid toxicity as a result of reduced metabolism and clearance of the drug.

Patients with CKD also have a tendency towards bleeding complications and anemia. The kidney produces erythropoietin, which is a hormone that stimulates the production of red blood cells. Patients with CKD will tend to have platelet dysfunction as well, which may be related to the electrolyte abnormalities that exist when the kidney is not functioning properly. For these reasons, close attention must be paid to a patient's bleeding, and local hemostatic measures should be used when appropriate [3].

Liver Disease

Liver disease is most commonly the result of infectious disease and/or alcohol abuse. Hepatitis, or inflammation of the liver, is usually the result of a viral infection and can be either acute or chronic. Cirrhosis, typically caused by alcohol abuse, leads to scarring in the liver, which has the effect of both reducing the number of functional hepatocytes, and also causing obstruction to the normal flow of blood through the liver. This results in reduced effectiveness of the liver's metabolic functions, as well as the backup of blood through the portal venous system. The portal venous system backs up into the splenic vein, and eventually the spleen, as well as esophageal veins.

Table 1.23 Management of patients with liver disease

Preoperative CBC, Coags, BMP, LFTs
Consider consultation with patient's physician for medical optimization
Anxiety reduction techniques
Limit the amount of surgery done at each visit if bleeding is a problem
Local hemostatic measures
Avoid Tylenol and other drugs with hepatic metabolism/elimination
Ensure that bleeding is under control prior to discharge. Swallowing a large amount of blood could lead to hepatic encephalopathy. Counsel these patients on the importance of returning to the office if they have prolonged or excessive bleeding

It is also important to understand the normal functions of the liver in order to understand how these disease processes can impact the body. The liver is responsible for many critical functions in the body, including manufacture of clotting factors, creating and secreting bile, detoxification of chemicals and drugs, excretion of chemicals and drugs through bile, cholesterol metabolism, production of important oncotic proteins including albumin, and converting ammonia to urea, among several other things. All of these important functions can be affected by hepatitis and cirrhosis. Risks of liver disease include increased risk of bleeding due to both clotting factor abnormalities and thrombocytopenia, increased toxicity to drugs, fluid shifts with ascites, and toxicity from ammonia. Preoperative laboratory evaluation will be critical, including liver function tests, complete blood count, and a coagulation panel. Interestingly enough, even in a patient whose lab tests appear to be within reasonable limits, patients with liver disease tend to still have difficulty with clotting, more so than their labs would suggest. It is wise to use adjunctive local hemostatic agents in these patients. It is also important to remember the risk that swallowed blood can have in these patients. Hemoglobin will be broken down by bacteria in the gut creating nitrogenous waste in the form of ammonia, which is typically detoxified to urea by the liver. A poorly functioning liver can lead to ammonia build up in the blood, which is particularly toxic to the brain. This can result in hepatic encephalopathy. The congestion of blood in the liver and resultant backup of blood into the spleen can cause excessive sequestration of platelets leading to thrombocytopenia. Pooling of blood in the esophageal veins can lead to varices. If these varices rupture, in a patient who often has a concomitant coagulopathy, the end result is often fatal. Patient's with end stage liver disease can have so many abnormalities and risks they certainly must be approached with caution, and consultation with the patient's physician is advised (Table 1.23).

Hematological Disorders

Fortunately, serious hematological conditions are quite uncommon. Most of the time, patients will present with a diagnosis of a hematological disorder, or at least a family history of one. However, many patients undergoing oral surgery are young, and may never have had a surgical procedure before. It is quite possible that a seemingly healthy patient has an inherited coagulopathy of which they are unaware.

Table 1.24 Management of patients with hematologic disorders

Consult with the patient's hematologist to create a hemostasis plan prior to performing surgery
Obtain preoperative CBC and Coags
Arrange for transfusion of blood products prior to surgery if necessary. This may necessitate performing the procedure in the hospital
For patients with von Willebrand Disease, particularly Type 1, administration of DDAVP preoperatively is often effective. If DDAVP is used, patient needs to have free water restriction
Hemophilia will likely require transfusion of blood products
Use local hemostatic measures including sutures, electrocautery, gelfoam, collagen plugs, oxidized cellulose, aminocaproic acid, topical thrombin, etc.
Monitor the wound to ensure complete hemostasis prior to discharge
Avoid NSAIDs and aspirin postoperatively

This makes it very important to ask every patient about bleeding history, including easy bruising, frequent nose bleeds, heavy menstrual flow, or prolonged bleeding following minor injuries such as cuts from shaving. A significantly suspicious history should be enough to evaluate that patient with laboratory tests (such as a complete blood count and coagulation panel) prior to surgery. Management will most often be related to the nature of the laboratory abnormalities (Table 1.24).

The most common inherited coagulopathy the oral surgeon will see is von Willebrand Disease (vWD). This is either a deficiency or qualitative defect in von Willebrand factor (vWF). Von Willebrand factor is made in the endothelium and is released in response to endothelial injury. Von Willebrand factor then acts to bind to collagen as well as platelets, and promote blot clot formation. Von Willebrand factor has also been found to stabilize factor VIII, so that factor VIII levels may be low in these patients. The end result, of course, is a patient with higher risk of bleeding.

There are three subtypes of von Willebrand disease. Type 1 is a quantitative deficiency of vWF. Type 2 vWD is characterized by relatively normal amounts of vWF, but there is a qualitative problem, where the vWF is not effective. Type 3 is characterized by an absence of vWF and is the most severe. Type 1 vWD is the most common. Typical treatment for this involves preoperative administration of DDAVP (Desmopressin). In addition to its antidiuretic effects, DDAVP causes the release of vWF from the endothelium. DDAVP, in conjunction with local hemostatic measures, is often all that is necessary. It is important to take note that this does not work for most patients with Type 2 or Type 3 vWD. It is also important to educate patients on the need for free water restriction after receiving DDAVP due to the antidiuretic effects.

Hemophilias are less common and result from inherited abnormalities or deficiencies of certain clotting factors. This can lead to serious bleeding complications, and should typically be managed by making a preoperative and postoperative plan with the patient's hematologist before undergoing surgery. There are also pro-thrombotic disorders, such as antiphospholipid antibody syndrome, which can put patients at risk for having deep venous thrombosis or pulmonary emboli after major surgery. These patients are often managed with anticoagulant medications and it should be verified that they are in the appropriate therapeutic range prior to undergoing elective surgery. Usually these drugs do not need to be stopped, and one must consider the risk of bleeding versus the risk of the patient experiencing a thromboembolic event.

Endocrine Disorders

Diabetes Mellitus

Diabetes mellitus is the most common endocrine disorder affecting patients in the dental office. Diabetes is a disorder of glucose metabolism and is related to either a deficiency in insulin production or decreased sensitivity to the effects of insulin. Insulin is one of the main anabolic hormones in the body, and helps to stimulate protein synthesis, uptake of glucose, and storage of energy in the forms of fats, glycogen, and protein. Diabetes is classified as either Type I or Type II. Type I is typically early onset, often seen in children, and is most commonly the result of autoimmune destruction of the pancreatic beta cells, which produce insulin. This causes a decrease, or absence, of insulin production and release in response to a spike in blood glucose. Insulin is critical for the regulation of glucose levels in the blood and helps to facilitate glucose uptake into the cells and out of the bloodstream. Absence (or very low levels) of insulin will result in elevated blood glucose levels. If not well managed, blood glucose can get high enough that the kidneys cannot reabsorb all the glucose from the urine and glycosuria will result. Within the urine, glucose acts as an osmotic diuretic. This will cause polyuria, dehydration, and as a result polydipsia. Patients are also missing the anabolic effects of insulin and will typically have breakdown of proteins and lipids. Lipid catabolism will ultimately result in the production of ketone bodies, which in conjunction with dehydration from high blood glucose levels are responsible for the well-known condition of diabetic ketoacidosis. This is a serious condition often requiring hospitalization and inpatient treatment.

Type II diabetes, on the other hand, is typically a result of decreased insulin production, decreased sensitivity of the tissue receptors to insulin, or a combination of both. This condition is more commonly adult onset. It is often associated with obesity, and there is a strong genetic component as well. Patients with Type II diabetes are at risk of a developing a different condition known as hyperosmolar hyperglycemic state. This can cause severe electrolyte and fluid disturbances and may have symptoms similar to diabetic ketoacidosis. The first outward sign is usually altered mental status, and this may progress into seizures, coma, and even death. While hyperosmolar hyperglycemic state is quite rare, diabetics have other risks related to oral surgery. If blood sugar is not well controlled, as monitored by hemoglobin A1c levels, diabetic patients have increased risk of infection, and decreased efficiency of wound healing. There is also the potential complication of acute hypoglycemia, particularly in patients who are insulin dependent. If NPO prior to a procedure, patients may inappropriately still take a dose of morning insulin while failing to put any glucose into their body. This can precipitate a medical emergency. Even when told to eat a normal breakfast ahead of surgery, many patients are nervous and do not feel like eating much of a breakfast. In any diabetic patients showing signs of hypoglycemia, including hunger, confusion, dizziness, diaphoresis, hypotension, tachycardia, or agitation, blood glucose should be checked preoperatively. Any patients with hypoglycemia should be given an oral

Table 1.25 Management of patients with diabetes mellitus

Defer elective surgery until patients have optimized glucose control
Aggressively treat infections. Diabetics will typically benefit from both surgical drainage and antibiotics
Remind patient to eat breakfast prior surgery
For patients who must be NPO, consult patient's physician for alterations to oral hypoglycemic and/or insulin
Check blood glucose prior to surgery
Monitor vitals throughout surgery
Avoid excessively long appointments
Have a source of glucose, such as apple juice, readily available
Maintain frequent communication with the patient to ensure they are coherent and feeling well
Encourage returning to normal PO intake postoperatively, or continue to modify oral hypoglycemic medications and/or insulin as instructed by the patient's physician

load of glucose such as apple juice or orange juice if able, with IV dextrose available for patients who may be too obtunded to tolerate oral fluids.

It is therefore important to establish a preoperative plan with the patient's physician, particularly in patients who are insulin dependent (Table 1.25). Temporary mild hyperglycemia is preferable to hypoglycemia in the perioperative period. Therefore, it is important for patients undergoing a procedure with local anesthesia to be encouraged to eat a normal meal, and if they don't have as much of an appetite as usual, to decrease the insulin dose they receive. In patients who will need to be NPO, the physician should be consulted for a plan regarding the change in the insulin regimen. Often times patients may not feel up to eating after surgery as well, so providers must take into account that some of the longer acting insulin formulations will have peak activity after the surgery, but patients may still be avoiding food due to factors related to the surgical procedure such as pain or bleeding.

Diabetic patients are also typically less tolerant of infections, and have more difficulty resolving infections. Poorly controlled diabetics are also more susceptible to infections in the first place. Even in a well-controlled diabetic, once an infection begins, this will often lead to wild spikes in blood sugar and poor glucose control. That, in turn, can lead to impaired leukocyte function, which only serves to further decrease the body's ability to fight off the infection. Diabetic patients with purulent infections should be managed aggressively with both surgical drainage and antibiotic therapy. In advanced infections, consideration should be given towards hospitalization for better control over blood glucose levels and more frequent monitoring of the potential spread of the infection.

Thyroid Disorders (Hypothyroidism and Hyperthyroidism)

Hypothyroidism is another commonly seen disorder in the oral surgeon's office. Fortunately, this is typically diagnosed and managed appropriately by the patient's primary care provider. Thyroid hormone is one of the major regulators of the body's metabolism, and decreased thyroid hormone production results in slowed

Table 1.26 Management of patients with thyroid disorders

Defer elective surgery until thyroid condition is well controlled
Patients who are hypothyroid do not typically require any specific modifications to treatment if they are appropriately managed with supplemental thyroid hormone
For patients who are hyperthyroid:
Monitor vitals during surgery
Watch for signs of thyrotoxicosis
Limit epinephrine

metabolism. Symptoms include fatigue, weight gain, joint pain, and changes in the quality and vibrancy of the skin, hair, and finger nails. As part of a head and neck exam, it is possible for the oral surgeon to palpate a thyroid abnormality or conduct a comprehensive review of systems and assist in the diagnosis of a thyroid condition.

Hyperthyroidism is less common, but it can potentially cause a more serious complication. Thyrotoxicosis is an acute state of excess thyroid hormone that can lead to increased body temperature, diaphoresis, and tachycardia. If untreated, this condition could potentially be fatal. Fortunately, it is rare, but surgeons should be on the lookout for signs or symptoms that could indicate hyperthyroidism. Common signs and symptoms of hyperthyroidism include weight loss, palpitations, tachycardia, heat intolerance, and changes to the skin and hair. Patients with Grave's Disease, an autoimmune over-activation of the thyroid gland, will also often have exophthalmos, or bulging eyes, as a result of increased volume of orbital fat. Table 1.26 details some considerations for the management of patients with thyroid disorders.

Neurological Conditions

One of the unfortunate effects of patients living longer is the increase in incidence of neurologic conditions such as dementia and stroke. These conditions can be very variable in their presentations, with nearly no disability to complete disability. It is often helpful to have a friend or family member present during the consultation, and it is also important to determine if the patient has any power of attorney or a conservator who will be responsible for consenting and signing for the patient. The patient's level of comprehension should be evaluated, and arrangements may need to be made to have the patient watched postoperatively to ensure that proper instructions are being followed. Patients with significant dementia may have difficulty understanding the nature of their dental disease, and why they are in the office at all. They should be given frequent reassurance and reminders of why they are in the office and what is being done. This generally helps with cooperation and compliance during the procedure. Some patients may not be able to tolerate in-office procedures at all, and may be better suited for the hospital with anesthesia provided by a medical anesthesiology (Table 1.27).

Seizures are another neurologic condition that may have implications for oral surgery. An accurate history is critical in establishing the patient's risk for a seizure during or following a surgery. The patient should be questioned about the frequency

Table 1.27 Management of patients with dementia

Preoperative consultation with patient and their care-giver or power of attorney
Medical consultation may be necessary to obtain a complete medical history
Speak to the patient and do not ignore their opinions or questions during the consultation or during the procedure
Specify legally who needs to give consent for the procedure, and obtain consent from that person
Anxiety reduction techniques
Keep procedures short
Use frequent conversation and re-orientation during procedure
Avoid surprises
Ensure that the patient will have a competent person to help them postoperatively to ensure post-op instructions are being followed
Consider general anesthesia in the hospital setting when necessary

Table 1.28 Management of patients with seizures

Defer elective surgery until seizures are well controlled
Identify and avoid any possible triggers including medications, dehydration, stress, and lack of sleep
Review recent labs or order new labs if patient is on a medication that can cause agranulocytosis or aplastic anemia
Anxiety reduction techniques
Consider IV sedation with administration of benzodiazepines

and type of seizures they have, what medications they are on, and how compliant they are with those medications. Some of these medications can have serious side effects including agranulocytosis and/or aplastic anemia. Patients should be asked if they are followed with any blood tests and results of those tests should be reviewed. Fortunately, those major side effects are rare. Patients who are well controlled with medications often do not need any specific modifications for office-based procedures. IV anesthesia may even help to decrease risk of seizures, particularly if the provider uses a benzodiazepine as part of the sedation regimen. Management considerations for patients who suffer from seizure disorders are listed in Table 1.28.

Musculoskeletal Conditions

Musculoskeletal conditions are not often of major concern for the dentist or oral surgeon. Patients should be questioned as to the nature of their injury or condition, and asked what exacerbates it and what alleviates it. Often, a discussion with the patient and some common sense regarding positioning can help to make patients comfortable for their procedures. There is also the consideration of patients with prosthetic total joints. This has been an area of some discourse in recent years. A joint recommendation came out from the ADA and AAOS (American Academy of Orthopaedic Surgeons) in the early 2000s stating that antibiotic prophylaxis for dental procedures was not indicated for most patients with a total joint replacement.

However, a few years later, the AAOS reversed its position and suggested that antibiotic prophylaxis was recommended for all patients with total joint replacements undergoing invasive dental procedures. The dental community had concerns about this recommendation, as it did not seem to be based on any new data. The ADA felt the existing data set supported no need for antibiotic prophylaxis. The most recent recommendation from AAOS is for limited use of prophylactic antibiotics prior to dental procedures on a case specific basis and discussion with the patient of the risks of prophylaxis versus no prophylaxis [2] (Table 1.29). Given this scenario, most oral surgeons will defer to the orthopedic surgeon's recommendation and proceed according to their wishes.

Osteoporosis is another musculoskeletal condition that will affect the oral surgeon. Many patients have been treated with bisphosphonates, biologics, or other medications that carry a risk for inducing MRONJ (medication-related osteonecrosis of the jaws) (Table 1.30). In patients treated with low doses of these medications for osteoporosis, the risk of developing MRONJ from dental surgery is quite low. Typically, if the patient has been treated with the medication for shorter than 3 years, the risk is even lower (<1% risk). Some clinicians suggest a drug holiday, which is a reasonable consideration for elective surgery. There currently is no strong evidence for or against this, but many people feel it makes logical sense, even without the evidence. If surgery is urgent, the surgeon should proceed and discuss the risks with the patient. The patient should know that this condition may be chronic and never resolve fully. In patients who have received higher doses of these medications for the treatment of bone metastases or cancer-related problems, every attempt should be made to avoid unnecessary surgery, particularly in the posterior mandible [4]. If surgery must be done, the patient should be counselled about the risks. Some providers suggest perioperative antibiotics and chlorhexidine mouth rinse to attempt to optimize the oral environment to achieve gingival coverage of the bony socket.

Table 1.29 Antibiotic prophylaxis in patients with total joint replacements

According to the 2015 ADA guidelines: In general, it is no longer recommended to provide antibiotic prophylaxis to patients with total joint replacements
Patients with specific risk factors such as immunosuppressant medications or previous joint infections can be considered with the orthopedic surgeon on a case by case basis

Table 1.30 Management of patients on bisphosphonates or other antiresorptive or antiangiogenic medications

If it is known that a patient is going to be put on these medications, a comprehensive oral evaluation and any necessary surgery should be completed prior to starting the medications
Consult with the patient's physician to discuss a drug holiday, particularly in patients who have been on high doses for cancer or those who have been on the drugs greater than 3 years
In patients on high doses for cancer treatments, avoid surgery if at all possible. Consider endodontic treatment even on non-restorable teeth

Cancer

Cancer is an extremely broad topic with many different kinds of cancer and widely variable medications, treatments, and systemic effects. There are, however, some general themes that hold true for most cancers. Regardless of where it originates in the body, cancer results from a malfunction of the cellular apparatus designed to regulate cell replication and tissue growth. The cell then begins to replicate in a rapid and uncontrolled manner. This then leads to the accumulation of additional mutations and abnormalities because of the rapid and unregulated replication process. As mutations and abnormalities accumulate, somewhere along the way, cells begin to dedifferentiate and lose certain characteristics of the original tissue.

Eventually, they evolve the potential to invade and metastasize, causing damage to other tissues throughout the body.

The process of a cancerous tumor growing requires a significant amount of energy. Patients will often present with unexpected weight loss without dieting or increasing exercise. This can lead to malnourishment, and compromise the body's ability to heal following surgery. Many of the drugs used to treat cancers are very toxic and cause suppression of the immune system. This leads to additional compromise to healing, and can also increase the risk of infection. Certain cancers, or drugs, may affect the patient's blood counts resulting in significant anemia or thrombocytopenia. This could put the patient at risk for significant bleeding. Any patient actively undergoing treatment for cancer should prompt a call to the treating physician for a discussion about the risks of oral surgery. Elective surgery should be delayed until the patient is in a more optimal physical state. Timing of urgent procedures should be discussed carefully and timed around the chemo or radiation regimen to attempt to optimize the patient's health on the day of surgery and for the initial recovery. Modifications may need to be made regarding the treatment regimen immediately following surgery to allow for initial healing. There is no way to make these decisions without consultation with the oncologist. A list of considerations for the management of a patient with cancer is provided in Table 1.31.

Table 1.31 Management of patients with cancer

Delay elective surgery until patient is not in active treatment if possible
Spend some time to familiarize yourself with the specific type of cancer and issues that may arise
Patients may have severe abnormalities with blood counts and electrolytes
Obtain preoperative CBC, Coags, BMP
Optimize patient's nutrition preoperatively when possible
Local hemostatic measures when necessary
Consultation with patient's physician to determine if any alterations may be made to chemo or radiation regimens
Expect delayed healing and higher risk of infections. Consider prophylactic antibiotics
Frequent follow up until surgical site has healed completely

Table 1.32 Management of patients with drug abuse history

Obtain an accurate history alone with the patient. Do not be judgmental
Stress the important of knowing what a patient is on because of the potential dangers of drug interactions
Communicate well with the patient and let them know that they may still be awake if they attempt an office sedation. If that is not acceptable to them, perhaps consider general anesthesia in the hospital
Determine a postoperative pain control plan before surgery, and stick to it. Many times, it is beneficial to avoid narcotic medications
Do not operate on someone who is impaired. They cannot consent to the procedure, and may have unpredictable reactions to medications and unpredictable behavior
Anxiety reduction techniques
Consider use of long acting local anesthetics for pain control to reduce need for narcotics

Drug Abuse

Drug abuse, or drug abuse history, is another condition that is unfortunately becoming more common in the United States (Table 1.32). Marijuana use is being legalized throughout the country, and opiate abuse is now a significant public health crisis. Given this environment, oral surgeons should not be surprised to see young patients who are regularly using drugs, or with a history of drug abuse now in recovery. Drug abuse is a very challenging condition to manage safely because many times a patient will not disclose the full extent of their drug habits to the surgeon. It is therefore the surgeon's duty to extract this information from the patient. It is important to ask them privately, in a non-confrontational way, and to emphasize the importance of this information. If they know that a serious interaction may take place, which could be debilitating or fatal, they may be more likely to disclose the behaviors. Elective surgery should be delayed on patients who are under the influence. They cannot legally give consent to procedures, and their behavior and ability to cooperate may be unpredictable.

Patients with a history of drug abuse can be a challenge as well. Prior opiate abuse can permanently alter the neurological system and the interpretation of pain within the brain. It may be difficult to obtain adequate local anesthesia, and they may be resistant to the effects of medications commonly used for IV sedation or office-based general anesthesia. Postoperative pain management must be considered and discussed with the patient preoperatively. Many patients may not want narcotic medications, or may contractually be prohibited from taking them from a rehabilitation program. A frank discussion should be had prior to undergoing surgery, so that all expectations regarding drugs and pain management are clear to both parties ahead of time. This should be documented.

Pregnancy

From time to time, pregnant women will present to the dental office in need of surgical care. Pregnancy carries both a risk to the developing fetus and to the mother. Many physiologic changes occur during pregnancy including increased fluid

Table 1.33 Management of a pregnant patient

Avoid elective procedures until after pregnancy is over
If procedures must be done, defer to third trimester if possible
Use minimal amount of radiation possible. Opt for PA's rather than a Panorex. Use lead shields to reduce radiation exposure as much as possible
Consult with the patient's obstetrician for specific recommendations
Lidocaine is generally safe, although some obstetricians prefer to avoid the use of epinephrine
Use the minimal number of medications possible
Avoid IV sedation or general anesthesia
Generally avoid the use of N_2O which is known to increase risk of spontaneous abortion with prolonged exposure
Avoid supine position late in pregnancy, use additional pillows to help position the patient comfortably
Ibuprofen should be avoided, particularly late in the pregnancy
Tylenol and narcotics are generally safe to use but verify any medications to be given with respect to potential fetal risk category and by discussion with the patient's obstetrician

volume, edema, increased heart rate and cardiac output, and decreased efficiency of the lungs to name a few. There is also the concern of injury to the developing fetus. Certain drugs and radiation are known to cause damage to a developing child. There are critical periods during development when exposure to radiation or drugs could be especially damaging, possibly causing birth defects or cognitive deficiencies. Therefore, any elective surgery should be deferred until after delivery. If a surgery must be done, every effort should be made to delay the procedure until after the first trimester. If that is not possible, radiographic examination should be as limited as possible with lead drapes over the rest of the body. Lidocaine is safe for use in pregnancy, but many obstetricians request limiting the dose of epinephrine. IV sedation or general anesthetic should not be considered. While a short-term exposure to nitrous oxide has not been specifically indicated in pregnancy complications, chronic exposure to nitrous oxide has been linked to higher rates of spontaneous abortion. For this reason, many clinicians advise avoiding nitrous oxide during pregnancy. Positioning may be difficult, particularly late in the third trimester, as the uterus grows in size and pushes upward on the diaphragm and may obstruct the inferior vena cava. Keeping the patient in a more upright position with a pillow under the right hip may help to improve the patient's comfort, as well as their ability to breathe and return venous blood to the heart. A summary of the management of pregnant women is provided in Table 1.33.

Office-Based Anesthesia Evaluation

One of the special privileges that oral surgeons have is the ability to provide surgical care in a private office with general anesthesia. It is no surprise that a large number of patients have intense fears of dental work. These fears are probably second to only one other fear: dental extractions. To be able to provide patients with the option of going to sleep is a wonderful service to many patients who would not tolerate or seek care otherwise. Therefore, it is important to protect this privilege, but even more important to protect the health of the patients. Of all the things that

Table 1.34 Evaluation for office-based anesthesia

Obtain a thorough medical history, including family history of anesthetic complications
Patients with significant cardiac, pulmonary, renal, and hepatic conditions are typically not good candidates for office-based anesthesia
Be wary of patients with current drug abuse or drug abuse history
Consult with a patient's physician when appropriate
Conduct a thorough airway examination including assessment of facial hair, dentition, neck mobility and size, tongue size, mouth opening, Mallampati score, scars from prior neck surgery, thyromental distance, and patient's BMI
If a patient is not a good candidate for office anesthesia, do not allow them to pressure you into putting them in an unsafe position. Even if it is not what they want, often it would be better to do the procedure with local, or in the hospital with a medical anesthesiologist

oral surgeons do in the office, administering general anesthesia can lead to the most devastating consequences, including death. In the vast majority of cases that result in adverse outcomes, patient selection has played a significant role. The evaluation of each individual patient must be done carefully and thoughtfully to determine if they are truly a candidate for office-based anesthesia (Table 1.34).

In assessing a patient, we must determine their risk of an adverse outcome. One portion of this assessment is to evaluate their general health and physiologic reserve. Cardiac and pulmonary conditions that reduce a patient's ability to compensate for stress and changes in hemodynamic status are a significant contraindication. Liver and kidney disease can lead to fluid shifts and electrolyte imbalances and those patients may not tolerate general anesthesia well. They can also lead to changes in metabolism and elimination of drugs leading to over-sedation. Bleeding disorders may cause excessive intraoral bleeding, which can become an airway obstruction or irritant. A family history of anesthesia complications such as malignant hyperthermia may need to be explored prior to a patient's first anesthetic experience.

The second part of this assessment is to anticipate potential problems and evaluate how effective emergency procedures would be. The most common issue oral surgeons will face during a non-intubated anesthesia is airway management. The practitioner providing the anesthesia must ask himself or herself, "If I need to bag mask ventilate, or intubate this patient, could I do it?" The airway exam is critical and should include an assessment of facial hair, dentition, neck mobility, tongue size, mouth opening, Mallampati score, ability to protrude the lower teeth beyond the upper teeth, neck size and girth, scars from prior neck surgery, and thyromental distance. Patient's BMI should be noted, and the distribution of the adipose tissue also should be considered. If the patient has a significant amount of mass in the upper body, around the chest, shoulders, and neck, this can make ventilation and intubation very challenging. Anxious patients will put pressure on the doctor to provide the services they want because they may not understand the risks. It is important to do a thorough and objective assessment of each patient regardless of the pressure one might feel to please a patient. When patient factors make office-based anesthesia an unrealistic solution, outpatient surgery in the hospital may be the best choice. This may still allow the patient the comfort of being asleep, while being in the safest setting with a secure airway and backup safety equipment and personnel readily available.

References

1. Jette M, Sidney K, Blumchent G. Metabolic Equivalents (METS) in exercise testing, exercise prescription, and evaluation of functional capacity. Clin Cardiol. 1990;13:555–65.
2. American Dental Association. 2018. https://www.ada.org/en/member-center/oral-health-topics/antibiotic-prophylaxis. Accessed 10 Dec 2018.
3. Jover-Cerveró A, Bagán JV, Jiménez-Soriano Y, Poveda-Roda R. Dental management in renal failure: patients on dialysis. Med Oral Patol Oral Cir Bucal. 2008;13(7):419–26. http://www.medicinaoral.com/medoralfree01/v13i7/medoralv13i7p419.pdf.
4. American Association of Oral and Maxillofacial Surgeons: Position Paper on Medication Related Osteonecrosis of the Jaw – 2014 Update. 2014. https://www.aaoms.org/docs/govt_affairs/advocacy_white_papers/mronj_position_paper.pdf. Accessed 12 Dec 2018.

Facial Assessment

2

Amir Tadros, Mohammad Banki, and Elie M. Ferneini

Introduction

Facial cosmetic surgery is becoming increasingly popular and more acceptable in society today. The concept of beauty has its cultural and generational differences, however certain facial proportions and balancing anatomic contours are universally accepted as aesthetically attractive. It is critical that a cosmetic surgeon understands the patient's cosmetic goals, along with the tools available to analyze facial symmetry, proportions, and anatomy to have a successful result through surgical or nonsurgical procedures. The surgeon must also be able to recognize preoperatively the deviations from accepted proportions of beauty and communicate to the patient the limitations related to the facial anatomy and available therapeutic modalities. Due to the vast surgical and nonsurgical therapies available today, the surgeon should also be able to recognize which therapy can be employed to obtain the desired changes, along with their limitations and risks. Having a mutual understanding of what cosmetic changes can be achieved predictably and safely between the surgeon and patient is paramount to a successful result.

A. Tadros
Division of Oral and Maxillofacial Surgery, School of Dental Medicine, University of Connecticut, Farmington, CT, USA
e-mail: atadros@uchc.edu

M. Banki (✉)
Artistic Contours, Warwick, RI, USA

E. M. Ferneini
Beau Visage Med Spa, Greater Waterbury OMS, Cheshire, CT, USA

E. M. Ferneini, M. T. Goupil (eds.), *Office-Based Maxillofacial Surgical Procedures*, https://doi.org/10.1007/978-3-030-22371-7_2

Anatomic Landmarks

- Frankfort Horizontal plane—imaginary horizontal line extending from the external auditory meatus through the inferior orbital rim. The Frankfort line is important in the analysis of the lateral profile as it provides a frame of reference for measurements to be recorded (Fig. 2.1).
- Trichion—anterior hairline in the midline of the forehead
- Orbitale—the most inferior point on the infraorbital rim
- Glabella—the most prominent point of the forehead above and between the eyebrows
- Nasion—the depression point at the bridge of the nose where the frontal and nasal bones meet
- Radix—depression at the root of the nose that corresponds to the nasofrontal suture
- Sellion—junction where bone and cartilage meet on the nasal dorsum
- Rhinion—soft tissue landmark that correlates to the sellion
- Nasal Tip—most anterior projection of the nose on the profile
- Subnasale—junction of the columella and upper lip.
- Stomion—central portion of the interlabial gap
- Stomion superius—lowest point of the vermilion of the upper lip
- Stomion inferius—highest point of the vermilion of the lower lip
- Labrale superius—vermilion border of the upper lip
- Labrale inferius—vermilion border of the lower lip
- Pogonion—most anterior point on the chin
- Menton—most inferior soft tissue point on the chin
- Gnathion—the point between the pogonion and the menton
- Gonion—the angle of the mandible where the ascending ramus becomes the body of the mandible

Facial Proportions

When evaluating the face, it is helpful to divide it into segments in order to assess the individual components. One method is to divide into three horizontal segments: the upper facial third extends from the trichion to the glabella, the middle third is from the glabella to the subnasale, and the lower third is from the subnasale to the menton (Fig. 2.2b). This is called the Da Vinci method and it allows to evaluate facial height [1].

Another method allows us to evaluate facial width and that is to divide the face into vertical fifths: lateral projection of the helix to the lateral canthus, lateral canthus to medial canthus, and the intercanthal distance (Fig. 2.2a). The segments should all be equal in distance.

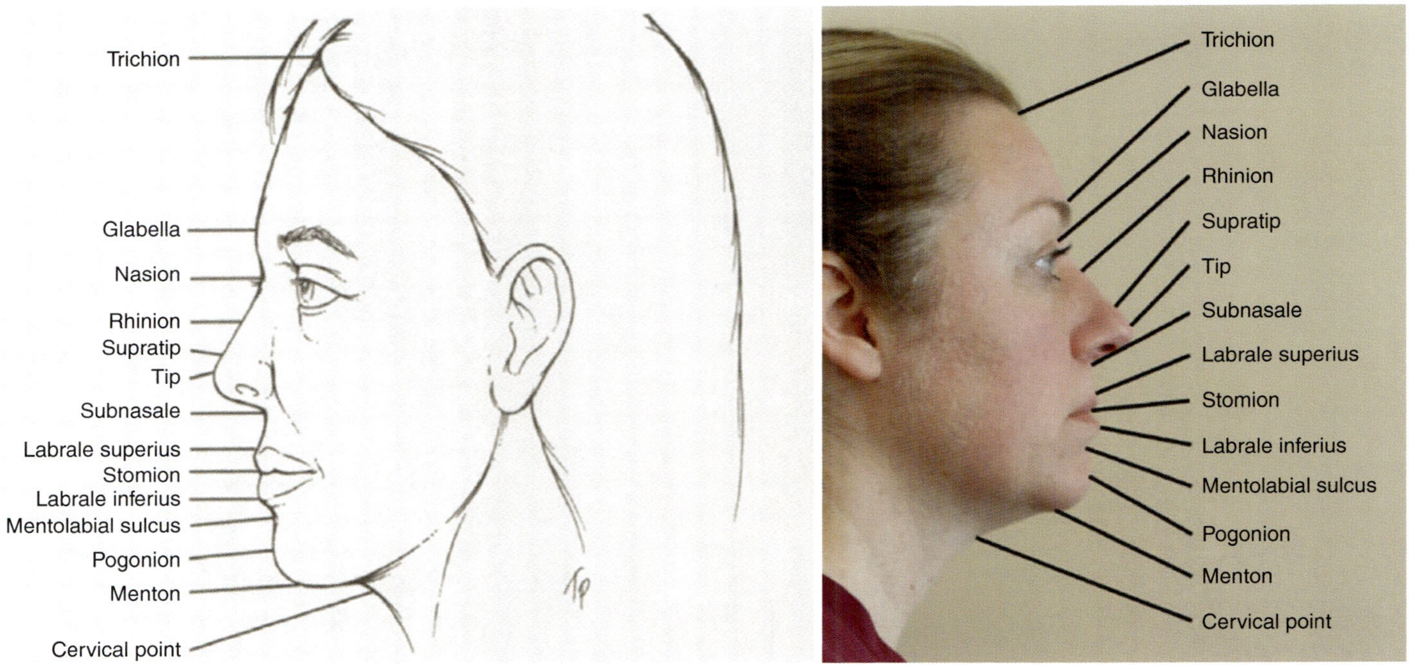

Fig. 2.1 Soft tissue anatomic landmarks on a profile view. Images citation: Ferneini, E., Bennett, J. Perioperative Assessment of the Maxillofacial Surgery Patient (p. 491–492). Cham, Switzerland: Springer 2018

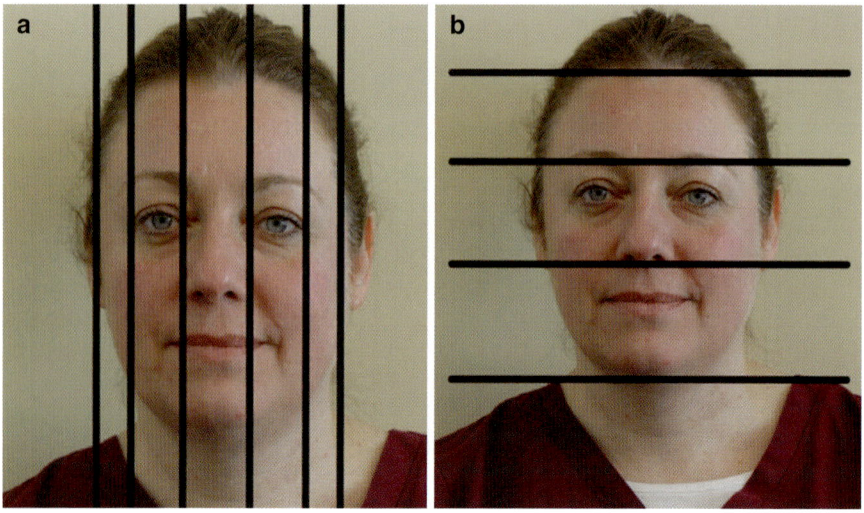

Fig. 2.2 (**a**) Vertical lines passing through the medial canthus, lateral canthus, and helix divide the face into vertical fifths. (**b**) Horizontal lines passing through the hairline, glabella, subnasale, and menton divide the face in horizontal thirds: Images citation: Ferneini, E., Bennett, J. Perioperative Assessment of the Maxillofacial Surgery Patient (p. 492). Cham, Switzerland: Springer 2018

Forehead

The forehead can significantly affect the appearance of other facial structure such as the eyes and nose and thus plays a huge role in esthetics. It constitutes the upper third of the face and the boundaries extend from the trichion down to the glabella. It should have a gentle convexity when viewed from the lateral profile with an ideal nasofrontal angle of 115–135° [2]. The nasofrontal angle is created by the intersection of lines tangent to the glabella and the nasal dorsum (Fig. 2.3).

A receding hairline can lead to the appearance of an elongated forehead, while loss of collagen and connective tissues will lead to rhytid (wrinkle) formation. Horizontal rhytids will form in a pattern that is perpendicular to the vertical fibers of the frontalis muscle [3].

Eyebrows

The medial aspect of the eyebrow should not extend past a vertical lined drawn from the lateral nasal ala through the medial canthus of the eye (Fig. 2.4), while the lateral brow is limited by an oblique line drawn from the nasal ala to the lateral canthus [4] (Fig. 2.5a). The medial and lateral ends should also be in the same plane [4]. Brow apex in women lies superior to the lateral limbus (Fig. 2.5b).

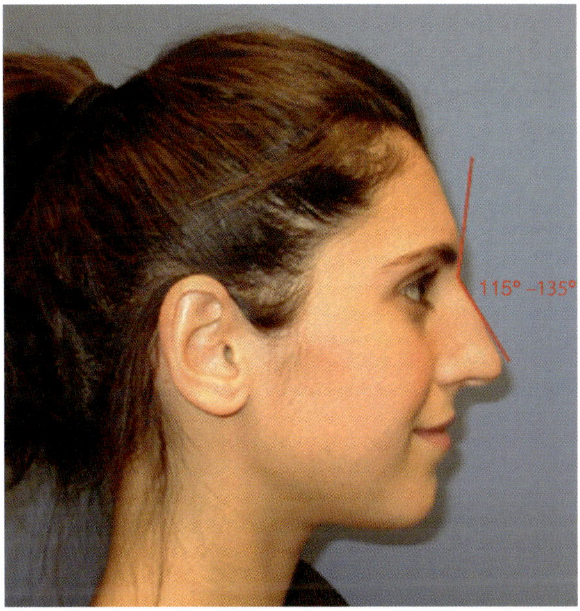

Fig. 2.3 The nasofrontal angle is created by the intersection of lines tangent to the glabella and the nasal dorsum. Image Citation: Ferneini, E., Castiglione, C., Banki, M. Complications in Maxillofacial Cosmetic Surgery (p. 28). Cham, Switzerland: Springer 2018

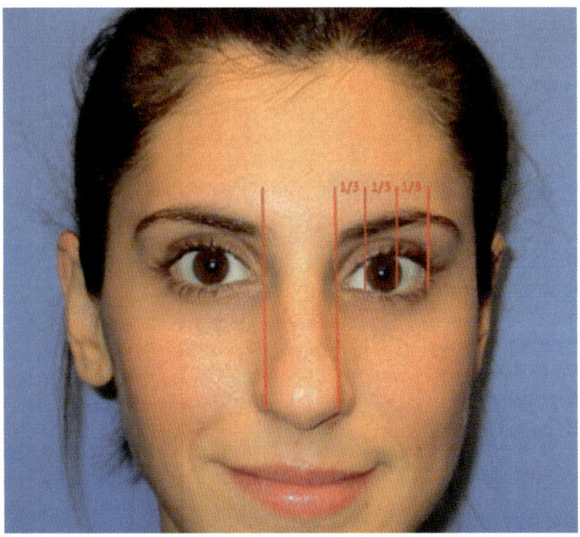

Fig. 2.4 The eye is divided into three vertical regions by vertical lines through the lateral canthus, lateral limbus, medial limbus, and medial canthus. Vertical lines drawn through the lateral nasal tip and medial canthi create the medial border of the eyebrow. Image Citation: Ferneini, E., Castiglione, C., Banki, M. Complications in Maxillofacial Cosmetic Surgery (p. 30). Cham, Switzerland: Springer 2018

There are gender differences with regard to eyebrow shape and position that surgeons must take into consideration. In males, eyebrows are ideally at the level of the superior orbital rim and have a much gentler curve [5]. In contrast, female eyebrows are 1 cm above the superior orbital rim and have a steeper upward curvature with the apex corresponding to the lateral limbus [5].

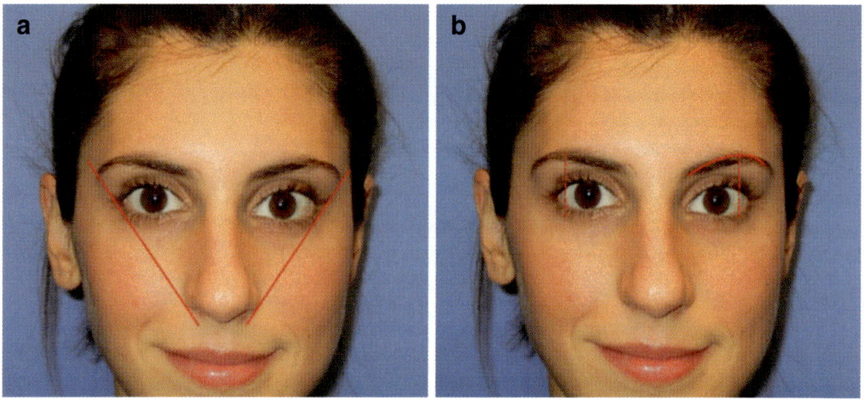

Fig. 2.5 (**a**) An oblique line drawn from the nasal ala to the lateral canthus outlines the lateral border of the brow. (**b**) Brow apex lies superior to the lateral limbus. Image Citation: Ferneini, E., Castiglione, C., Banki, M. Complications in Maxillofacial Cosmetic Surgery (p. 29). Cham, Switzerland: Springer 2018

Adverse surgical outcomes include over-depression or over-elevation of the eyebrows. Over-depression of the brow can lead the patient to appear tired or sleepy while an over-elevation can make them appear overly surprised [2]. Aging can also lead to brow ptosis causing a "grumpy" look by crowding the eyes.

Eyes

When looking at a face, humans spend more time looking at the person's eyes than any other facial structure. Therefore, the eyes can contribute a great deal to the overall esthetics of the face. The eye can be divided into three regions: medial canthus to medial limbus, medial limbus to lateral limbus, and lateral limbus to lateral canthus [3]. These three regions should be equal in width.

Furthermore, the width of an individual eye as measured from the medial canthus to the lateral canthus should constitute one-fifth of the overall facial width. The intercanthal distance should also make up another one-fifth of the distance. Average intercanthal distance is about 30 mm [5]. Increased (hypertelorism) or decreased (hypotelorism) intercanthal distance can distract from the esthetics of the rest of the face.

The periorbital features can greatly affect the appearance of the eye. A canthal tilt where the lateral tilt is superior to the medial canthus exudes youthfulness and vibrance while a superior medial canthus is a sign of aging and fatigue. The lateral canthus should generally be 2–4 mm superior to the medial canthus [1, 3].

The upper eyelid should cover 1–2 mm of the iris superiorly, while the lower eyelid should be at the level of the inferior limbus [6]. The upper eyelid should have an acute medial angle with a gentle curve laterally. Ptosis of the upper eyelid can occur due to a variety of reasons (trauma, aging, etc.) and can give the appearance of being tired and sleepy. In situation like these, a blepharoplasty can be performed where excess skin is removed from the upper eyelid in order to create more tension in the eyelid and prevent it from drooping over the eye.

The lower eyelid is continuous with cheek. With the descending of the malar fat that is common with aging, the demarcation becomes more apparent as the facial bone is more pronounced [5]. Fat grafting or cheek fat pad elevation are surgical options to blend the junction and create a once again smooth transition [6].

Nose

The central location of a nose on the face makes it a critical part of facial esthetics. The esthetic ideals of a nose are influenced by a patient's facial anatomy, age, own desires, ethnicity, and cultural values. Generally, the nose should be positioned in the middle third of the face length. Nasal length, nasal tip position, and rotation are some of the aspects analyzed in nasal esthetics.

From the lateral profile view, the radix is the deepest part of the nose and marks the transition point from the glabella to the dorsum of the nose [2]. The dorsum of the nose, referred to as the bridge of the nose, runs from the radix to the nasal tip. From the frontal view, the dorsum should draw an aesthetic line that narrows in from the medial border of the eyebrows along the lateral nose bone, before curving out along the nasal tip [3, 7]. In the lateral view, the dorsum should follow a smooth continuous line from the glabella to the nasal tip (Fig. 2.6a, b). Keeping the anatomy of the nose and adjacent structures in mind, the average measurements of an ideal nose are as follows: nasofrontal angle is 115–135°, nasolabial angle is 95–110° for women and 90–95° for men, nasofacial angle is 30–40°, and nasomental angle is 120–132° [1, 2, 4].

Through worm's eye view, the nasal tip and bilateral ala form an equilateral triangle (Fig. 2.7). The ideal width of the nose at the base of the alar margins should be equidistant to the intercanthal distance between two medial canthi. If the triangle is divided into three horizontal columns, the nostrils should occupy two-thirds of the columns at the base of the triangle and the tip of the nose should occupy the top one-third tip of the triangle [7].

There is no ideal shape of the dorsal aesthetic lines, but it is integral for a graceful appearance that the lines run smoothly parallel through the nasal bridge and slightly taper out as they approach the nasal tip. Even a slight discrepancy or interruption in the tracking of aesthetic lines along the nose can cause the nose to appear asymmetrical and unbalanced [2, 8]. A common correction of the nose is a reduction of the dorsal hump, which is a result of large nasal bones and/or septum. While men might prefer a nose with a small dorsal hump, women tend to prefer a straight dorsum or sometimes even a slightly concave dorsum [8]. Some other common corrections to the nose include narrowing of a widened nasal bridge and septoplasty to address a deviated septum. These corrections involve manipulating the position of the medial and lateral crural and septal cartilages within the base of the nose to create a more narrow, straight nose.

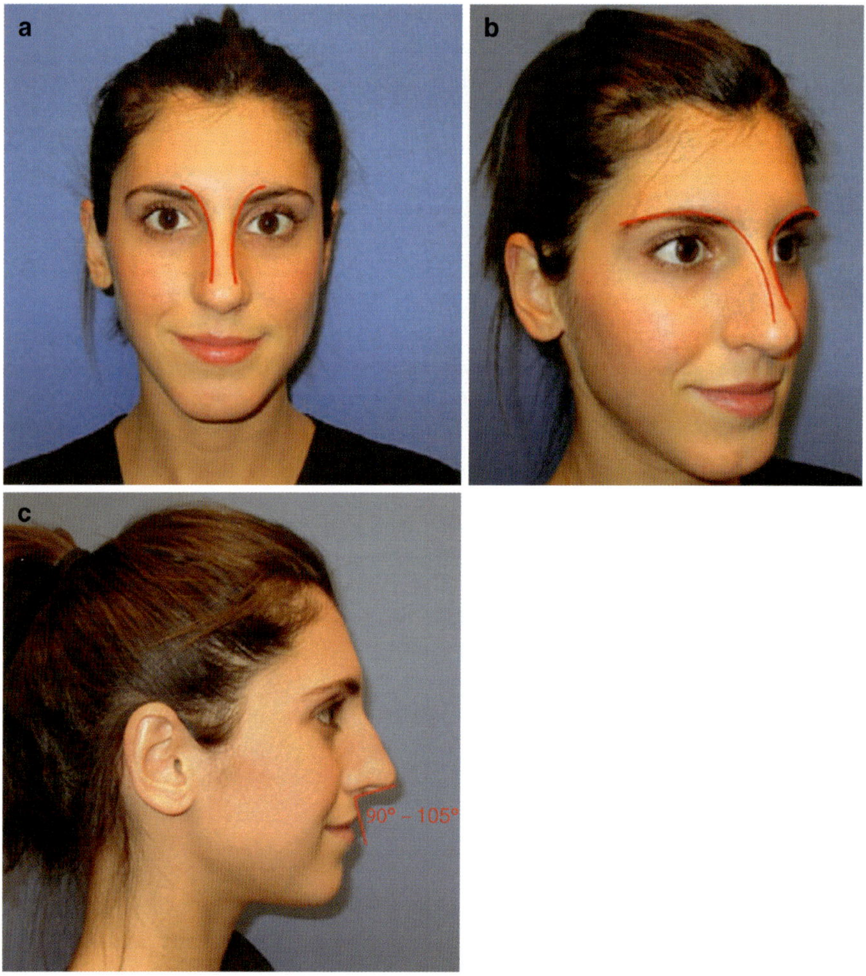

Fig. 2.6 (**a**) The medial margin of the superior orbital rim forms the brow tip aesthetic line as it curves medially along the lateral basal bone. (**b**) The brow tip aesthetic line should frame the eyebrows and follows a smooth curve trajectory before straightening to form the contours of the nasal dorsum. (**c**) The nasofrontal angle from the profile view

Lips

The lips can reflect the age of a person, as more full and luscious lips give a person an appearance of youthfulness while flatter, longer, and less defined lips are telling signs of aging [7]. The lips are located within the lower one-third of the face. The upper lip is measured from the subnasale to stomion, and makes up one-third of the total lip height. The lower lip and chin are measured from stomion to gnathion and make up the second two-thirds of the lip height.

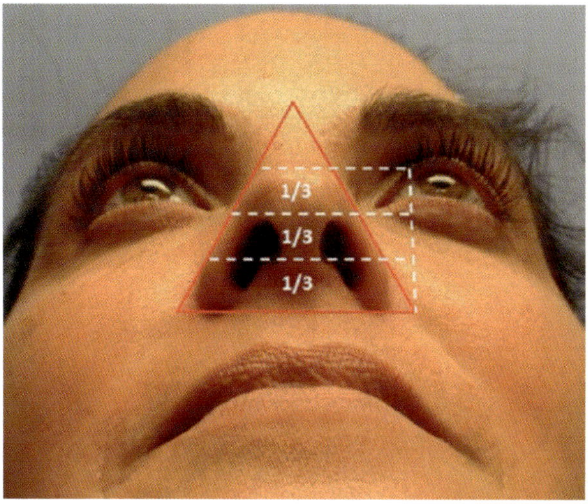

Fig. 2.7 The columella is divided into three equal zones: upper lobular, middle, and basal zones. The nasal tip and bilateral alar rims form a triangle. The nostrils should make up two-thirds of the length of the columella, with the nasal tip making up the final third. The ideal width of the nose corresponds to the intercanthal distance. Image Citation: Ferneini, E., Castiglione, C., Banki, M. Complications in Maxillofacial Cosmetic Surgery (p. 29, 31). Cham, Switzerland: Springer 2018

The ideal width of the lips is determined by drawing a vertical line from the medial limbus down, which should intersect the lateral most edge of the oral commissures. The philtra columns extend from Cupid's bow to the columella (Fig. 2.8a, b).

Lip projection is a common assessment used to determine ideal position of lips by drawing a line from the subnasale to pogonion. The upper lip should be around 3.5 mm anterior to that line and the lower lip should be around 2.2 mm anterior to the same line [5]. Also, the lower lip height should be twice the size of the upper lip [4]. As we age, the projection of the lip decreases due to perioral tissue changes and volume loss in the lips. With age the lips become thin, vermilion border rolls inward, and upper lip lengthens and droops down [7]. Common lip and perioral rejuvenation to restore youthfulness include surgical and nonsurgical procedures that utilize hyaluronic acid, dermal fillers, and non-ablative lasers.

Chin

The chin is demarcated superiorly by the labiomental sulcus, inferiorly by the menton, and should make up two-thirds of the height of the lower facial third. Vertical chin height can be altered by loss of teeth and resorption of the mandibular ridge leading to changes in the appearance of the lower lip as well as the contours of the neck [4].

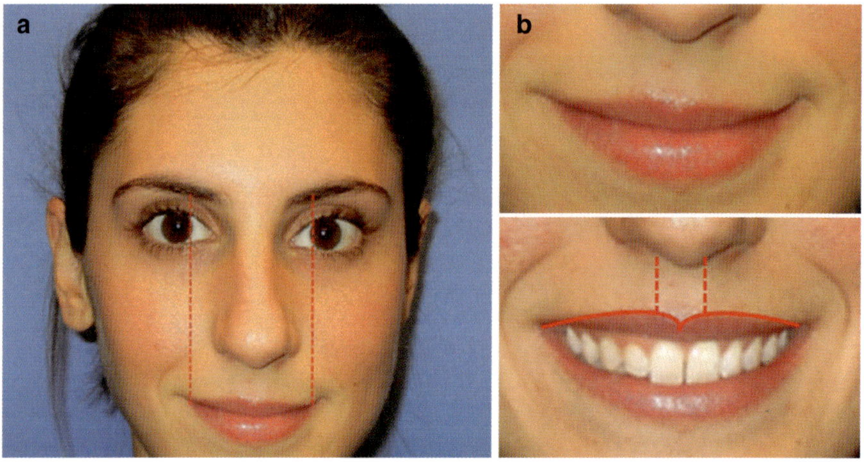

Fig. 2.8 (**a**) A vertical line drawn from the lateral edge of the oral commissure should be in line with the medial limbus. (**b**) The philtra columns extend from Cupid's bow to the columella. Image Citation: Ferneini, E., Castiglione, C., Banki, M. Complications in Maxillofacial Cosmetic Surgery (p. 27, 33). Cham, Switzerland: Springer 2018

Chin projection is evaluated in the lateral profile by the angle formed by a line drawn from glabella and subnasale and a line drawn from subnasale to pogonion. The angle should be 11° [2, 7].

While evaluating a patient for a small or "weak" chin, it is important to differentiate between microgenia and micrognathia. Microgenia can be corrected for with a genioplasty alone. However, micrognathia will generally be associated with malocclusion as well and may require orthognathic surgery to advance the mandible and achieve proper chin projection [2]. Fillers and botulinum injections are other viable options for chin enhancement.

Neck

While technically not part of the face, the neck can still influence facial esthetics by affecting the contours of the chin and lower face. The cervicomental angle is formed by a horizontal line drawn from the menton to the innermost point between the submental area and neck (cervical point) and a vertical line drawn from the pogonion to the glabella [4, 9] (Fig. 2.9). The ideal cervicomental angle is acute and is ideally between 85° and 95° with acceptable ranges of 90–110°. Skin laxity that occurs with aging leads to loss of definition around the mandible and an obtuse cervicomental angle [2, 7]. A SMAS face-lift technique can be used to create a tauter look and restore youthful appearance.

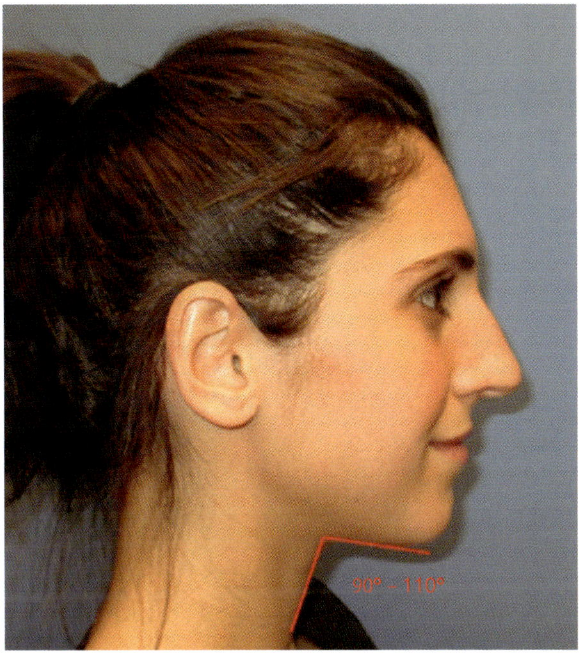

Fig. 2.9 The cervicomental angle is created by two intersecting planes: the horizontal plane from the menton to the cervical point, and the vertical plane parallel to the neck. Image Citation: Ferneini, E., Castiglione, C., Banki, M. Complications in Maxillofacial Cosmetic Surgery (p. 34). Cham, Switzerland: Springer 2018

Ears

The superior aspect of the ear should align with the eyebrow, while the inferior part should be at the level of the nasal ala. Ear width should be 50–60% of the length, and ear length should be approximately the same as the length of the nose. The long axis of the ear should be posteriorly inclined 15–30° and should be parallel to the long axis of the nasal dorsum. The angle between the helix and the mastoid skin is 20–30° and the distance is 15–25 mm. [4, 9].

References

1. Ferneini E, Bennett J. Perioperative assessment of the maxillofacial surgery patient. Cham, Switzerland: Springer; 2018.
2. Ferneini E, Castiglione C, Banki M. Complications in maxillofacial cosmetic surgery. Cham: Springer; 2018.
3. Nahai F. The art of aesthetic surgery: principles and techniques, three volume set. 2nd ed. Boca Raton: CRC Press; 2012.
4. Karimi K, Adamson P. Patient analysis and selection in aging face surgery. Facial Plast Surg. 2011;27(1):5–15. Web
5. Truswell W. Surgical facial rejuvenation: a road map to safe and reliable outcomes. New York: Thieme Medical; 2009. Print
6. Papel ID, Frodel JL. Facial plastic and reconstructive surgery. 4th ed. New York: Thieme; 2017.

7. Warren RJ, Neligan PC. Plastic surgery, Aesthetic surgery, vol. 2. 3rd ed. Philadelphia, PA: Saunders; 2013.
8. Azizzadeh B, Reilly M. Dorsal hump reduction and osteotomies. Clin Plast Surg. 2016;43(1):47–58.
9. Zimbler MS, Ham J. Aesthetic facial analysis. In: Cummings head and neck surgery. St. Louis: Mosby; 2015.

Office-Based Laboratory Indications and Interpretation

3

Benjamin Noblitt

Part I: The Basics

Basics of Laboratory Testing

In the very early years of medicine the practitioner had to rely solely upon their physical exam to diagnose and subsequently treat disease. The physical exam has become no less important in today's day and age, but the use of the laboratory and the various tests that they can run has greatly augmented diagnostic ability and accuracy.

Physical exam findings are fundamental to every healthcare practitioner. Most diseases can be diagnosed on history and physical exam, or at the very least an appropriate differential can be obtained. Some would argue that this is the core skill set required to be an effective healthcare practitioner. While advances in medicine have made small improvements in the physical exam, there have been enormous advances in the laboratory setting. This has allowed the practitioner to gain an enormous increased ability to effectively diagnose disease.

Calibration is key. Calibrating a history and physical exam is near impossible; the way one practitioner performs an examination will be different from how another practitioner performs their exam. Additionally, the patient history is invaluable to diagnosis, but it also has the same built-in variance—there is no way to standardize physical exam and patient history. In contrast to this, the laboratory has the ability calibrate and standardize their results.

In summary, the history and physical exam are still, and should always be the foundation of diagnosis and the development of a differential. However, the laboratory can help provide additional, reliable, and repeatable information to the practitioner that they would not be otherwise able to obtain.

B. Noblitt (✉)
University of Cincinnati Oral and Maxillofacial Surgery, Cincinnati, OH, USA
e-mail: NoblitBN@ucmail.uc.edu

E. M. Ferneini, M. T. Goupil (eds.), *Office-Based Maxillofacial Surgical Procedures*, https://doi.org/10.1007/978-3-030-22371-7_3

Understanding the Laboratory: Statistics

It is vital to understand the statistical nuances of laboratory tests. No single lab test is perfect, and there will likely never be one. As such, some tests are more reliable than others, some provide greater diagnostic ability than others, and some rely on the history and physical exam of the patient before they are of any use. It is well beyond the scope of this chapter to cover the statistical world involved with the laboratory, but a few key points will be covered.

Pre-test probability is the probability that a patient will have either a positive or negative result PRIOR to having the test performed. This number is based on epidemiological data, but is more commonly determined based on the practitioner's experience.

For example, if a patient has a history of chronic kidney disease, it is reasonable to determine that the patient will likely have an elevated creatinine. This means that if they take a blood sample, and the laboratory tests the blood creatinine, there is a *high* pre-test probability of measuring an *elevated* creatinine value.

The value in this knowledge is most easily seen when an unexpected lab value is obtained. For example, let's say we see an 18-year-old, lean, muscular varsity soccer player come to the office. For some reason a blood test is drawn (ignore the reason why) which presents a hemoglobin of three. This lab value is likely false due to such a low pre-test probability based on the scenario given. Hemoglobin levels that low will translate into physical exam findings that are in opposition to how the patient presented. The patient here is a very healthy athlete that would not be able to physically perform at his level with a hemoglobin of three. The value of this knowledge is being able to see that the most likely scenario is a false lab result. This would direct the practitioner to send a new set of laboratory specimens instead of working the patient up for profound anemia.

There is little use in attempting to calculate the actual pre-test probability of a lab test. It is more important for the practitioner to simply understand the idea that common diseases are common, and that the lab values should fit the clinical presentation of the patient.

Tests can be sensitive and/or specific.

Tests that are very **sensitive** can be used to **rule out** disease when the test is negative. This is because a sensitive test is good at detecting a value when there is one present. Unfortunately, they also can tend to give false positive results. The important point is that a very sensitive test will rarely be negative when a positive value is present. This means that if a very sensitive test is negative, one can rest assured that the disease process is NOT likely to be present.

Tests that are very **specific** are used to **rule in** disease when a test is positive. This is because a specific test has high requirements for detecting a value when one is present. Unfortunately, since they are so specific they also tend to give negative results even when a positive value is present. The important point is that very specific tests will rarely give positive results when there is no positive value. This means that if a very specific test is positive, one can rest assured that the disease process IS likely to be present.

Very few tests have both high sensitivity and specificity. It is important to know the limitations of any lab value or test before treating the results of any test as truth.

Understanding the Laboratory: Diagrams

Many common labs are presented in a shorthand format called a fishbone diagram. There are multiple variations in these diagrams, but the two common examples (Figs. 3.1 and 3.2) are presented below for the sake of familiarity:

Understanding the Laboratory: Nothing in Isolation

Tests should not be interpreted in isolation. Each lab value should be interpreted in conjunction with the clinical exam and history of the patient. For example, if a patient presents with an elevated white blood cell (WBC) count, a practitioner might have a differential diagnosis including a possible infection. The patient then reveals that that they have chronic asthma and take inhaled corticosteroids as needed. With this added history, the elevated WBC is now understood to be the result of the corticosteroids, not an infection or other such cause. If the lab test was interpreted alone, it would have led down an erroneous pathway. Laboratory tests should be ordered based on the practitioner's evaluation of the clinical exam and history, not the other way around.

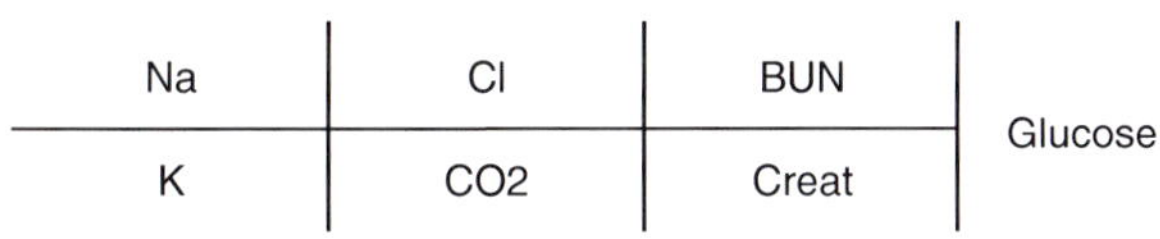

Fig. 3.1 Electrolytes: cations, anions, urine, and sugar

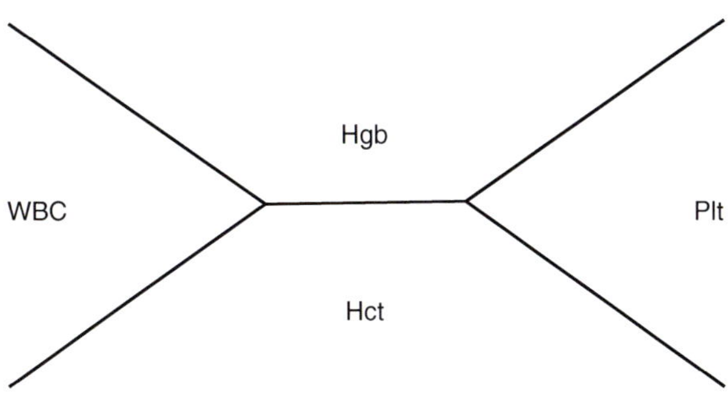

Fig. 3.2 CBC: white blood cell count, hemoglobin, hematocrit, and platelets

Understanding the Laboratory: Time Frame

Lab values can represent either a single point in time or an average over a block of time. For example, if someone has their blood glucose measured, it will show what the blood glucose is at that single moment. If the blood glucose is measured again a few hours later, it will likely be a very different number. Other tests can represent a longer period of time. For example, the hemoglobin A1c number allows the practitioner to get an idea of what the average blood glucose levels looked like for a patient over the last 60–90 days. It is important to know the timeframe of the lab tests being interpreted.

Understanding the Laboratory: Reference Ranges

Reference ranges for a lab value will vary from region to region, and even sometimes from hospital to hospital. These variations are typically not significant but are enough to create a "gray zone" for interpretation. Furthermore, reference ranges typically will be different for children and adults, men and women, etc. Note that children and pregnant women are especially prone to having different reference ranges than that of the general population.

Understanding the Laboratory: Blood Tests

The body is composed of many different tissues (bone, muscle, cartilage, etc.), fluids (blood, urine, CSF, saliva, etc.), and compartments (intracellular, extracellular, etc.). Laboratory tests can be associated with each one of these, but some are more common than others. The most common lab tests are from blood (more specifically venous blood), urine, and soft tissue. Venous blood has a different composition than that of arterial blood, so it is important to know the difference. Systemic arterial blood is coming from the heart and lungs and is fully oxygenated while venous blood is oxygen depleted. Also, venous blood is usually full of metabolic waste as it washes the waste products from the tissue bed it is coming from (with exception of the renal veins). It is the practitioner's responsibility to know and understand these differences when it comes time to interpret the laboratory results they requested.

Part II: Common Labs Drawn for Office-Based Procedures

Complete Blood Count: WBC, RBC, Hgb, Hct, and Plt

The complete blood count (CBC) is a common set of labs that are used to assess the cells in the blood. These tests are usually automated tests that physically count the number of cells per unit of volume to give a concentration of each cell type.

CBC	
WBC	9.1
RBC	4.50
Hemoglobin	13.7
Hematocrit	41.7
Platelets	254

Fig. 3.3 A common example presentation of the CBC with normal range values. Note that many labs auto populate these panels with other readings such as the mean corpuscular volume (MCV), red cell distribution width (RDW), mean corpuscular hemoglobin concentration (MCHC), etc. Also note that units are implied if not given

The CBC is one of the most common lab panels ordered because the lab values it utilizes can be used as proxies for the body's immune status, hemodynamics, and hemostasis. If the practitioner has reason to suspect any issue with these, a CBC would be warranted.

The CBC can come in many different formats, but the essentials of a CBC are noted below (Fig. 3.3).

White Blood Cells (WBC) Count

Common reference range: 3.8–10.8 × 10^3 cells/μL [1]

This test looks at the concentration of circulating white blood cells in the blood. WBCs are the immune system's work horses and are used in the immune response to facilitate the body's immune function. Elevated numbers (leukocytosis) can be indicative of many things such as infection, a response to medications, or a disorder of the bone marrow. Depressed numbers (leukopenia) can indicate a viral infection, cancers of the bone marrow, autoimmune disorders, a response to a medication, or even severe infections. In the setting of clinical swelling, an elevated WBC is often a diagnostic sign of infection.

Red Blood Cells Count (RBC)

Common reference range for males: 4.2–5.8 × 10^6 cells/μL [1]

Common reference range for females: 3.8–5.1 × 10^6 cells/μL [1]

This test looks at the concentration of circulating red blood cells in the blood. RBCs are used to carry oxygen from the lungs to the tissues of the body. This test is often paired with other tests such as the hemoglobin and hematocrit mentioned later in this chapter because the RBC count alone is not very diagnostic. On its own, elevated numbers can indicate bone marrow disease, heart disease, lung disease, dehydration, or a response to medications. Similarly, decreased numbers can indicate anemia, nutrient deficiency, kidney injury, bone marrow disease, or even a response to medications.

Hemoglobin (Hgb)

Common reference range for males: 13.2–17.1 g/dL [1]

Common reference range for females: 11.7–15.5 g/dL [1]

This test looks at the amount of hemoglobin in the blood. Hemoglobin is carried inside the RBCs and is the substrate to which oxygen is carried in the blood. As mentioned earlier, this is one of the tests that is commonly paired with the RBCs to give a better idea of the oxygen carrying capacity of the blood. Elevated hemoglobin values have similar causes to that of elevated RBC counts; bone marrow disease, heart disease, lung disease, dehydration, or a response to medications. Decreased levels of hemoglobin can have many causes including various anemias, chronic bleeding, heavy menstrual cycles, cancer, nutrient deficiency, kidney injury, bone marrow disease, hypothyroid, or even a response to medications. A sedated patient with a low hemoglobin will likely have a low oxygen reserve and will desaturate quickly and easily.

Hematocrit (Hct)

Common reference range for males: 38–50% [1]

Common reference range for females: 35–45% [1]

The hematocrit is the ratio of total RBC volume to total blood volume after centrifugation. For this reason, some people refer to this as the packed-cell volume (PCV) test. In general, elevated Hct counts can be caused by dehydration, or any other cause of elevated RBCs. Decreased hematocrit counts can be from any cause of decreased RBCs or increased blood volume such as the administration of IV fluids.

Platelets (Plt)

Common reference range: 140–400 × 10^3/μL [1]

This test looks at the concentration of platelets in the blood. Platelets are the first responders to an injury and are essential in hemostasis. They form a platelet plug during primary hemostasis and subsequently initiate secondary hemostasis. Elevated platelet counts (thrombocytosis) can be caused by acute bleeding, splenectomy, cancer, or infections. Decreased platelet counts (thrombocytopenia) can be caused by sequestration of platelets in the spleen, bone marrow disease, certain immune related diseases, or even a response to medications. Low platelet counts are often associated with easy bruising, prolonged bleeding, mucosal bleeding, and petechia.

Coagulation Studies: PT, INR, aPTT

If a surgeon has reason to suspect a disorder in hemostasis, it is likely that they will order a coagulation panel. Assessment of the coagulation process can alter the treatment planning and surgical process used by the practitioner, making this another very common panel (Fig. 3.4).

Most coagulation panels consist of the following:

Coagulation Panel	
PT	24.2
INR	2.40
aPTT	41.8

Fig. 3.4 A common example of the coagulation panel. Note that this example shows a patient who is on warfarin with a prolonged PT, elevated INR, and prolonged aPTT. Also note that units are implied if not given

Prothrombin time (PT)

Common reference range: 11.6–14.4 s [1]

Prothrombin is a coagulation factor that is used in the extrinsic pathway (tissue factor pathway) of the coagulation cascade (as opposed to the PTT which uses the intrinsic pathway). The PT looks at the time it takes to clot after clotting is initiated. The test is timed and is reported in seconds. The more seconds means a lower ability to clot, while fewer seconds means a higher ability to clot. This test is commonly used to assess the coagulation of a patient with liver damage (prothrombin in made in the liver) or for someone who is on blood thinners such as warfarin. If a patient has liver disease or is on such a blood thinner, one would expect longer durations to clot.

International Normalized Ratio (INR)

Common reference range: 0.9–1.1 [1]

Normal therapeutic range: 2.0–3.0 [2]

High-risk therapeutic range: 2.5–3.5 [2]

The INR is the more common presentation of the PT time. The reason is that small variations in the materials used in the lab can provide substantial differences in the duration of clotting and thus can greatly affect the PT duration. To remove this variation, the lab can run a reference test to act as a baseline time to clot specific to that lab's materials. The ratio of the sample clot time to the reference clot time is reported as the INR. The INR can then be consistently compared from patient to patient regardless of where the INR was performed. If a surgery patient presents with an elevated INR, practitioners will sometimes often request a reduction of the INR by the patient's physician prior to surgery. Note that the risks (such as an embolism) and benefits of lowering the INR have to be taken into consideration prior to altering the patient's regimen. The upper INR limit before surgery is held is typically provider specific, but an INR of 2.8 is a common ballpark figure. Note that the INR can change in as little as 24–48 h, so an INR the day before surgery can sometimes be prudent.

Activated Partial Thromboplastin Time (aPTT)

Common reference range: 24.3–33.1 s [1]

The aPTT is used to measure the intrinsic pathway of the coagulation cascade, as opposed to the PT (which uses the extrinsic pathway). This test is similar to the

PT in that it is timed in seconds. The "activated" portion comes from an activator being added to a regular PTT test to reduce the overall time of the test (roughly takes half as along). Additionally, this test is often paired with the PT in order to assess the full coagulation cascade. Prolonged aPTT can be the result of hemophilia, von Willebrand disease, liver disease, lupus anticoagulant, or even a response to medications. Similar to a prolonged PT and elevated INR, a prolonged aPTT will indicate prolonged bleeding from surgical intervention.

Glucose Assessment: Blood Glucose and Glycosylated Hemoglobin

Blood Glucose (BG)

Common reference range for fasting blood glucose: 70–100 mg/Dl [1]

Blood glucose levels are probably the most common in office lab measured. Blood glucose is most commonly measured with a finger stick test chairside. This is done quickly with a high rate of accuracy and is usually tolerated well by the patient. Additionally, it can often be added onto other blood tests (such as the CBC) after they are drawn to avoid a finger stick.

Both high and low blood sugars are of concern. Elevated blood sugars are associated with chronic issues such as neuropathy, retinopathy, macroangiopathy, etc. One such concern that is very relevant to the surgeon is the immunosuppression and impaired wound healing. Chronically elevated blood sugars impede circulation as well as the immune response. Because of this, diabetics can take longer to heal and recover from surgical insult than those with more normalized blood sugar levels. The more elevated the blood sugar, generally the greater the impairments [3].

Low blood sugars are more of an acute concern. Hypoglycemia starves tissue of essential nutrients and can be fatal. Because of this, hypoglycemia must be treated if it is suspected. Common symptoms of hypoglycemia include tachycardia, pallor, shakiness, confusion, blurred vision, etc. [3].

Many diabetic patients know what it feels like to be hypoglycemic. It is always prudent to ask the patient if they know how their body reacts to being hypoglycemic and to let the provider know if they feel they are becoming hypoglycemic. Note that a patient can still be hypoglycemic even if they show no symptoms.

The use of 10–15 mg of carbohydrates is a good starting point for glucose levels below 70 [3]. Orange juice or soda is a good source of these sugars. If an IV has already been placed, the provider can consider crystalloid solution with 5% dextrose as well. 10–25 g of IV dextrose is usually a good dose (20–50 mL of 50% dextrose solution or 200–500 mL of a 5% solution) [4].

Glycosylated Hemoglobin (A1c)

Common reference range chart (Fig. 3.5) [5]:

Glycosylated hemoglobin also known as hemoglobin A1C, HbA1c, or just A1c help give an estimate of the average blood glucose level over the last 60–90 days.

Fig. 3.5 This chart shows the hemoglobin A1c with its associated blood glucose levels. Note that these are the average blood glucose level over the past 60–90 days

HbA1c	Associated Blood Glucose
5%	97 mg/dL
6%	126 mg/dL
7%	154 mg/dL
8%	183 mg/dL
9%	212 mg/dL
10%	240 mg/dL
11%	269 mg/dL
12%	298 mg/dL
13%	326 mg/dL
14%	355 mg/dL

The basic premise is that glucose will bind to the hemoglobin in the blood at different rates based on its concentration. Since the average life span of the red blood cell is about 90–120 days, the A1c can give an estimate of the average blood glucose over about 60–90 days [3].

Note that the blood glucose variability is not covered by the A1c, only the average value. This means that someone with relatively consistent blood glucose and someone with highly variable blood glucose can average the same A1c number despite these differences.

Assessment of Pathology: Culture and Sensitivity, Biopsy with Permanent Stain, and Immunofluorescence

Culture and Sensitivity

Cultures can be separated from most laboratory tests because most tests look at molecular values whereas cultures are attempting to harvest living organisms. Many lab tests can be completed in a matter of minutes or hours, but this is not the case for cultures. Cultures are analogous to a farmer growing livestock. Because of this, cultures tend to take more time to produce results that that of most other lab tests. These results are on the order of days to weeks.

Another important aspect is that some bacteria require very specific environments to grow. Unfortunately, the environment of the culture is often quite different than the environment of the sample, so not all bacteria/fungi are able to be cultured.

The second part is the sensitivity portion of the test. Sensitivity is based on the culture specimen. If the organism is able to be cultured the lab can then test to see which antibiotics the organism is susceptible to. This is most useful when the offending organism has developed resistance to certain medications. This can allow for better understanding of the treatment options available to the practitioner.

Note that the culture process usually can take several days, so empiric treatment should be started before the results of the study comes back.

Not all infections necessitate a culture and sensitivity. Many localized infections can be treated with minor interventions. However, larger and more aggressive infections should cause the practitioner to think about the utility of a culture and sensitivity.

If a culture and sensitivity are to be obtained, it is recommended to have the patient swish with chlorhexidine mouthwash for 30 s prior to obtaining an oral sample. Additionally, it is best to limit contamination and all attempts at obtaining purulent discharge only should be made.

Biopsy with Permanent Stain

Biopsies are another very common procedure in the office. This is covered in greater depth in sect. History and Physical, Chap. 8. Biopsies are sent when clinical history and physical exam are not sufficient to provide a diagnosis. When the biopsy is sent, it should be sent with a clinical history, either radiographs or radiographic read of the lesion, and a differential diagnosis. This will help the pathologist interpret the histopathology.

The foundation of histopathology is the permanent stain. The most common stains are hematoxylin and eosin (H&E). There are many other stains available and most of them are lesion or cell specific.

Note that frozen sections can also be sent but are not as common in the office-based setting. The general reason for this is that frozen sections are mainly used to assess surgical margins. It can often take some duration of time for the results of the frozen section to return with results, and in that time the surgeon can continue to operate or wait for the results. Most surgeries of this nature are often done in the operating room, though not always.

Immunofluorescence

Many pathologies of the oral and maxillofacial region are immune modulated. Immunohistochemistry has largely been based on the application of antibodies with florescent markers on them that can bind to certain tissues. Very similar to permanent stain, this allows the practitioner to know where the lesion in question is having an immune-mediated reaction within the tissue layers. This location is diagnostically important.

The most common form of immunohistochemistry is the immunofluorescence stain. These stains should not be employed alone, but in conjunction with standard H&E preparations.

The most common pathologies on the differential that would warrant immunofluorescence staining would be the immune-mediated diseases (such as pemphigus vulgaris or pemphigoid).

Two main methods exist, direct and indirect immunofluorescence. The direct method uses antibodies labeled with fluorescein that came from another source (usually rabbits) that directly bind to the tissue in question. The indirect method uses the patient's serum antibodies and binds them to a test tissue with known substrates. These bound antibodies are then washed with fluorescein-labeled antihuman immunoglobulins. The direct method is more sensitive and more diagnostic [6].

Gender Specific Assessment: Urine Pregnancy

Urine Pregnancy (u preg)

One group of patients that is distinct from all others is pregnant women. Medications and treatments can have different effects on them when compared to nonpregnant patients. Pharmacodynamics and pharmacokinetics are different as well due to altered volumes of distribution, blood enzymes, etc. Additionally, physical manipulation is different because of the mass effect of the fetus in the abdomen.

Due to delicate state of the fetus, they are prone to injury from medications. For this reason, most medications have distinct classifications based on their safety to the fetus.

Many women will not show their pregnancy on clinical exam. Additionally, some women would not know they are pregnant until a few weeks into their pregnancy. This means that many women who do not appear to be pregnant could be.

For all of these reasons, the urine pregnancy test should be performed before any invasive procedure or administration of medications on all women of childbearing age.

If this is not feasible, any women of childbearing age should sign a waiver indicating there is no possibility of being pregnant. The risks of the procedure while being pregnant should also be reviewed with the patient.

The urine pregnancy tests look for human chorionic gonadotropin (hCG) in the maternal urine. HCG can be detected as early as 6 days after ovulation following implantation on some ultrasensitive tests. Most urine pregnancy tests are very accurate depending on the timing of the test [7].

Any woman with a positive pregnancy test should be worked up and treated as though she is pregnant.

References

1. Clinical Laboratory Reference Ranges. http://laboratory.uchealth.com/tests/reference-ranges-pdf/. 2015. Accessed 1 Sept 2018.
2. Padilla O. Normal Laboratory Values. Merck Manual. 2018. https://www.merckmanuals.com/professional/appendixes/normal-laboratory-values/blood-tests-normal-values#v8508814. Accessed 1 Sept 2018.
3. Abubaker AO, Lam D, Benson KJ. Oral and maxillofacial secrets. 3rd ed. Amsterdam: Elsevier; 2016.
4. Medscape dextrose (Rx). Medscape, LLC, New York. 2018. https://reference.medscape.com/drug/d50w-dglucose-dextrose-342705. Accessed 1 Sept 2018.
5. Nathan D, et al. Translating the A1C assay into estimated average glucose values. Diabetes Care. 2008; 31:1473–1478. http://care.diabetesjournals.org/content/31/8/1473. Accessed 1 Sept 2018.
6. Marx RE, Stern D. Oral and maxillofacial pathology: a rationale for diagnosis and treatment. 2nd ed. Berlin: Quintessence Pub; 2012.
7. Cole L, Ladner D, Byrn F. The normal variabilities of the menstrual cycle. Fertil Steril. 2009;91:522–7.

Local Anesthesia

4

Christy Lottinger and Julie McNeish

Introduction

It wasn't until the late 1800s when surgeons and dentists alike began to use cocaine as a topical analgesic to perform surgical procedures painlessly on conscious patients. Prior to this development, painful procedures would require the use of general anesthetic agents, most often ether, developed in 1846 by a dentist by the name of W.T.G. Morton who first publicly demonstrated its effectiveness by performing a tooth extraction of a patient under its influence [1]. However, general anesthesia carries inherent risks to the patient and can prove to be impractical, particularly in an outpatient setting. Notable advancements over the following decades would include the addition of vasoconstrictor to local anesthetic solutions, the concept of nerve blockade, the development of the modern syringe, and the introduction of several synthetic analogs of cocaine, which would prove to be safer and more efficacious as local anesthetics [2].

The ability to provide temporary sensation loss intraoperatively without the need for general anesthetic agents provides a safe and comfortable working environment that is the cornerstone of many office-based oral and maxillofacial surgical procedures. In oral surgery, local anesthesia is frequently employed as the primary surgical anesthetic for minimally to moderately invasive procedures on conscious patients via infiltration or nerve blockade. Additionally, it may be used even in the setting of more global anesthetic agents for the control of postoperative pain and, if compounded with a vasoconstrictor, the provision of hemostasis at the surgical site.

C. Lottinger · J. McNeish (✉)
University of Connecticut Oral and Maxillofacial Surgery, Farmington, CT, USA
e-mail: lottinger@uchc.edu; jmcneish@uchc.edu

E. M. Ferneini, M. T. Goupil (eds.), *Office-Based Maxillofacial Surgical Procedures*, https://doi.org/10.1007/978-3-030-22371-7_4

Anesthetic Options

Topical

Although topical anesthetics are commonly used to improve patient comfort prior to injection of local anesthesia, there is some utility for its solo use for small procedures such as gingivectomy, extraction of exfoliating deciduous teeth in children, and the biopsy of superficial mucosal lesions, as well as for the relief of oral lesions such as aphthous ulcers. Topical anesthetics are transferred through the mucous membrane by diffusion over a period of 30 s to 2.5 min depending on site of administration, and they penetrate only to a depth of 2–3 mm, thus limiting their usefulness to the block of sensation in the surface mucosa [3, 4]. They should be applied in small quantities to mucosa dried with gauze at the proposed site of needle penetration. Once applied the topical should remain in place for at least 2 min to allow diffusion across the mucous membrane [5]. Because their action requires diffusion across this distance, they typically require higher concentrations to achieve clinical effect than injected anesthetic agents. Additionally, they may not contain vasoconstrictors and may undergo rapid vascular uptake. Therefore, care must be taken to avoid over administration resulting in local and systemic toxicity, particularly when used in conjunction with injected local agents. The two most commonly used topical anesthetics in dentistry, lidocaine and benzocaine, are not water soluble and therefore poorly absorbed into circulation, which reduces the likelihood of toxicity [4]. However, compound agents, which employ a combination of topical anesthetic agents with or without vasoactive agents, have been implicated as potentially harmful if used without caution due to their low therapeutic index, variations in composition, and difficult dosing [6].

Benzocaine is most commonly used supplied in either the spray or gel form, although gel patches, ointments, and solutions are also on market. This agent is an ester local anesthetic that is mostly insoluble in water and poorly absorbed into systemic vasculature, therefore making systemic toxicity clinically irrelevant. However, methemoglobinemia secondary to topical application of benzocaine has been documented, so care must be taken especially in elderly and neonatal populations. There have also been a few reports of allergic reaction after the use of topical benzocaine with the incidence of contact dermatitis being about 2% in the North American literature [5, 6–9].

Lidocaine, perhaps the most well-known and common form of topical anesthetic in both dentistry and medicine, is also found in many different forms but is most commonly utilized in sprays and gels. Additionally, viscous lidocaine solutions can be found in concentrations of 0.5%, 1%, and 2% and may be used topically for the relief of multiple conditions including radiation mucositis and aphthous ulcers as well as in preparation for instrumentation of the airway [10]. It should be noted that systemic absorption is greater with the water-soluble form and care must be taken to avoid overdose especially in the pediatric population [5]. Due to lidocaine being an amide the risk of allergy is low, with incidence of allergy being about 0.7% in the North American literature [11].

Eutectic Mixture of Local Anesthetics (EMLA) is an emulsion of 2.5% lidocaine and 2.5% prilocaine in the form of a eutectic oil that has the ability to penetrate intact skin. As such, it has been popularized for its use in venipuncture, especially in children, as well as a topical anesthetic agent for a variety of minor soft tissue procedures. For proper administration, a quarter-sized amount of EMLA cream should be applied to the desired site and covered with an occlusive dressing, such as a Tegaderm, for at least 60 min for adequate loss of sensation [12]. Maximum effect can be expected to occur at 2–3 h. Superficial dermal anesthesia lasts approximately 1 h after removal of the cream [5]. EMLA appears to be a potent topical anesthetic when used on oral mucosa as well, although this use remains "off-label," as the manufacturer guidelines state that EMLA is indicated for intact skin and genital mucous membranes only [13–16]. It is important for the practitioner to keep in mind that the use of compound topical anesthetics may pose a significant risk of toxicity due to their varying composition, difficult dosing, and low therapeutic index. Therefore, caution should be exercised in their use, particularly when used in conjunction with injected local anesthetic [6].

Injectable Local Anesthetics

There are a variety of local anesthetic agents on the market with varying properties that allow for variation in their timing on onset, duration of action, diffusibility, and maximum allowable dose. Therefore, the choice of anesthetic will depend upon the demands of the patient and procedure. Currently, anesthetic agents available in North America that are available in dental cartridges are lidocaine, mepivacaine, bupivacaine, articaine, and prilocaine. These anesthetics are all amide-type local anesthetics, almost all of which are packaged with the addition of a vasoconstrictor, either epinephrine or levonordefrin. The addition of vasoconstrictor serves to counteract the vasodilating properties of local anesthetic agents, thereby increasing their duration of action and minimizing the risk of systemic toxicity by slowing their absorption into the systemic vasculature. Because of the risk of systemic toxicity for all local anesthetic agents, the practitioner must take care to select the proper anesthetic for the given procedure and consider the weight-based maximum allowable dose of the particular agent to be employed, keeping in mind that maximum allowable doses may be altered in the medically compromised, debilitated, or elderly patients. Additionally, effectiveness of local anesthetic administration can be heavily dependent on accuracy and method of administration, individual patient response, and tissue conditions. The lowest dose necessary to achieve the desired clinical effect should always be employed to limit the risk of side effects and systemic toxicity.

While there are several choices for local anesthetic on the market, lidocaine is the most widely used in both dentistry and medicine and has been considered the "gold standard" since its introduction in 1943. When used for local infiltration, the onset of anesthesia is less than 2 min, and dental pulpal anesthesia can be expected for at least 1 h, with soft tissue anesthesia duration up to 2.5 h. Lidocaine is also frequently administered to achieve nerve blockade, where average time of onset is between 2 and 4 min, resulting in pulpal and soft tissue anesthesia for 90 min and approximately 3 h, respectively [17].

Mepivacaine, which is pharmacologically similar to lidocaine, has much less potent vasodilating properties and can therefore be found in 3% concentration without the addition of vasoconstrictor. This preparation is commonly used where adrenergic agonism is not desirable, as in patients with severe ischemic heart disease. However, while mepivicaine and lidocaine perform similarly when packaged with the addition of vasoconstrictor, "plain" mepivacaine has been shown to have inferior success in terms of duration and depth of anesthesia compared to lidocaine with epinephrine and is best reserved for short procedures where profound pulpal anesthesia is not required [18]. Prilocaine is another amide-type anesthetic available on the market in a 4% concentration as both a "plain" preparation without addition of vasoconstrictor and a local anesthetic compounded with epinephrine. 4% prilocaine may similarly be used in patients where the use of vasoconstrictor is not desirable but is perhaps more commonly used in its topical preparation, as in EMLA, which is previously discussed. Of note, prilocaine has been implicated in the development of acquired methemoglobinemia through a metabolite (orthotoluidine) that inhibits the methemoglobin reductase pathways. Peak levels of methemoglobin occur 3–4 h after administration and may manifest as weakness, tachycardia, respiratory distress, nausea, and vomiting and can be fatal if not promptly identified and treated.

Bupivacaine is another common local anesthetic agent frequently used in both dentistry and medicine. Due to its high liposolubility, bupivacaine has a higher potency compared to lidocaine, which may be responsible for its potential for cardiotoxicity, particularly at higher doses [19–21]. Nonetheless, bupivacaine is a useful anesthetic at therapeutic doses that can achieve a duration of pulpal anesthesia anywhere from 90 to 180 min and soft tissue anesthesia up to 9 h. As such, this anesthetic is valuable for lengthy procedures and in the provision of provision of post-op pain control, which can mitigate or even obviate the need for postoperative opioid analgesics in some patients.

Articaine, another commonly used anesthetic in dentistry, has found popularity only recently in the United States since its approval in 2000. Articaine has a unique molecular structure that increases its liposolubility, and therefore it is able to diffuse quickly through both hard and soft tissue. The duration of onset of articaine is short, approximately 1–9 min, and there is some evidence that it has a superior anesthetic effect compared to lidocaine on buccal infiltration in both the maxilla and the mandible [22–25]. It may additionally be able to achieve palatal anesthesia in the maxilla with buccal administration alone, sparing patients painful palatal injections [26]. However, 4% articaine has been implicated in increased incidence of neurosensory disturbances when employed for nerve blockage and should therefore be avoided for this use.

Lastly, prilocaine with another amide-type local anesthetic available in dental cartridges as a 4% concentration both without epinephrine and as a solution with 1:200,000 epinephrine. Prilocaine is another amide-type anesthetic available on the market in a 4% concentration as both a "plain" preparation without addition of vasoconstrictor and a local anesthetic compounded with epinephrine. 4% prilocaine may similarly be used in patients where the use of vasoconstrictor is not desirable but is perhaps more commonly used in its topical preparation, as in EMLA, which is previously discussed. Of note, prilocaine has been implicated in the development of acquired methemoglobinemia through a metabolite (orthotoluidine) that inhibits the methemoglobin reductase pathways. Peak levels of methemoglobin occur 3–4 h after administration and may manifest as weakness, tachycardia, respiratory distress, nausea, and vomiting and can be fatal if not promptly identified and treated [27, 28].

Intraoral Anesthetic Techniques

Local Infiltration

Local infiltration of local anesthetic agents is commonly used for a variety of intraoral and extraoral procedures including soft and hard tissue biopsy, the extraction of teeth, and the repair of lacerations. To achieve pulpal anesthesia of the maxillary or mandible teeth, anywhere from 25 gauge to 30 gauge needle is used to penetrate the oral mucosa at the height of the mucobuccal fold as the lip is drawn taught. The needle need only be advanced approximately 2–3 mm, and the desired amount of local anesthesia can then be deposited, and the needle withdrawn. On the skin, the technique of local infiltration entails the deposition of local anesthetic into the submucosal tissue directly adjacent to or at the site of required intervention. It is the preferred technique for small areas on the face and areas that cannot be easily anesthetized by nerve blockade, such as the scalp.

Inferior Alveolar Nerve Block (IAN)

After the mandibular division of the trigeminal nerve passes through the oval foramen, it branches into the auriculotemporal, inferior alveolar, and lingual nerves in the infratemporal fossa. Only the inferior alveolar nerve enters the bony mandibular canal that courses through the mandible from mandibular foramen, located at the medial aspect of the mandibular ramus, to the mental foramen, most commonly located apical to the mandibular premolar teeth. At the mental foramen, the inferior alveolar nerve emerges as the mental nerve, supplying sensation to the skin of the lip, the chin, and anterior mucosal membranes and gingiva [29].

Typically, blockade of the inferior alveolar nerve is at the mandibular foramen prior to its entry into the mandibular canal, which serves to anesthetize the structures distal to this point—the body of the mandible, the buccal mucoperiosteum, and the mucous membranes anterior to the mental nerve. However, blockade can be achieved further anteriorly at the mental foramen to anesthetize only the more anterior structures. This will be discussed later.

The inferior alveolar nerve supplies sensation to the mandibular teeth as well as the chin and lower lip by virtue of the anterior mental branch. Because of its wide zone of distribution to include all of the mandibular teeth, plus the relative difficulty of local infiltration of local anesthetic in the mandible that would obviate the need for nerve blockade, the inferior alveolar nerve block is essentially indispensable in the field of dentistry. Despite some commentary, there is no absolute contraindication to bilateral IAN blocks. However, a large area of soft tissue anesthesia associated with bilateral inferior alveolar nerve blockade can be associated with patient anxiety, as the sensation of speaking and swallowing are altered, although the mechanisms are not. There is also a risk of inadvertent injury to anesthetized soft tissue in the form of lip biting, which is of greater concern in the pediatric population and in patients with developmental delay. These injuries may occur in as many as 18% of children and are more common in young children, although children 12 years and older are still at a risk of about 7%. However, the rate of injury has not been shown to significantly differ between patients receiving unilateral versus bilateral nerve blockade [30, 31].

Technique: A long, 32 mm, 25 or 27 gauge needle is required for this block. The patient is ideally placed into a slightly reclined position with the mandibular occlusal plane approximately parallel to the floor. The patient is then asked to open their mouth as wide as possible. In patients who have trismus, often seen with infection and trauma, this can be challenging. With the nondominant hand, the coronoid notch is palpated with the index finger and the thumb is placed intraorally on the ascending ramus. This hand will also aid in retraction of the soft tissue. Alternatively, a retractor can be used in the nondominant hand to retract the cheek laterally. The pterygomandibular raphe is identified with the patient's mouth in an open position. The barrel of the syringe is positioned at the contralateral corner of the patient's mouth, at approximately the area of the contralateral premolar teeth, and the needle is inserted into the buccal mucosa just lateral to the pterygomandibular raphe and approximately 1 cm superior to the mandibular occlusal plane (See Fig. 4.1). At initial insertion into the mucosa, a small amount of anesthetic can be infiltrated to aid in comfort. The needle should then be advanced until the medial aspect of the mandible is encountered, typically about 20–25 mm. If bony resistance is met prior to 20 mm, the needle is either positioned too anteriorly or posteriorly on the ramus. To correct an inadvertent anterior position, retract the needle slightly and move the syringe barrel toward the midline and advance again until mandible is contacted. To correct an inadvertent posterior position, retract the needle slightly and move the syringe barrel lateral over the molars and advance again until mandible is contacted. Once the medial mandibular ramus is contacted, the needle should be withdrawn about 1 mm, aspiration is performed to insure the tip of the needle is not placed within the vasculature, and approximately ¾–1 cartridges (or 1.5–1.8 cc) of anesthetic is then deposited slowly, over a period of approximately 30–60 s. The needle is then withdrawn, and anesthetic is allowed to achieve maximal effect prior to the initiation of any surgical procedure.

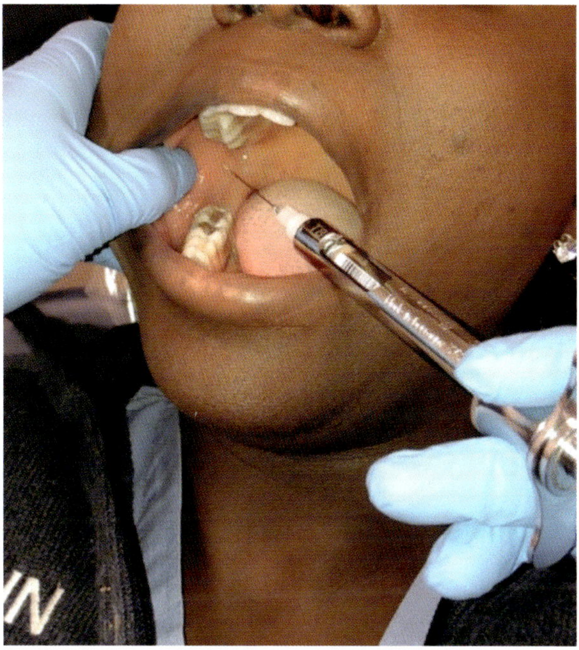

Fig. 4.1 Inferior alveolar nerve block

Lingual Nerve Block

Like the inferior alveolar nerve, the lingual nerve is a division of the mandibular branch of cranial nerve V. However, unlike the inferior alveolar nerve, the lingual nerve divides from the mandibular branch prior to entry into the mandibular canal. At the level of the mandible, the lingual nerve is approximately 1 cm in front of the mandibular foramen. Due to its proximity to the desired location of the inferior alveolar nerve block, this is the preferred site of blockade of the lingual nerve. Farther distally, the lingual nerve will pass within the soft tissue between the medial aspect of the mandible and the medial pterygoid muscle. It is often seen in close association with the mandible at the region of the mandibular third molar prior to its anteromedial turn above the mylohyoid muscle and into the inferior surface of the tongue [32]. As it supplies sensation to the lingual gingiva and mucosa of the mandible as well as the anterior 2/3 of the tongue, it is commonly anesthetized for procedures including mandibular extractions, mandibular tori removal, and tongue biopsies.

Technique: The technique and approach is the same as for the IAN block but after contacting the mandible the needle is withdrawn until about half of the needle is exposed, approximately 1 cm full centimeter. Aspiration is again performed to prevent inadvertent administration of anesthetic into the vasculature, and ¼–1/2 cartridges (or 0.5–1 cc) of local anesthetic is slowly deposited. The needle is then withdrawn, and anesthetic is allowed to achieve maximal effect prior to the initiation of any surgical procedure.

Buccal Nerve Block

The buccal nerve is yet another branch of the mandibular division of the trigeminal nerve that carries sensory fibers to the mandibular buccal gingiva and mucosa and overlying skin of the cheek. As such, it is desirable to anesthetize the buccal nerve in preparation for surgical procedures involving the posterior mandible, such as mandibular third molar removal. It is not necessary to anesthetize this nerve for surgical manipulation of the anterior aspect of the mandible or for the extraction of anterior teeth, as the zone of innervation of the buccal nerve does not extend this far anteriorly.

Technique: Armamentarium and patient positioning are identical to that of the inferior alveolar and lingual nerve blocks. The ipsilateral buccal soft tissues should be retracted with the nondominant hand or a retractor. Place the barrel of the syringe at same side of the area that requires anesthesia. Enter the soft tissue parallel to the plane of the mandibular teeth distal and buccal to the last molar. At initial insertion into the mucosa, a small amount of anesthetic can be infiltrated to aid in comfort. The needle only needs to be advanced approximately 2–3 mm to insure its location in the submucosa. Again, aspiration is performed, and a small amount of local anesthetic is deposited—approximately a quarter of a dental cartridge (or about 0.5 cc).

Mental Nerve Block

The mental nerve block is utilized when anesthesia of only the anterior mandibular teeth or mucoperiosteum or lower lip is required. As previously discussed, posterior mandibular anesthesia will require inferior alveolar nerve blockade.

Similar to the inferior alveolar nerve blockade at the mandibular foramen, a 27G or 25G needle is used. Because the depth of penetration required for blockade at the mental foramen is less than at the mandibular canal, a shorter needle, which is 19 mm when utilizing a dental needle, typically can be used, although this is not mandatory. Otherwise, armamentarium and patient positioning are similar to inferior alveolar nerve blockade. Trismus does not prevent conduction of the mental nerve block, and a semi-closed position of the patient's mouth can make administration easier due to laxity of the labial tissue.

Technique: The ipsilateral buccal soft tissues should be retracted with the nondominant hand or a retractor. Place the barrel of the syringe at same side of the area that requires anesthesia. A gloved finger can be used to palpate the depth of the mandibular buccal fold along the premolar region for the mental foramen, but palpation is not always possible. Imaging can also aid in identifying the location of the mental foramen. Once landmarks are identified, the needle should be advanced into the depth of the mucobuccal fold, angled toward the mandible, to a depth of about 5–6 mm. Again aspirate to ensure the needle is not retained within a vessel, and if negative, slowly deposit approximately ½ a cartridge of local anesthetic (or approximately 1 cc). After withdrawing the needle, pressure may be applied for 1–2 min at the depth of the sulcus to facilitate entry of the local anesthetic into the mandibular foramen. After dissipation of the initial bolus of local anesthetic, this procedure can be conducted again with the remaining local anesthetic in the cartridge for a total administration of a full dental cartridge (or 1.8 cc).

Posterior Superior Alveolar Nerve Block

The posterior superior alveolar nerve is a major sensory branch of the maxillary nerve that enters the maxilla at the posterior aspect of the maxillary tuberosity and supplies sensation to the maxillary molars as well as the mucosal membranes and gingiva. Because of the presence of a middle superior alveolar nerve in a portion of the patient population, the posterior superior alveolar nerve block will not always anesthetize the mesiobuccal root of the maxillary first molar, resulting in a failure of anesthetize of the maxillary first molar in approximately 9% of patients [33].

Technique: Prior to administration, the patient should be placed in a recumbent position with their back at approximately a 60° angle to the floor. The patient should be instructed to open their mouth partially, as tautness of the cheek associated with wide opening may make retraction difficult. The patient may also be instructed to turn their head opposite the site of anesthetic administration to facilitate visualization of the posterior maxilla. Either a short (1.9 cm) or long (3.2 cm) needle may be utilized, keeping in mind that a long needle will only require insertion about half the length of the needle. The ipsilateral buccal soft tissues should be retracted with the nondominant hand or a retractor, and the barrel and needle of the syringe are directed in a straight line that is angled 45° superiorly, posteriorly, and medially, to enter the soft tissue at the mucobuccal fold above and distal to the maxillary second molar. Advance the needle about 10–14 mm and aspirate. Aspiration is imperative here, as there is rich vascularity in the area posterior to the maxilla. If aspiration is negative, slowly deposit ½–1 cartridge (0.9–1.8 cc) of local anesthetic. If aspiration is positive, it is recommended to withdraw and redirect the tip of the needle 1–2 mm and aspirate once again. If blood within the cartridge obscures the results of subsequent aspiration, the cartridge should be replaced, and nerve blockade should be reattempted with a fresh cartridge.

Infraorbital Nerve Block

The infraorbital nerve is a division of the maxillary nerve (cranial nerve V2) that supplies sensory innervation to the lower eyelid, upper lip, side of the nose, and maxillary anterior teeth definitively from the central incisor to the canine including the periodontium and alveolar bone, but often anesthetizes the premolars as well. The infraorbital nerve gives rise to both the anterior and middle superior alveolar nerves that supply innervation to the maxillary teeth from central incisor to as far posteriorly as the mesiobuccal root of the maxillary first molar. The anterior, middle, and posterior alveolar nerves form a dental plexus called the superior dental plexus. The infraorbital nerve finally exits the infraorbital foramen on the anterior aspect of the maxilla and can be approached for nerve blockade via a transoral or transfacial approach. We will discuss the intraoral approach here.

Technique: Armamentarium and patient positioning is similar to the posterior superior alveolar nerve block. The infraorbital notch can be first palpated, as inferior to it is the infraorbital foramen. The ipsilateral buccal soft tissues should be retracted with the nondominant hand while placing the nondominant thumb at the infraorbital foramen. Enter the soft tissue at the mucobuccal fold buccal and anterior to the region of the lateral canine to first premolar. The needle is advanced until bone is contacted which should be palpable with the thumb of your nondominant hand as previously described. Aspiration is performed prior to deposition to ½–1 cartridge (0.9–1.8 cc) of local anesthetic.

Greater Palatine Nerve Block

The greater palatine nerve is a branch of the pterygopalatine ganglion that descends through the greater palatine canal and exits the foramen of the same name on the posterior hard palate, where it then traverses anteriorly to supply sensory innervation to the hard palate as far forward as the anterior teeth. Blockade of this nerve will result in anesthesia of the hard palate and its overlying soft tissue as far anteriorly as the canine tooth. The greater palatine nerve communicates anteriorly with the nasopalatine nerve, which supplies sensation palatal to the maxillary incisors and canine. Therefore, palatal anesthesia is more reliable in the posterior region with a greater palatine nerve block, as anterior teeth may require nasopalatine nerve blockade.

Technique: Prior to administration, the patient should be placed in a recumbent position with their back at approximately a 60° angle to the floor similarly to the PSA and infraorbital blocks. The patient should be instructed to open their mouth fully. Either a 27G or 25G short needle may be used. The greater palatine foramen is identified as a depression just distal to the maxillary second molar at the junction of the horizontal hard palate and the more vertically oriented alveolus. Typically, pressure is applied over the foramen, using the end of a dental mirror or a cotton tip applicator, as the needle is inserted to ameliorate the pain of injection. The barrel of the syringe should be placed at the contralateral side (See Fig. 4.2). The needle is advanced 2–3 mm into the mucosa overlying the foramen, aspiration is performed, and a small quantity of local anesthetic is slowly injected, just until blanching is observed overlying the site of administration.

Nasopalatine Nerve Block

The nasopalatine nerve is a branch of the maxillary division of the trigeminal nerve that exits the nasopalatine canal to innervate the palatal aspect of the anterior maxilla and is useful for anesthesia of the maxillary incisors and canines.

Technique: Injection can be directed posterior to the incisive papilla, which is the area of raised palatal tissue between the central incisors (See Fig. 4.3). Similarly to the greater palatine nerve block, pressure can be applied overlying the site of

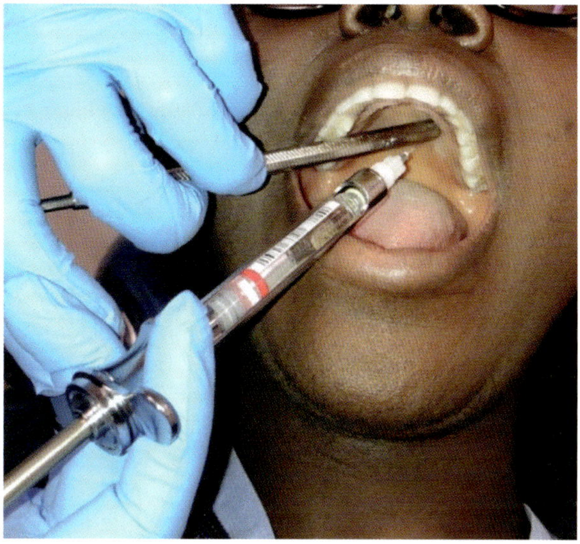

Fig. 4.2 Greater palatine nerve block

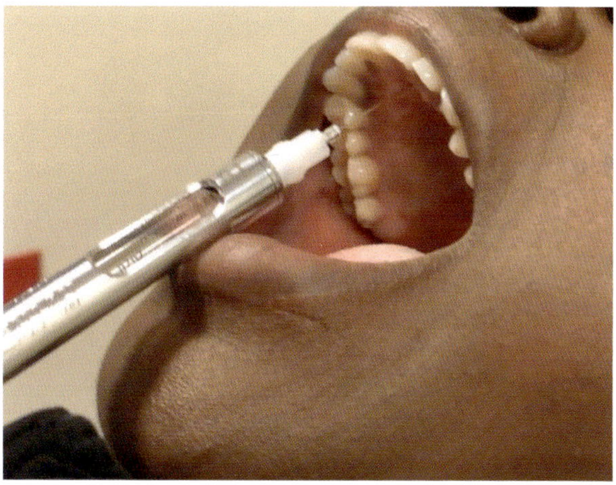

Fig. 4.3 Nasopalatine nerve block

injection with the end of a dental mirror or a cotton tip applicator to attenuate the pain on needle insertion. Alternatively, some practitioners prefer injecting into the papilla between the two maxillary central incisors in a buccal to palatal direction after local infiltration on the buccal aspect of the maxilla, as this may be more easily tolerated.

Transfacial Anesthesia

Frontal Nerve Block

The frontal nerve block is also referred to as the supraorbital or supratrochlear block. The frontal nerve is the largest branch of ophthalmic nerve, which is the first division of cranial nerve V (trigeminal nerve), and it is responsible for sensory innervation to the ipsilateral middle portion of the forehead, medial upper eyelid, medial nasal skin, conjunctiva and lacrimal apparatus [34]. The most terminal branches of the frontal nerve are the supraorbital and supratrochlear nerves. The supraorbital nerve exits from the supraorbital foramen (~27 mm from the facial midline), whereas the supratrochlear nerve exits more medially from the orbit (~17 mm from midline) [34, 35]. These nerves can be addressed separately or in one injection. When both nerves are anesthetized, it results in anesthesia of the forehead, upper eyelid, bridge of nose, and scalp. Blockade of the supraorbital and/or supratrochlear nerves is frequently employed in the repair of lacerations of the brow (See Fig. 4.4).

Technique: Palpate the superior orbital rim for the supraorbital notch which is located at the medial 1/3 of the orbital rim. Once the notch is palpated, the skin at this site should be cleansed with an alcohol or prep swab and given appropriate time to dry. A 25G needle should be inserted just through the thick skin of the brow and directed medially. The nondominant hand should be placed slightly inferior to the superior orbital rim to minimize inferior infiltration of local anesthetic toward the upper eyelid. Aspiration is performed, and anesthetic is deposited in the subcutaneous tissue overlying the supraorbital notch or foramen. About 1–2 mL per site is sufficient for profound anesthesia.

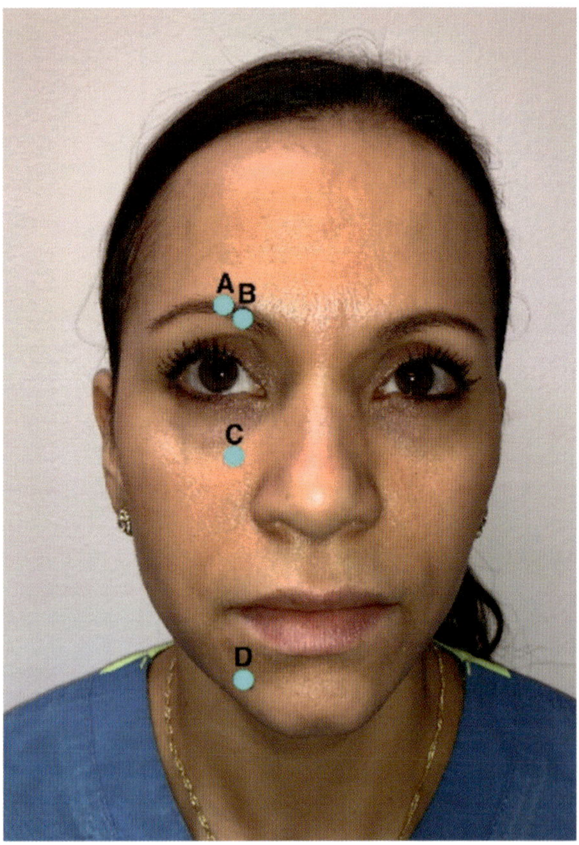

Fig. 4.4 Transfacial nerve blocks; (**a**) supraorbital nerve, (**b**) supratrochlear nerve, (**c**) infraorbital nerve, (**d**) mental nerve

Infraorbital Nerve Block (Transfacial)

Important anatomy: The infraorbital nerve block as previously discussed in this chapter can be performed from either an intraoral or transfacial approach. The infraorbital nerve is a branch of the maxillary nerve, with is the second division of cranial nerve V, and is responsible for sensory innervation of the ipsilateral lower eyelid, lateral aspect of the nose, cheek, and upper lip. Literature does not show that one approach is superior to the other, but the intraoral approach is often subjectively preferred [36].

Technique: Palpate the inferior orbital rim to find the orbital notch. The infraorbital foramen is about 1 cm inferior to the notch and 3 cm lateral from the midline of the face and is typically a palpable concavity. The skin should be cleaned with an alcohol or prep swab and given appropriate time to dry. A 25G needle should be inserted at this level until contact with bone. The needle can then be withdrawn about 1 mm. Aspiration is performed, and if negative local anesthetic is slowly deposited.

Mental Nerve Block

Important anatomy: The mental nerve block as previously discussed in this chapter is another block than can be performed from both an intraoral and transfacial approach. The mental nerve is a terminal branch of the inferior alveolar nerve, which is the third division of cranial nerve V, and is responsible for sensory innervation of the ipsilateral anterior teeth and buccal mucous membranes anterior to the mental foramen, as well as the lower lip.

Technique: Palpate the mandible to find the mental foramen. This is difficult to do. The foramen is in the middle of the superior and inferior mandibular borders lateral to where the chin ends. You can confirm location by approximating where the premolars are in the mouth. The skin should be cleaned with an alcohol or prep swab and given appropriate time to dry. A 25G needle should be directed posteriorly and inserted anterior to the suspected site of the foramen. The needle can be advanced until contact with bone. The needle can then be withdrawn about 1 mm. Aspiration is performed, and if negative local anesthetic is slowly deposited.

Superficial Cervical Nerve Block

Important Anatomy: The cervical plexus comprises the ventral rami of the first four cervical spinal nerves that arise from C1 to C4 and give off both cutaneous and muscular branches. The superficial cervical nerve block targets the cutaneous branches where as a deep cervical nerve block targets the muscular branches. The superficial cervical plexus includes the greater auricular nerve, the transverse cervical nerve (also known as the cutaneous cervical nerve), lesser occipital, and the supraclavicular nerves. These nerves provide sensation from the mandible to the clavicle [37]. Therefore, blocking this nerve can be useful in soft tissue injuries of the neck and ear requiring laceration repair. Neck dissections typically require both a superficial and deep cervical nerve block.

Technique: First, the patient should be placed in a supine position. The patient should be asked to contract their sternocleidomastoid (SCM) by asking the patient to lift their head against pressure applied to their forehead. The posterior border should then be marked with a marking pen. Next, the midline between the mastoid proceed and the prominent tubercle of C6 should be marked along the previous demarcated line. This point, also known as Erb's point, is the estimate for where the cervical plexus emerges (See Fig. 4.5). A long 25G needle is directed anteriorly and superficially. Aspiration is performed, and if negative local anesthetic is slowly deposited. The local anesthetic is often distributed in three directions: superior, perpendicular, inferior, all placed from the same needle insertion point. Typically, about 5 cc of local anesthetic in each direction is needed for profound anesthesia [37].

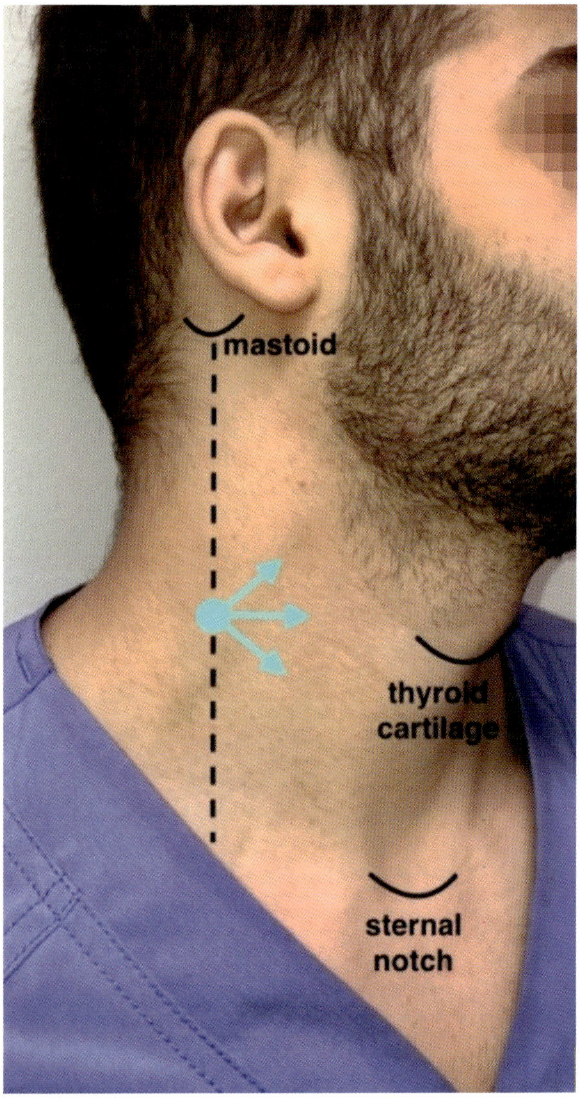

Fig. 4.5 Superficial cervical nerve block

Field Blocks

Field blocks are ways of providing local infiltration in the subcutaneous tissue to cover a larger area. Local anesthetic is injected along the perimeter of the operative field which usually consists of four walls. These blocks are utilized in areas where the operative field is innervated by multiple nerves. They serve an important role in aesthetic procedures in which the deposition of a large amount of local anesthesia can easily distort the soft tissue [38].

Ear

The nerves that provide sensation to the ear are the greater auricular, lesser occipital, auriculotemporal nerves, and the mastoid branches of the lesser occipital nerve. Using a long needle, 10 mL of local anesthetic is infiltrated superficially around the ear to create a circular or rhomboid shaped block [37, 38] (See Fig. 4.6).

Nose

The nerves that provide sensation to the nose are the infratrochlear nerve, infraorbital nerve, and the external branch of the anterior and posterior ethmoidal nerves. Using a long needle, 10 mL of local anesthetic is infiltrated superficially around the nose to create a "U"- shaped block (See Fig. 4.7).

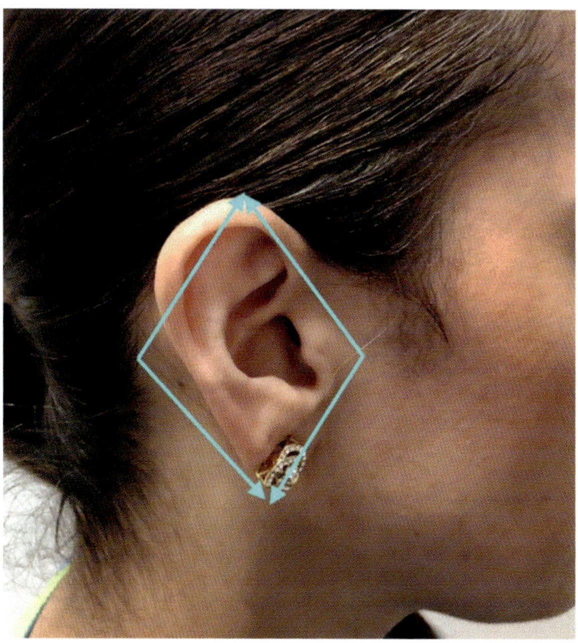

Fig. 4.6 Field block for the ear

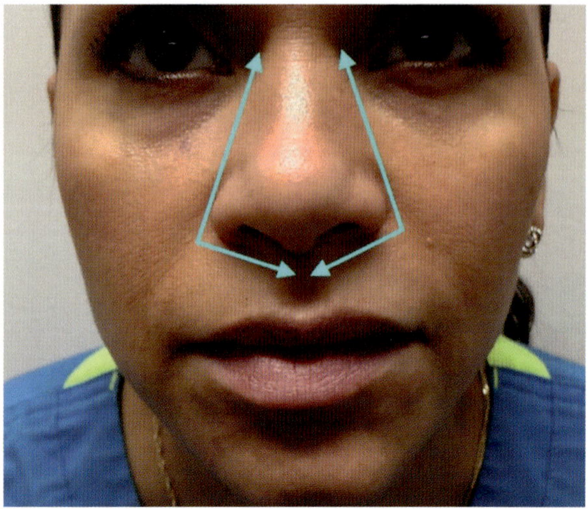

Fig. 4.7 Field block for the nose

Complications

The statistics regarding the incidence of complications from the administration of local anesthesia for dental procedures are not well reported on but may be anywhere from 4% to 26% and are generally transient and relatively minor [39–41]. A 1997 study by Daublander et al. of 2731 patients evaluated by questionnaire after receiving dental anesthesia reports only a 4.5% incidence of complication, 0.07% of which were severe adverse events [39]. It can be reasonably assumed from the prolific use of local anesthetic agents in the field of dentistry and oral surgery that they are safe, effective, and reliable. However, the injection or administration of any drug is not without risk, and the prudent practitioner should be well aware of the potential adverse events as well as the appropriate strategies for their management.

Local Complications

Paresthesia

The most common cause of paresthesia associated with the administration of local anesthesia is with a mandibular nerve block. The incidence of trigeminal nerve injury varies wildly in the literature, although it is probably between 1:20,000 and 1:785,000 [42]. It is also believed that all but 10–15% of these patients recover full sensation over the course of a few days, up to several months after the procedure [43]. Paresthesia may be caused from mechanical injury from the needle, pressure secondary to edema or a hematoma, or from neurotoxicity of the local anesthetic agent. As discussed previously, there may be an association with certain local anesthetic agents and higher incidence. When paresthesia does occur, a neurosensory exam should be performed and repeated at each follow-up in order to document the extent and degree of injury. Steroids and NSAIDs may be useful in treating acute nerve injury by alleviating edema around the affected nerve but do little to improve persistent paresthesia beyond 10 days after injury. Painful dysesthesias that do not resolve within 1–2 weeks after injury may be treated with tricyclic antidepressants or gabapentin, but these medications are for symptom relief only [43].

Prolonged Anesthesia and Soft Tissue Injury

Particularly in children and in the mentally disabled, prolonged soft tissue anesthesia can result in inadvertent biting of the tongue, lips, or cheek, resulting in minor to potentially severe soft tissue damage in the form of laceration, ulceration, and/or contusion. Even in the normally mentating adult, self-inflicted trauma is a complication of dental treatment under local anesthesia if care is not taken to prevent it. The treatment for soft tissue as a result of inadvertent self-mutilation is generally aimed at treating and protecting the affected soft tissue until sensation is restored. Largely, the focus is on prevention such as the use of shorter acting local anesthetics and/or reversal agents such as phentolamine mesylate (OraVerse), which results in return to normal sensation in about 50–60% normal recovery time [44, 45].

Hematoma

Hematomas result from injection into an area of high vascularity, such as the pterygoid plexus while performing posterior maxillary infiltration or a PSA block. Bleeding is generally self-limited, and goals of initial treatment are to achieve hemostasis via pressure and minimize inflammation by application of an ice pack. The patient should be evaluated in 24–48 h and reassured that while hematoma is often accompanied by trismus and bruising, these affects generally resolve on their own in 1–2 weeks (80, 81). The frequency of hematoma formation after injection is higher with maxillary posterior injections, but the overall incidence is around 0.1% [46].

Trismus

Trismus is an uncommon complication of local anesthetic injection, but it has been known to be associated with inferior alveolar nerve blocks and posterior maxillary injections. The likely etiology is intramuscular edema and hemorrhage, both of which are worsened by multiple needle passes [47]. Treatment is aimed at addressing pain and inflammation and improving range of motion, often with NSAIDs, moist heat, and physiotherapy.

Palsy of CN VII

Palsy of the facial nerve is possible with injection of local anesthetic and most often presents immediately but can present in a delayed fashion, typically within hours to days. The common etiology is inadvertent local anesthesia administration into the parotid gland, as from a mandibular nerve block where the practitioner has injected too posteriorly [48]. On clinical presentation, patients will display unilateral facial weakness on the side of injection. Immediate palsy of the facial nerve after administration of local anesthesia is a result of direct blockade of neural conduction and should resolve within a few hours, depending on the duration of action of the local anesthetic agent.

Systemic Complications

Overdose

The maximum dosages of local anesthetic agents provided by the manufacturer in accordance with the FDA and ADA are generally weight-based and formulated for the "average" patient. These suggested dosages do not take more specific patient considerations into account; therefore, some patients may experience signs of local anesthetic systemic toxicity at lower doses than the proposed maximum dose. Overdose of local anesthesia may occur even when local anesthesia is properly administered in appropriate amounts, but it is more likely to occur with intra-arterial injection or with dosages exceeding the recommended maximum.

In the early stage of local anesthetic toxicity, the patient may complain of tinnitus, lightheadedness, and circumoral tingling. Initial cardiovascular and central nervous system response to local anesthetic toxicity is excitatory, but what follows is a generalized depression phase characterized by myocardial depression, ectopic cardiac rhythms, bradycardia, and hypotension [41]. Respiratory and circulatory collapse are the end-points of severe local anesthetic overdose and present a dire situation for the patient.

Management of local anesthetic overdose will depend on the severity of the reaction and is aimed at providing support to the patient until symptoms subside, or help arrives. The practitioner should administer supplemental oxygen to the patient and monitor their vital signs carefully while continuing to assess the patient's airway, breathing, and circulation. Tonic-clonic convulsions are common with overdose and should be treated accordingly.

Methemoglobinemia

Methemoglobinemia is a condition that results from a dysfunction in hemoglobin molecules that impairs their ability to bind oxygen [49]. In dentistry, the most common causes of acquired methemoglobinemia are application of topical anesthetics such as benzocaine and the injection of prilocaine, in which peak levels of methemoglobin occur 3–4 h after administration [28]. Mental changes such as headache, fatigue, and syncope may be noted at methemoglobin levels of 20–30%, and physiologic signs of tachypnea, tachycardia, dysrhythmia, and seizure may be evident at concentrations above 30%. At further increased blood concentrations of methemoglobin, lethargy and stupor can occur, and levels above 70% are often fatal if untreated [50].

A diagnosis of methemoglobinemia should be considered in a cyanotic patient that is unresponsive to administration of supplemental oxygen with unexplained decreased SpO_2 despite adequate ventilation. Another hallmark feature is a chocolate-brown appearance of the arterial blood and cyanosis in the face of a falsely elevated SoO_2 reading. Upon diagnosis or high suspicion, immediate treatment should be instituted in the form of 1% methylene blue 1–2 mg/kg administered over a period of 5–10 min, which can be re-dosed after 1 h up to a maximum of 7 mg/kg.

Allergy

True allergy to local anesthetic is estimated to account for only 1% of all adverse reactions during dental anesthesia, and 80–90% of these cases are allergic contact dermatitis. In patients suspicious for anesthetic allergy, a challenge test, whereby a small amount of local anesthetic is deposited into the mucosa as the patient is monitored for adverse effects, is thought to be the best strategy to determine if an allergic response is present [51]. Challenge testing carries a risk of anaphylaxis, however, and therefore should be undergone with caution, in a setting with a proper emergency response team, and with continuous monitoring. For patients with true allergy to local anesthetics, 1% diphenhydramine has been used as an alternative to more traditional local anesthetic agents with reportedly good success and no cross-reactivity [52].

Summary

Local anesthetic administration is technically easy to perform in either an office or hospital based setting alone or in conjunction with sedation and allows for the comfortable completion of a variety of oral and facial procedures. There are several local anesthetic agents available to the practitioner that lend themselves to a variety of uses. Complications associated with the administration of local anesthesia are uncommon and almost always self-limiting, but adverse effects are possible and must be closely surveilled for. As such, judicious and cautious use of any drug is the standard of care in both medicine and dentistry.

References

1. Calatayud J, Gonzalez A. History of the development and evolution of local anesthesia since the coca leaf. Anesthesiology. 2003;98:1503–8.
2. Nathan J, Asadourian L, Erlich MA. A brief history of local anesthesia. Int J Head Neck Surg. 2016;7(1):29–32.
3. Meechan JG. Intra-oral topical anaesthetics: a review. J Dent. 2000;28(1):3–14.
4. Golan DE, Tashjian AH, Armstrong EJ, et al. Principals of pharmacology: the pathophysiology basis of drug therapy. 2nd ed. Philadelphia: Wolters Kluwer; 2012. p. 157–8.
5. Malamed SF. Handbook of local anesthesia. 6th ed. St. Louis: Mosby; 2013. p. 69–73.
6. Kravitz ND. The use of compound topical anesthetics: a review. J Am Dent Assoc. 2007;138(10):1333–9.
7. Guerriero SE. Methemoglobinemia caused by topical benzocaine. Pharmacotherapy. 1997;17(5):1038–40.
8. Aronson JK. The international encyclopedia of adverse drug reactions and interactions. In: Meyler's side effects of drugs. 16th ed. Amsterdam: Elsevier Science; 2016.

9. Marks JG Jr, Belsito DV, DeLeo VA, et al. North American contact dermatitis group patch-test results, 1996–1998. Arch Dermatol. 2000;136:272–3.
10. Boyce RA, Kirpalani T, Mohan N. Updates of topical and local anesthetic agents. Dent Clin North Am. 2016;60(2):445–71.
11. Mackley CL, Marks JG Jr, Anderson BE. Delayed-type hypersensitivity to lidocaine. Arch Dermatol. 2003;139(3):343–6.
12. Rogers TL, Ostrow CL. The use of EMLA cream to decrease venipuncture pain in children. J Pediatr Nurs. 2004;19(1):33–9.
13. Vickers ER, Punnia-Moorthy A. A clinical evaluation of three topical anaesthetic agents. Aust Dent J. 1992;37(4):267–70.
14. Bernardi M, Secco F, Benech A. Anesthetic efficacy of a eutectic mixture of lidocaine and prilocaine (EMLA) on the oral mucosa; prospective double-blind study with a placebo. Minerva Stomatol. 1999;48(1-2):9–43.
15. Munshi AK, Hegde AM, Latha R. Use of EMLA: is it an injection free alternative? J Clin Pediatr Dent. 2001;25(3):215–9.
16. AstraZeneca. 2013. EMLA Cream 5% Consumer Medicine Information. Available at www.aspenpharma.com.au/product_info/cmi/CMI_Emla.pdf. Accessed 26 Oct 2017.
17. Prescribing information: 2% Xylocaine dental with epinephrine, Cambridge, Ontario, Canada. Densply Pharmaceutical. Revised December 2011.
18. Su N, Liu Y, Yang X, et al. Efficacy and safety of mepivacaine compared with lidocaine in local anaesthesia in dentistry: a meta-analysis of randomised controlled trials. Int Dent J. 2014;64(2):96–107.
19. Tanz RD, Heskett T, Loehning RW, et al. Comparative cardiotoxicity of bupivacaine and lidocaine in the isolated perfused mammalian heart. Anesth Analg. 1984;63(6):549–56.
20. Pitkanen M, Feldman HS, Arthur GR, et al. Chronotropic and inotropic effects of ropivacaine, bupivacaine, and lidocaine in the spontaneously beating and electrically paced isolated, perfused rabbit heart. Reg Anesth. 1992;17(4):183–92.
21. Bourne E, Wright C, Royse C. A review of local anesthetic cardiotoxicity and treatment with lipid emulsion. Local Reg Anesth. 2010;3:11–9.
22. Ogle OE, Mahjoubi G. Advances in local anesthesia in dentistry. Dent Clin North Am. 2011;55(3):481–99.
23. Malamed SF, Gagnon S, Leblanc D. Efficacy of articaine: a new amide local anesthetic. J Am Dent Assoc. 2000;131(5):645–2.
24. Katyal V. The efficacy and safety of articaine versus lignocaine in dental treatments: a meta-analysis. J Dent. 2010;38(4):307–17.
25. Shurtz R, Nusstein J, Reader A, et al. Buffered 4% articaine as a primary buccal infiltration of the mandibular first molar: A prospective, randomized, double-blind study. J Endod. 2015;41(9):1403–7.
26. Vahatalo K, Antila H, Lehtinen R. Articaine and lidocaine for maxillary infiltration anesthesia. Anesth Prog. 1993;40(4):114–6.
27. Kreutz RW, Kinni ME. Life-threatening toxic methemoglobinemia induced by prilocaine. Oral Surg. 1983;56(5):480–2.
28. Rehman HU. Methemoglobinemia. West J Med. 2001;175(3):193–6.
29. Juodzbalys G, Wang HL, Sabalys G. Anatomy of mandibular vital structures. Part I: mandibular canal and inferior alveolar neurovascular bundle in relation with dental implantology. J Oral Maxillofac Res. 2010;1(1):e2. Published 2010 Apr 1
30. College C, Feigal R, Wandera A, et al. Bilateral versus unilateral mandibular block anesthesia in a pediatric population. Pediatr Dent. 2000;22(6):453–7.
31. Chi D, Kanellis M, Himadi E. Lip biting in a pediatric dental patient after dental local anesthesia: a case report. J Pediatr Nurs. 2008;23(6):490–3.
32. Sittitavornwong S, Babston M, Denson D, et al. Clinical anatomy of the lingual nerve: a review. J Oral Max Surg. 2017;75(5):926.e1–9.
33. Singla H, Alexander M. Posterior superior alveolar nerve blocks: a randomised controlled, double blind trial. J Maxillofac Oral Surg. 2014;14(2):423–31.

34. Mariman K, Shanmugasundaram N, et al. Regional anesthesia in faciomaxillary and oral surgery. J Pharm Bioallied Sci. 2012;4(Suppl 2):S264–9.
35. Rathmell JP, Pollack GJ. Chapter 18: Nerve blocks for the head and neck. In: Hadzic A, editor. NYSORA textbook of regional anesthesia and acute pain management. New York: McGraw-Hill; 2007.
36. Lynch MT, Syverud SA, Schwab RA, Jenkins JM, Edlich R. Comparison of intraoral and percutaneous approaches for infraorbital nerve block. Acad Emerg Med. 1994;1:514–9. https://doi.org/10.1111/j.1553-2712.1994.tb02543.x).
37. Niamtu J. Local anesthetic blocks of the head and neck for cosmetic facial surgery, Part V: techniques for the head and neck region. Cosmet Dermatol. 2005;18(1):65–8.
38. Salam G. Regional anesthesia for office procedures: Part I. head and neck surgeries. Am Fam Physician. 2004;69(3):585–90.
39. Daublander M, Muler R, Lipp MDW. The incidence of complications associated with local anesthesia in dentistry. Anesth Prog. 1997;44(4):132–41.
40. Kaufman E, Goharian S, Katz Y. Adverse reactions to local anesthesia. Anesth Prog. 2000;47(4):143–38.
41. Moore P, Hersh EV. Local anesthetics: pharmacology and toxicity. Dent Clin North Am. 2010;54(4):587–99.
42. Moore PA, Haas DA. Paresthesias in dentistry. Dent Clin North Am. 2010;54(4):715–30.
43. Moon S, Lee S-J, Kim E, et al. Hypoesthesia after IAN block anesthesia with lidocaine: management of mild to moderate nerve injury. Restor Dent Endod. 2012;37(4):232–5.
44. Tavares M, Goodson M, Studen-Pavlovich D, et al. Reversal of soft-tissue local anesthesia with phentolamine mesylate in pediatric patients. J Am Dent Assoc. 2008;139(8):1095–104.
45. Hersh EV, Moore PA, Papas AS, et al. Reversal of soft-tissue local anesthesia with phentolamine mesylate in adolescents and adults. J Am Dent Assoc. 2008;139(8):1080–93.
46. Kuster CG, Udin RD. Frequency of hematoma formation subsequent to injection of dental local anesthetic in children. Anesth Prog. 1984;31(3):130–2.
47. Stone J, Kaban L. Trismus after injection of local anesthetic. Oral Surg Oral Med Oral Pathol Oral Radiol. 1979;48(1):29–32.
48. Cummings DR, Yamashita DR, McAndrews JP. Complications of local anesthesia used in oral and maxillofacial surgery. Oral Maxillofacial Surg Clin North Am. 2011;23(3):369–77.
49. Hall DL, Moses MK, Weaver JM, et al. Dental anesthesia management of methemoglobinemia-susceptible patients: a case report and review of the literature. Anesth Prog. 2004;51(1):24–7.
50. Trapp L, Will J. Acquired methemoglobinemia revisited. Dent Clin North Am. 2010;54(4):665–75.
51. Berkun Y, Ben-Zvi A, Levy Y, et al. Evaluation of adverse reactions to local anesthetics: experience with 236 patients. Ann Allergy Asthma Immunol. 2003;91(4):342–5.
52. Pavlidakey PG, Brodell EE, Helms SE. Diphenhydramine as an alternative local anesthetic agent. J Clin Aesthet Dermatol. 2009;2(10):37–40.

Oral Sedation

5

Christopher Haxhi and Michael T. Goupil

Introduction

Dental anxiety and fear are not novel concepts to even the most novice dental professional. Dental phobia can cause patient populations to avoid regular dental care throughout their lifetime. This in turn causes a compounding effect and necessitates ultimately more extensive treatment by general practitioners and more referrals to the oral and maxillofacial surgeon for disease control and restorative work. In this modern era, where, culturally, there is more emphasis on comfort, feelings, and avoiding situations that may be uncomfortable, the demand for sedation in dentistry and oral surgery has increased exponentially. Sedation in dentistry has become, to some, an expectation. To adequately treat patients who may otherwise refuse basic dental care, and for commercial success, the practitioner should be familiar with oral sedation methods. This same concern can be expanded to other healthcare situations where patients can exhibit anxiety when undergoing non-dental, office procedures. This chapter is designed to familiarize clinicians with their sedation medication arsenal, the pharmacologic effects of these drugs, and techniques for safely providing oral sedation. The goal of oral sedation is to relieve dental phobia and increase compliance during the treatment time.

When choosing a route of administration and a sedative agent, the clinician must assess the associated risks. In addition, a comprehensive medical evaluation should be completed on each patient regardless of whether a patient will receive sedation or not. However, the information gathered from the medical assessment will help in the decision-making process as to the most appropriate sedative medication is prescribed. The foundations of medical assessment were discussed in the first chapter of this section.

C. Haxhi
UCLA Oral and Maxillofacial Surgery Department, Los Angeles, CA, USA

M. T. Goupil (✉)
University of Connecticut School of Dental Medicine, Farmington, CT, USA
e-mail: mtgoupil@comcast.net

E. M. Ferneini, M. T. Goupil (eds.), *Office-Based Maxillofacial Surgical Procedures*, https://doi.org/10.1007/978-3-030-22371-7_5

The Spectrum of Sedation

While this chapter will focus on oral conscious sedation in the dental office, in order to understand the effect this technique will have on a patient it is necessary to understand the varying degrees of sedation and anesthesia, especially the fluidity between levels. The American Society of Anesthesiologists regards the varying levels of sedation as a continuum. **Minimal Sedation** is defined as anxiolysis and is "a drug-induced state during which patients respond normally to verbal commands" [1]. At this level of anxiolysis, the patient's cognition and motor reflexes will be impaired; however, the dosage of medication is not high enough to produce any cardiac or respiratory effects. The next level along the continuum is **Moderate Sedation**, also referred to in dentistry as "Conscious Sedation" and is defined as a "drug-induced depression of consciousness during which patients respond purposefully to verbal commands, either alone or accompanied by light tactile stimulation" [1]. Again, as in minimal sedation, there is no effect on the airway or respirations and usually cardiac function is preserved [1]. The appropriate usage of oral medications will yield this mild to moderate sedation and will be the focus of this chapter. When combined with profound local anesthesia this can facilitate the effective delivery of dental care or other office procedures. Local anesthesia is discussed in Chap. 4 of this section. Progressing along the continuum of sedation, **deep sedation/analgesia** is a "drug-induced depression of consciousness during which patients cannot be easily aroused but respond purposefully following repeated or painful stimulation" [1]. At this deep level it becomes variable from patient to patient whether respiratory function is impaired, and a patient at this level may require assistance in maintaining their airway and/or ventilations. This level is usually achieved in the outpatient clinical setting via intravenous administration of anesthetic medications. However, given that this is defined as a continuum, inappropriate administration of oral sedative agents pre- or perioperatively can result in a patient being pushed past moderate sedation and into deep sedation. With excessive levels of sedation, respiratory and cardiovascular complications can arise and the dentist or surgeon administering the sedation should be ready to recognize and manage the situation. The clinician should be prepared with the appropriate skill set and armamentarium to **rescue** the patient. Rescue is defined as the intervention to manage airway and advanced life support [1]. A patient should be returned to the intended level of sedation as it is inappropriate to continue any procedure at a level deeper than intended and discussed with the patient in the informed consent process. The last level of sedation is **general anesthesia**; it is a "drug-induced loss of consciousness during which patients are not arousable, even by painful stimulation" [1]. This level of anesthesia is achievable by either intravenous or inhaled anesthetics, and the anesthesia received in a hospital operating room is the classic prototype of this level. A protected airway, i.e., endotracheal tube, is not always necessary; however, the patient will have impaired respiratory function and may require advanced techniques to deliver breaths.

With a deeper understanding of the levels of sedation and the often hazy boundaries between them, it should be clear to the clinician as to what should be the goal of oral conscious sedation (mild to moderate sedation). The choice in sedative drugs delivered should be based on the desired level of sedation combined with patient and procedure specific factors. The additional levels of anesthesia and routes of delivery highlighted in this section are described in Chap. 6 of this section.

Advantages vs. Disadvantages

As sedation dentistry becomes more and more popular, due to successful advertising, depictions in popular culture, and increased access to care, it becomes important for the clinician to integrate the patient's current medical condition, level of anxiety, and scope of treatment to be rendered in deciding which modality of sedation to administer, i.e., nitrous inhalation, oral, intramuscularly, or intravenous. In order for the clinician to develop a decision-making algorithm, it is important for the clinician to be aware of the advantages and disadvantages of the methods of delivery. Oral sedation is always worth consideration when treatment planning a patient's care as the method of administration is accepted by the general population [2]. This is due to the oral route being the most prevalent method of administration for medications and also the relative ease of administration of the drugs through the p.o. (per oral) route [2]. Dental anxiety can be exacerbated by apparatuses for delivery of inhalational agents or intravenous needles. Intravenous (IV) line placement has the potential for syncopal responses in those with dental phobia pertaining to needles. Oral medications are relatively lower cost than those of the IV variety [2]. Additional advantages of the p.o. route of administration are the decreased incidence of adverse reactions and decreased severity of the adverse reactions [2].

Most medications taken orally undergo an extensive first pass metabolism requiring quite substantial dosages of the medication in order to cause toxicity. Of course, the dosages to produce an effect can vary based on age, sex, ethnicity, and genetics. The intravenous route bypasses the mechanisms of first pass metabolism and has a sharper curve of titration. It is important to understand that oral sedative drugs can lead to adverse effects, including but not limited to anaphylaxis or cardiovascular; however its incidence is much less common [3]. As alluded to previously in this section, there is no special equipment needed for the sedation, i.e., needles and syringes [2]. This again helps with patient anxiety and, equally important, from an operations standpoint cuts down on preparation and recovery time, cost, and other practices that decrease efficiency and productivity. An important point must be made that a patient will usually still be under the effect of the medication after completion of the procedure and will require some recovery and cannot leave without an escort. As of the writing of this chapter, there are no specialized education requirements for oral sedation in the dental office, which is another advantage [2].

Oral medications can be administered at home before the patient arrives to the office; however, this brings up one of the major disadvantages of oral sedation in dentistry, which is patient compliance [2]. Patient compliance becomes an issue with both actual dosing and perioperative factors. Patients often forget to take their medication, do not follow the instructions for dosing, or do not take it at the recommended time interval. Any clinician with patient's requiring antibiotic prophylaxis can attest to the problems of patient compliance.

Drugs

This upcoming section will be a brief survey of the drugs used for oral conscious sedation. There are multiple classes of medications that a practitioner should be aware of and have in their arsenal. These classes include benzodiazepines, histamine blockers (H1), and opioids [4]. The chapter will go through their pharmacology, dosing, and warnings including specific examples of each class. There are other categories of oral drugs (i.e., chloral derivatives); however, much of their use is historical and will not be discussed for ease and speed of reference for the clinician.

Benzodiazepines

Benzodiazepine drugs are subdivided into two categories based on effect: antianxiety and sedative-hypnotic. Both categories belong to a larger group of antianxiety and sedative-hypnotic which include other drugs which are not benzodiazepines. The antianxiety drugs are CNS depressants and can provide relief of anxiety without altering a patient's alertness, responsiveness, or motor function, making them a viable option for patients with mild to moderate dental phobia [5]. The sedative-hypnotic drugs produce either a calming effect (sedation) or inducing a sleep-like state (hypnosis) depending on the dose amount of the drug administered [5]. Benzodiazepines are considered first-line medications for most procedural sedations in the outpatient clinic [4]. The main reasons behind this are the high therapeutic index and the shallow dose-response curve [4]. Therapeutic index is "the range of doses at which a medication is effective without unacceptable adverse events" [6]. A high therapeutic index will mean that there is a wide range of doses that can produce the desired effect without toxicity. A dose-response means "that a dose required to produce minimal to moderate sedation is well below that required to produce hypnosis" [3]. The magnitude and duration of effect is dependent on patient specific factors including age, medication history, and health history [7]. For example, drug clearance of benzodiazepines in elderly patients is slower than younger patients and total elimination will thus take longer [7]. The benzodiazepine class of drugs is relatively safe and toxic effects would require very high dosages.

Mechanism of Action

The benzodiazepine class of drugs work to enhance the effects of the inhibitory neurotransmitter gamma-aminobutyric acid (GABA). GABA has inhibitory effects on neurons throughout the central nervous system by binding "GABA receptors" and opening chloride channels on the neuronal membrane. This leads to an influx of chloride and hyperpolarizes the cell membrane decreasing the likelihood of an action potential stimulating the neuron [4]. Benzodiazepine drugs bind the same GABA chloride channels at the $GABA_A$ receptor and increase the frequency of chloride channel activation in a GABA-dependent manner. Independent activation of these channels with benzodiazepines is not possible, drugs like propofol can open GABA chloride receptors independent of GABA [4]. The benzodiazepine drugs acts in a similar mechanism to the way that alcoholic beverages affect the central nervous system. It is not uncommon for patients to feel "drunk" after being given a dose of a benzodiazepine, either orally or intravenously.

Respiratory Effects

At appropriate doses, there is a very low likelihood of any significant respiratory depression with oral benzodiazepines. This makes them the agent of choice for most anxiety and phobia related issues, both in relation to dentistry and overall [8]. However, as with any CNS depressant there are reported cases of respiratory depression and one can never rule out this adverse effect [8]. In patients with respiratory disease, the stress of the dental appointment can trigger bronchospasm, in asthmatics or COPD populations, if severe enough. The reduction of anxiety by benzodiazepines can provide a protective mechanism [8]. Overall, the benzodiazepines are generally considered safe in regard to adverse respiratory effects, but still necessitate monitoring of a patient's pulmonary health preoperatively and breathing intraoperatively.

Cardiovascular Effects

Benzodiazepines have a similar safety profile between respiratory and cardiovascular systems. This class of medication has minimal cardiovascular effects in healthy patients. A study done in critically ill patients found that benzodiazepines, out of multiple classes of sedative drugs, provide the best amnestic profile while maintaining cardiac stability [9]. The study recognized that there is a risk for significant hypotension in patients who are already hemodynamically unstable [9]. Benzodiazepines are already employed in cardiac patients to reduce stress and anxiety issues that provide extra strain on the myocardium [8]. In the outpatient setting, in previously health patients with no history of heart disease, benzodiazepines are not only safe but also effective.

Hepatorenal Effects

Benzodiazepines are metabolized by the liver and their specific reactions varies based on formulation. Diazepam (Valium) is broken down into an active metabolite that persists with continued sedative properties [8]. Two benzodiazepines lorazepam and oxazepam are conjugated in the liver, which makes them water soluble, and they are excreted via the urine [4]. In patients with preexisting hepatic dysfunction or on medications that inhibit liver enzymes, clearance of the drugs may be prolonged [7]. In general, the benzodiazepines are considered among the safest sedative drugs with respect to hepatic function, especially in the setting of dental procedures when taken in a one-off scenario [8]. The clinician should consider smaller doses in the elderly, children, and those with hepatic dysfunction.

Central Nervous System Effects

As previously discussed in this section, benzodiazepines are central nervous system depressants. They potentiate the effect of the inhibitory neurotransmitter GABA. These effects are widespread and act at various centers of the brain to reduce emotions of fear, stress, anger, frustration, etc. This class of drugs is also well known and desired for their ability to create anterograde amnesia. An interesting phenomenon that has been noted in patients receiving benzodiazepines either orally or IV has been referred to as the paradoxical disinhibition. This phenomenon can cause aggression, talkativeness, emotional release, excitement, and excessive movement [10]. It is difficult to predict which patients will have this response and one study puts the incidence at approximately 1% of patients receiving benzodiazepines [10]. Some risk factors identified are patients with a history of psychological disturbance, history of alcohol abuse, children, and geriatric patients who are likely to be disinhibited by benzodiazepines [10].

It is a well-known fact the benzodiazepines are anticonvulsants and are not contraindicated in the use of the epileptic dental patient, as they may provide a protective role. The anticonvulsant effects are primarily when the drug is administered via the intravenous route. It should be noted that given their anticonvulsant properties, if ever flumazenil, the benzodiazepine reversal agent, was administered to a patient, even someone without a history of epilepsy, this patient is at risk for the onset of a seizure.

Contraindications

With a relatively favorable safety profile there are few contraindications to the use of benzodiazepines via the oral route. The main contraindications would be those with a history of anaphylaxis or hypersensitivity reaction to benzodiazepines, as well as, narrow-angle glaucoma [11].

Warnings

In addition to the contraindications, benzodiazepines can have adverse effects on patients, primarily if used chronically. The clinician should be aware of these even if the use is only for occasional surgery procedures. The most likely adverse effect that the practitioner may experience in the dental setting is transient or persistent psychomotor depression [12]. The patient will require an escort as the operation of an automobile or any other kind of equipment is inadvisable for patients that have taken a sedative. It also puts the patient at risk for falls and injuries due to this, which the provider may be held liable for. The primary concern for patients taking chronic benzodiazepine is the idea of tolerance and the drug history of the patient should be fully elucidated during the medical history taking [12]. Additionally, through chronic usage of benzodiazepines a patient can develop both psychological and physical dependence in patients [12]. Psychological dependence would see patients exhibiting drug seeking behaviors while physical refers primarily to withdrawal symptoms. Given that benzodiazepines act in a similar manner to alcohol, it is not difficult to understand the consequence of physical dependence. Concomitant use of benzodiazepines and alcohol is strongly advised against.

Pregnancy

Studies on diazepam have shown that is potentially a teratogen and should not be used in pregnancy [13]. There have been studies on diazepam usage in the third trimester that has been linked to floppy infant syndrome [13]. Additionally, there is concern of diazepam being linked to facial clefts in children [13]. Most of these studies, again, have investigated chronic usage of benzodiazepines. Most benzodiazepines have either a teratogenicity rating of either D or X. If considering oral surgical procedures in any pregnant patient, it is prudent to contact the obstetrician for consultation regarding the procedure and use of any drug.

Diazepam

Diazepam, marked as Valium, out of the other benzodiazepines that will be discussed in this chapter, is the oldest oral benzodiazepine and considered to be the model for oral benzodiazepine medications. Diazepam's effects are typical of the benzodiazepine group, which include anxiolysis, anterograde amnesia, sedation, anticonvulsant effects, and muscle relaxation [14]. The drug is lipophilic and absorption will be delayed with the concomitant ingestion of a moderately fatty meal [14]. In a fasted patient, between 90% and 100% of the drug is absorbed [14]. The peak plasma concentration is achieved approximately between 1 and 1.5 h [14]. Diazepam is highly bound to plasma proteins and so are its active metabolites and this drug and its metabolites cross the blood-brain barrier, the placental barrier, and into breast milk [14]. Due to the active metabolites, Valium has a long half-life, up to 48 h, according to the FDA. After it is broken down in the liver, the metabolized are conjugated and excreted in the urine [14]. Its use as a sedation agent has decreased in favor of drugs without active metabolites and shorter half-lives.

Availability: Valium is available for oral administration as tablets containing 2 mg, 5 mg, or 10 mg diazepam [14].

Dosing: To relieve anxiety, 2–10 mg, 2–4 times daily depending on the severity of the symptoms of anxiety [14].

Alprazolam

Alprazolam, belonging to the benzodiazepine family, is widely known and famous in popular culture as Xanax. It produces anxiolysis and amnesia and is indicated for anxiety and panic disorders [15]. It is quickly absorbed in the GI tract, reaches its peak plasma concentration between 1 and 2 h, and is approximately 80% bound to albumin in plasma [15]. The drug is metabolized by the CYP3A4 hepatic enzymes with no active metabolites and is excreted in the urine [15]. The CYP3A4 enzyme can be inhibited and induced by various medications, supplements, and foods, so a careful history should be taken. Patients with a history of alcohol abuse, geriatric, or with liver problems should be sedated with this medication with caution.

Availability: 0.25, 0.5, 1.0, or 2.0 mg tablets under the brand name Xanax [15].

Dosing: Initial dose of 0.25–0.5 mg given three times daily for patients with anxiety [15]. The dose may be increased to achieve a maximum therapeutic effect, at intervals of 3–4 days, to a maximum daily dose of 4 mg, given in divided doses [15].

Midazolam

Midazolam, previously branded as Versed, belongs to the sedative-hypnotic class of benzodiazepines, as opposed to the previously discussed antianxiety examples. It is available as both an IV and oral formulation and is the drug of choice in many surgical appointments. The drug induces sedation, anterograde amnesia, and anxiolysis. Midazolam is classified as a water-soluble benzodiazepine [16]. It is rapidly absorbed from the GI tract and produces drowsiness in about 30 min [16]. The time to peak plasma concentration in studies is approximately 20 min and its half-life is 1–5 h [16, 17]. Midazolam circulates bound to protein at approximately 95%-bound [17]. Oral Versed is commonly used by anesthesiologists in OR settings to facilitate preoperative preparations, including IV placement and induction of general anesthesia. It is a very short acting benzodiazepine which had made it popular among outpatient providers and dentists. It has favorability with those dealing with pediatrics, but it should not be used in pediatric populations below the age of 6 months.

Availability: Oral midazolam is available in a syrup that is 2.0 mg/mL [17].

Dosing: In patients between 6 months and 16 years old, 0.25–0.5 mg/kg PO (Max: 20 mg/dose) as a single dose 30–45 min before procedure [17].

Lorazepam

Lorazepam, branded under the name Ativan, is a long-acting benzodiazepine that is available in both oral and IV forms. It is a sedative-hypnotic benzodiazepine that when used in appropriate dosages has a tranquilizing effect with no impairment of cardiopulmonary function [18]. The bioavailability of the drug is approximately 90%, it is absorbed slower in comparison to the other medications discussed and will reach peak plasma concentration at 2 h [18]. A 2 mg oral dose will reach a peak plasma level of 20 ng/mL at 2 h [18]. Lorazepam will circulate at about 80% protein bound and its excretion half-life is 20 h [18]. It is excreted in the urine after conjugation and does not have active metabolites. Integrating the above data, lorazepam clearly has a long duration of action and should be considered in longer surgical procedures. As with the other benzodiazepines, use should be attenuated in geriatric patients.

Availability: Oral lorazepam tablets are available in 0.5 mg, 1 mg, and 2 mg tablets [18].

Dosing: The dosage of Ativan is 2–6 mg per day divided into multiple doses [18]. For anxiety, most patients require an initial dose of 2–3 mg/day given two times a day or three times per day [18].

Triazolam

Triazolam, marketed as Halcion, is another sedative-hypnotic benzodiazepine that is popular for dental clinical procedures. This hypnotic drug has a short half-life of 1.5–5.5 h; it reaches peak plasma concentration at 2 h and has peak plasma concentrations from 1 to 6 ng/mL when given in the p.o. formulation [19]. Additionally, it has no active metabolites and is excreted in the urine after conjugation by hepatic enzymes [19]. Its popularity is mainly due to its quick onset and short half-life. The safety profile and warnings are typical of the benzodiazepine group, which has been extensively discussed in this section. Due to its quick onset this makes it an ideal drug to be administered under supervision in the office setting.

Availability: Halcion is available in 0.25 mg tablet [19].

Dosage: The recommended dose for most adults is 0.25 mg before bedtime [19]. A dose of 0.5 mg should be used only for exceptional patients who do not respond adequately to a trial of a lower dose [19]. A dose of 0.5 mg should not be exceeded [19].

Name	Onset of Action	Elimination Half-Life	Peak Plasma Concentration	Active Metabolites	Excretion
Diazepam (Valium)	40 min	Up to 48 h	1–1.5 h	Yes	Urine
Alprazolam (Xanax)	60 min	6.3–26.9 h	1–2 h	No	Urine

Name	Onset of Action	Elimination Half-Life	Peak Plasma Concentration	Active Metabolites	Excretion
Midazolam (Versed)	30 min	1–5 h	20 min	No	Urine
Lorazepam (Ativan)	20–40 min	20 h	2 h	No	Urine
Triazolam (Halcion)	20–40 min	1.5–5.5 h	2 h	No	Urine

Histamine Blockers

Histamine blockers are drugs with a primary action that is intended to be involved in attenuating the allergic response in patients [20]. While its intended use is for this, this class of medications became well known for drowsiness and the induction of sedation [8]. These drugs soon became marketed for that purpose as well. The efficacy of sedation, especially in the setting of dental phobia and anxiety, is well below that of the benzodiazepines [4]. It is for this reason that antihistamine drugs are not recommended as the primary drugs for oral conscious sedations and why benzodiazepines take the top spot [4]. However, it is important to be aware of this class of drugs and how they work for instances in which patients cannot use drugs from another class of medication. You may consider histamine blockers in patients who have narrow-angle glaucoma and cannot tolerate benzodiazepines for example. The two main examples of H1 Blocker sedatives are hydroxyzine and promethazine.

Mechanism of Action

The main action of the H1 blockers is to prevent the allergic response in patients by acting as an antagonist at the histamine receptors. These histamine subtype 1 receptors are located throughout the CNS neurons, glandular cells, and smooth muscles [20]. Histamine granules, among other cytokines and inflammatory mediators, are released by mast cells in response to antigen and this histamine increases smooth muscle contractions in various organs (respiratory tract, GI tract) and increases vascular permeability which can cause a dangerous drop in blood pressure. One of the main side effects of this mechanism was sedation. The prevailing theory of the mechanism of action for this sedation is that, in the normal physiologic response, when histamine binds H1 receptors on neurons there is a partial depolarization of the neuronal membrane [21]. This partial depolarization increases the likelihood of excitation of the neurons. When there is a blockade of this depolarization it is likely that this contributes to the sedative effect of the drug [21]. It is important to understand that H1 receptor antagonists also likely exert their effect through non-selective and low affinity binding for muscarinic, adrenergic, and serotonergic receptors [21]. The final important point about the mechanism of H1 blockers is that they are independent of the GABA receptor channels that are targeted by the benzodiazepine medications [4]. This is important because an H1 blocker can be used to potentiate the effects of a benzodiazepine without administering more of the benzodiazepine [4]. These drugs are generally considered safe, with less potential for side effects than with benzodiazepines [4]. The major warnings and physiologic effects vary from drug to drug and will be discussed individually. The main drugs this section will cover are promethazine and hydroxyzine.

Promethazine

Promethazine, branded as Phenergan, is a phenothiazine derivative as well as an antihistamine and has long been used not only for sedation but also as an anti-emetic [8]. It has been available in the United States since 1951 and it is popular in the use of pediatric dental patients [8, 22]. Oral promethazine is readily absorbed and sedation can be appreciated within 20 min, with effects lasting between 4 and 6 h [23]. The drug is metabolized in the liver and excreted in the urine [23]. Of note, Phenergan is not addictive which differentiates it from the benzodiazepine class of drugs [5].

Availability: Phenergan is available in 12.5 mg, 25 mg, and 50 mg tablets [23].

Dosing: Pediatric sedation: 12.5–25 mg oral route at bedtime, Adults: 25–50 mg for preoperative sedation [23].

Warnings

Promethazine in dosages used for sedation do not induce an actual unconscious state (similar to general anesthesia) or incite any deficits in cardiovascular function, however, according to the manufacturer, there have been cases of fatal respiratory depression [5, 23]. There is a black box warning for Phenergan stating that the drug should not be used in children less than 2 years old due to fatal respiratory complications [23]. Additional warnings include the potential for extrapyramidal side effects, the lowering of seizure threshold, bone marrow depression, and it is a considered a Category C teratogen [5, 23]. It should also be noted that in geriatric patients with dementia and Alzheimer's disease antihistamines should be avoided [4].

Adverse Reactions

The most common adverse reactions from the use of promethazine are anticholinergic side effects including dry mouth and blurry vision, among others [23].

Hydroxyzine

Hydroxyzine, marketed as Vistaril, is another class of H1 blocker that is unrelated to promethazine. Its primary effects in addition to sedation are skeletal muscle relaxation, bronchodilation activity, antihistaminic, anti-emetic and analgesic effects

[24]. Hydroxyzine's onset is approximately 15–30 min with peak effect at about 2 h [8, 24]. The drug effects begin to decline after 3 4 h [24]. There is a very small side effect profile with this drug and there is a minimal effect on cardiovascular and respiratory function [24]. Hydroxyzine is the drug of choice in pediatric patients when compared to promethazine [22].

Availability: Vistaril is prepared as 25 mg and 50 mg tablets and as an oral suspension [24].

Dosing: Usual adult doses range from 50 mg to 100 mg [24].

Warnings

Hydroxyzine is contraindicated in pregnancy and nursing mothers [24]. It is also contraindicated in any patient with a history of hypersensitivity reaction to the drug [24]. A reduction in the dosing should be made when used with any analgesic (narcotic and non-narcotic) and barbiturates [24].

Adverse Reactions

Potential adverse reactions include transient drowsiness and dry mouth [24].

Opioid Sedation

Sedation with opioid medication is possible, however it is not routinely achieved via the oral route. Opioids produce primarily analgesia but can also have the effect of sedation, and respiratory depression [4]. The mechanism of action of opioids is as agonists of the mu and kappa opioid receptors [4]. Typically, opioid effects outside of analgesia are unpredictable when taken through the oral route, especially if there is no preoperative pain. Opioid induced sedation is primarily considered to be a side effect of the drug. The primary application of opioid administration in sedation is when administered via the intravenous route. An opioid in addition to a benzodiazepine has a synergistic effect to increase sedation, as well as to centrally blunt the pain response [4]. A multi-modal approach to deep sedations and general anesthetics is an important practice and limits the amount of each individual drug needed to produce a satisfactory effect. The drugs, techniques, and mechanisms behind intravenous sedation will be discussed in detail in Chap. 6 of this section. Due to the current opioid crisis these drugs should be used in caution.

Summary

The use of oral sedation is an excellent adjunct when performing surgical procedures in an outpatient clinical setting. They not only reduce patient anxiety, but they have an additional benefit of proving a more relaxing and safer environment for the surgeon. Benzodiazepines are predictably effective and carry minimal risk to the patient. No additional equipment is required for their use as patient monitoring can be accomplished with monitoring devices already available in the office (i.e., blood pressure cuff). The only downside to oral sedation is the requirement for a patient escort to transport the patient to and from the office and to watch them until the effects of the sedation wear off.

References

1. Committee on Quality Management and Departmental Administration. 2019. *Continuum of Depth of Sedation: Definition of General Anesthesia and Levels of Sedation/Analgesia | American Society of Anesthesiologists (ASA).* [online] Asahq.org. Available at: https://www.asahq.org/standards-and-guidelines/continuum-of-depth-of-sedation-definition-of-general-anesthesia-and-levels-of-sedationanalgesia.
2. Matear D, Clarke D. Considerations for the use of oral sedation in the institutionalized geriatric patient during dental interventions: a review of the literature. Spec Care Dentist. 1999;19(2):56–63. https://doi.org/10.1111/j.1754-4505.1999.tb01369.x.
3. Gill CJ, Michaelides PL. Dental drugs and anaphylactic reactions: report of a case. Oral Surg Oral Med Oral Pathol. 1980;50:30.
4. Becker D. Pharmacodynamic considerations for moderate and deep sedation. Anesth Prog. 2012;59(1):28–42. https://doi.org/10.2344/0003-3006-59.1.28.
5. Malamed S. Sedation. 6th ed. St. Louis, MO: Elsevier; 2018. p. 100–14.
6. Tamargo J, Le Heuzey J, Mabo P. Narrow therapeutic index drugs: a clinical pharmacological consideration to flecainide. Eur J Clin Pharmacol. 2015;71(5):549–67. https://doi.org/10.1007/s00228-015-1832-0.
7. Jacobi J, Fraser G, Coursin D, Riker R, Fontaine D, Wittbrodt E, et al. Clinical practice guidelines for the sustained use of sedatives and analgesics in the critically ill adult. Crit Care Med. 2002;30(1):119–41. https://doi.org/10.1097/00003246-200201000-00020.
8. Donaldson M, Gizzarelli G, Chanpong B. Oral Sedation: a primer on anxiolysis for the adult patient. Anesth Prog. 2007;54(3):118–29. https://doi.org/10.2344/0003-3006(2007)54[118:osapoa]2.0.co;2.
9. Darrouj J, Karma L, Arora R. Cardiovascular manifestations of sedatives and analgesics in the critical care unit. Am J Ther. 2009;16(4):339–53. https://doi.org/10.1097/01.pap.0000249925.76324.47.
10. Mancuso C, Tanzi M, Gabay M. Paradoxical reactions to benzodiazepines: literature review and treatment options. Pharmacotherapy. 2004;24(9):1177–85. https://doi.org/10.1592/phco.24.13.1177.38089.
11. Bounds CG, Nelson VL. Benzodiazepines. [Updated 2018 Nov 13]. In: StatPearls [Internet]. Treasure Island (FL): StatPearls Publishing; 2018 Jan. Available from: https://www.ncbi.nlm.nih.gov/books/NBK470159/
12. Gudex C. Adverse effects of benzodiazepines. Soc Sci Med. 1991;33(5):587–96. https://doi.org/10.1016/0277-9536(91)90216-y.
13. McElhatton P. The effects of benzodiazepine use during pregnancy and lactation. Reprod Toxicol. 1994;8(6):461–75. https://doi.org/10.1016/0890-6238(94)90029-9.
14. Valium [package insert] South San Francisco, CA: Roche Pharmaceuticals Inc.; 2016.
15. Xanax [package insert] New York, NY: Pfizer Pharmaceuticals Inc.; 2011.
16. Smith M, Eadie M, Brophy T. The pharmacokinetics of midazolam in man. Eur J Clin Pharmacol. 1981;19(4):271–8. https://doi.org/10.1007/bf00562804.
17. *Midazolam drug monograph, ClinicalKey. Elsevier.* [Available at] www.ClinicalKey.com. Accessed 18 Jan 2019.
18. Ativan [package insert] Bridgewater, NJ: Valeant Pharmaceuticals North America LLC; 2016.
19. Halcion [package insert] New York, NY: Pfizer Pharmaceuticals Inc.; 2016.

20. Baroody F, Naclerio R. Antiallergic effects of H1-receptor antagonists. Allergy. 2000;55:17–27. https://doi.org/10.1034/j.1398-9995.2000.00803.x.
21. Reiner P, Kamondi A. Mechanisms of antihistamine-induced sedation in the human brain: H1 receptor activation reduces a background leakage potassium current. Neuroscience. 1994;59(3):579–88. https://doi.org/10.1016/0306-4522(94)90178-3.
22. Wright GZ, McAulay DJ. Current premedicating trends in pedodontics. J Dent Child. 1973;40:185–7.
23. Phenergan [package insert] Philadelphia, PA: Wyeth Pharmaceuticals Inc.
24. Vistaril [package insert] New York, NY: Pfizer Labs; 2014.

Parenteral Sedation

6

Gregory Biron

Introduction

For the correct patient, office anesthesia provides relief from anxiety related to surgical procedures. Many oral and maxillofacial surgeons practice as operator-anesthetists, meaning, they perform anesthesia and surgery simultaneously. This unique practice requires an abundance of knowledge regarding airway physiology in order to maintain airway patency while also depressing consciousness. By the end of this chapter, the reader should appreciate the level of complexity involved in the operator-anesthetist model and understand basic anesthetic techniques.

The Initial Consultation

Medical History

Chapter 1 highlighted the medical and surgical history as a foundation for risk assessment prior to surgery. This chapter focuses specifically on conditions that affect the airway and delivery of anesthesia. A risk assessment should be conducted for each patient that will help guide the expected morbidity and mortality on an individual basis. A commonly utilized scoring system is the American Society of Anesthesiologists (ASA) physical status, which sets clear parameters as demonstrated in Table 6.1. Although this is a highly subjective system with moderate inter-rater variability, it can be helpful when deciding if a patient can handle the stress of a procedure and anesthesia [2]. Patients with an ASA physical status of I or II tend to have a large reserve and tolerate anesthesia, whereas a physical status of III or above are at risk for perianesthesia cardiac or respiratory events [3].

G. Biron (✉)
University of Pittsburgh Medical Center, Pittsburgh, PA, USA
e-mail: Birongs@upmc.edu

E. M. Ferneini, M. T. Goupil (eds.), *Office-Based Maxillofacial Surgical Procedures*, https://doi.org/10.1007/978-3-030-22371-7_6

Table 6.1 Excerpted from ASA Physical Status Classification System, 2014 of the American Society of Anesthesiologists

ASA Physical Status Classification System
I—A normal healthy patient
II—A patient with mild systemic disease
III—A patient with severe systemic disease
IV—A patient with severe systemic disease that is a constant threat to life
V—A moribund patient that is not expected to survive without the operation
VI—A declared brain-dead patient whose organs are being removed for donor purposes

A copy of the full text can be obtained from ASA, 1061 American Lane Schaumburg, IL 60173-4973 or online at www.asahq.org [1]

Table 6.2 Adapted from Chung F, Yegneswaran B, Liao P, et al. STOP questionnaire: a tool to screen patients for obstructive sleep apnea, *Anesthesiology*, 2008, vol. 108 (pg. 812–21) [6]

STOP-bang obstructive sleep apnea screening tool
S: Snoring: Do you snore loudly (loud enough to be heard through closed doors)?
T: Tired during the day: Do you often feel tired, fatigued, or sleepy during daytime?
O: Observed: Has anyone observed you stop breathing during your sleep?
P: Blood pressure: Do you have or are you being treated for high blood pressure?
B: BMI: BMI >35?
A: Age: Age over 50 years old?
N: Neck circumference: Neck circumference >40 cm?
G: Gender: Male?

Obstructive Sleep Apnea

Patients with obstructive sleep apnea (OSA) likely have multiple comorbidities including hypertension, cardiovascular disease, or metabolic disorders [4]. According to a study by Chung et al., 82% of men and 92% of women with moderate-severe OSA are undiagnosed [5]. Undiagnosed moderate-severe OSA can be identified by answering "yes" to at least five of the risk factors in the screening mnemonic "STOP-Bang," as described in Table 6.2 [4, 5]. Patients with high probability of OSA should be referred for further workup usually via polysomnography and optimization prior to elective anesthesia [7]. Patients with OSA often have increased opioid sensitivity resulting in worsening respiratory depression, as well as upper airway obstruction from relaxation and collapse of pharyngeal tissues. Well-managed OSA with continuous positive airway pressure (CPAP) and optimized comorbidities may actually be candidates for office anesthesia. CPAP compliant patients should be instructed to bring their device to the office and use for several days postoperatively [7]. If postoperative pain cannot be adequately treated with nonopioid pain medications or they are not compliant with CPAP, anesthesia with a secured airway should be considered [7].

Obesity

Obesity is divided into three classes: Class I (BMI 30–34.9), Class II (BMI 35–39.9), and Class III (BMI $\geq$ 40) [8]. The obese patient population presents with many similar office anesthesia difficulties as OSA discussed above. Other comorbidities resulting from obesity include hypertension, diabetes, and cardiovascular disease [8]. Morbidly obese patients generally are more sensitive to anesthetics and opioids, therefore, may lose airway reflexes and cause respiratory depression at an alarming rate [3]. Obese patients may be more difficult to ventilate due to excess soft tissues in the neck and pharynx [3, 9]. Evaluation prior to administering anesthesia can be assessed by weight or BMI, Mallampati score (Fig. 6.1), or neck circumference [9]. Obese patients, especially morbidly obese patients, may be safer to treat in a setting that provides a secured airway with help nearby in case of emergency [3]. Use caution in prescribing of opioids postoperatively due to risk of respiratory compromise [8].

Cardiorespiratory

Cardiac diseases most commonly encountered in the office include congestive heart failure, myocardial ischemia, and valvular heart disease [11]. Cardiac consultation may be indicated to assess severity of disease based on EKG, chest X-ray, echocardiogram, stress test, or physician recommendations prior to anesthesia. Respiratory diseases often encountered are asthma and chronic obstructive pulmonary disease (COPD). Consultation with physician may be indicated to determine disease severity based on prior hospitalizations and exacerbation, pulmonary function tests or chest X-ray. The functional capacity of a patient should be estimated at the consultation appointment to predict risk for cardiac and respiratory events in the perianesthesia period. A simple screening tool that can be used is metabolic equivalent of task (METs), which estimate energy expenditure based on activity level (Table 6.3). If the patient can exert 4–5 METs without symptoms, likely they will be able to tolerate surgery and

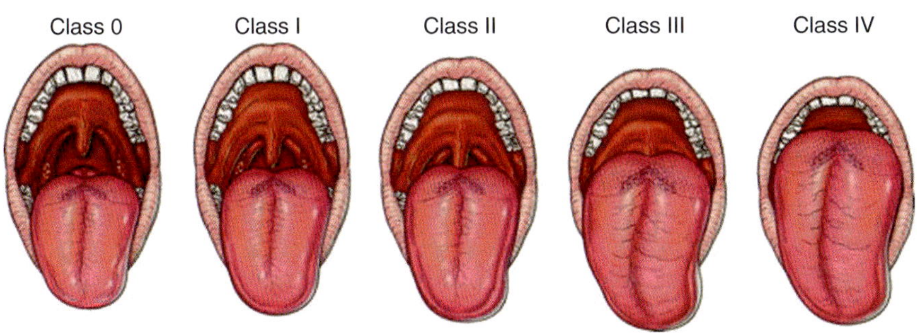

Fig. 6.1 Modified Mallampati Classification. Adapted from Finucane B, Tsui B, Santora A. Principles of airway management, 4th ed., New York, Springer, 2010 [10]

Table 6.3 Adapted from Freeman WK, Gibbons RJ (2009) Perioperative Cardiovascular Assessment of Patients Undergoing Noncardiac Surgery. Mayo Clinic Proceedings 84:79–90

Metabolic equivalent of task (MET)
1 MET: eat, dress, toilet, walk inside house
<4 MET: light work such as dusting or washing dishes
≥4 MET: climb flight of stairs, run short distance
>10 MET: strenuous sports such as football, basketball, skiing

anesthesia [4, 12]. Patients identified as high risk for adverse events may be referred for further workup and optimization or anesthesia may be completed in a hospital setting with an anesthesiologist.

Endocrine Disorders

The most common endocrine disorder that will be observed in the office is diabetes mellitus. Proper history should be obtained including compliance with medications and monitoring, most recent hemoglobin A1c, fasting glucose levels, or glucose tolerance test [11]. Gastroparesis is a common comorbidity; therefore, the surgeon should consider an extended NPO period and prophylactic H2 blockers to prevent acid reflux and aspiration [11]. Diabetic patients are known to have "silent" cardiovascular events due to neuropathy and cardiac consultation may be indicated [11]. Discuss insulin and oral hypoglycemic agent therapy with prescribing physician as doses may be adjusted to prevent hypoglycemia on the day of anesthesia [11].

Special Populations

Opioid Abuse

In the late 1990s, pain became known as "the fifth vital sign," and quality of patient care began to revolve around adequate pain control [13]. Increasing pressure on physicians to prescribe opioids for aggressive pain control led to a steady rise in misuse of the unnecessarily prescribed narcotics [13]. According to the U.S. Department of Health and Human Services, the opioid epidemic in the U.S. was declared a public emergency in 2017 [14]. This special population will be encountered frequently in the office, and it is the responsibility of the surgeon to formulate a safe and effective anesthetic plan. Opioid-sparing anesthetic techniques should be implemented rather than withholding opioids [15]. Opioids in the postoperative setting may be appropriate as inadequate pain control may act as a trigger to relapse into drug use [15]. The surgeon must not mistake drug-seeking behavior with inadequate pain control, a term referred to as pseudoaddiction [15, 16]. Increased doses of opioids may be required with chronic opioid use due to increased tolerance or opioid induced hyperalgesia [13, 17, 18]. A thorough history and physical must be obtained as chronic opioid users may have underlying cardiopulmonary disease, renal impairment, anemia, and adrenal hypertrophy [18]. Physical exam findings of acute opioid use include lethargy, pinpoint pupils, and slow respiratory rate [19].

Smoking

Cigarette smoking has many deleterious effects on the airway and cardiovascular system that negatively impacts office-based anesthesia [20]. The nicotine in cigarettes causes an endogenous release of catecholamines leading to increased blood pressure, heart rate, and peripheral vascular resistance [20]. Levels of carboxyhemoglobin are drastically increased in smokers, which prevent tissues from extracting the oxygen leading to chronic tissue hypoxia [20, 21]. Pulse oximeters are unable to detect the difference between oxyhemoglobin and carboxyhemoglobin; therefore, oxygen saturation will be overestimated [20]. Other negative respiratory effects include increased secretions, impaired mucociliary clearance, and increased reactivity of airways [20, 21]. Perianesthesia risk decreases if the patient quits smoking around 8 weeks prior to anesthesia and may actually be at higher risk if quitting less than 8 weeks prior to anesthesia [20]. For this reason, it is recommended that patients quit smoking at least 8 weeks prior to anesthesia [20].

Breastfeeding

There are few clinical trials that have been completed demonstrating clear recommendations regarding breastfeeding after receiving parenteral sedation; most information is based on expert opinion [22]. The consensus is that most commonly used sedation drugs are relatively safe while breastfeeding when used judiciously. Sedation should be scheduled early in the day and the mother is encouraged to breastfeed or pump before anesthesia to prevent breast engorgement [22]. Profound local anesthesia should be administered to decrease amount of systemic parenteral medications required [23]. Mothers undergoing office anesthesia with short-acting anesthetics and analgesics are encouraged to continue breastfeeding when alert and recovered from anesthesia [23]. Caution should be used with mothers of neonates at risk for apnea, hypotension, or hypotonia, as small amounts of drug in the breast milk can be harmful [22]. Codeine is not recommended in the breastfeeding mother as it is easily secreted into breast milk and is metabolized into morphine by the liver and may lead to sedating levels if the patient or child are rapid metabolizers [23].

Pregnant

In rare cases, such as emergencies, the pregnant patient may require sedation if pain and anxiety cannot otherwise be controlled [8]. The risk of medication teratogenicity must be weighed against harm to the patient if presenting issue is not dealt with. Local anesthesia with epinephrine has been shown to be safe during pregnancy and should be used in sufficient quantity to prevent endogenous release of epinephrine [8]. Little is known about the teratogenicity of opioids and benzodiazepines on the human fetus [8]. Risks involved with sedation include hypotension and decreased perfusion of the fetus, risk of aspiration from decreased gastric emptying and decreased lower esophageal sphincter tone, and airway edema leading to hypoxia, and preterm labor [8]. Consultation with the practitioner primarily caring for the pregnant patient should be obtained prior to administering anesthesia [8].

Table 6.4 Examples of pertinent findings within the anesthesia history

Anesthesia history
Difficult intubation or ventilation
Postoperative nausea and vomiting (PONV)
Anxiety
Delayed emergence
Delirium (emergence agitation)
Respiratory or cardiac events
Malignant hyperthermia
Pseudocholinesterase deficiency
Family history of adverse effects

Anesthesia History

The surgeon should inquire about prior anesthesia experiences including regional (local), minimal, moderate, deep, or general anesthesia. Many adverse events can be prevented or at least anticipated if identified at the consultation appointment. Genetic conditions such as malignant hyperthermia, although rare, can be life threatening if not diagnosed and treated early. Examples of pertinent findings within the anesthesia history can be found in Table 6.4.

Physical Examination

Cardiorespiratory Examination

Vital signs are obtained at the consultation appointment to provide a baseline for the patient, uncover potentially undiagnosed conditions, and allow for optimization prior to anesthesia. Vitals include blood pressure, heart rate, respiratory rate, and oxygen saturation. The heart should be auscultated to listen for arrhythmias or valvular disturbances. The lungs are auscultated to identify severity of chronic lung conditions or acute infections. Measurement of height and weight is important for drug dosing [4].

Airway Assessment

If the patient is low risk for anesthesia from a medical standpoint, the next step is the airway assessment. The surgeon must understand airway anatomy and identify key landmarks prior to administration of anesthesia. Relevant airway exam techniques can be found in Table 6.5 and further demonstrated in Fig. 6.1. The surgeon must be competent in mask ventilating a patient that has slipped into a deeper plane of anesthesia than intended or is experiencing desaturation for another reason as it can be lifesaving. Approximately 0.9–7.8% of the population is considered a difficult mask ventilation, which can be predicted based on the risk factors listed in Table 6.6 [24, 25]. Inadequate mask ventilation can lead to hypoxic brain damage or death due to poor oxygenation and ventilation, and aspiration of gastric contents. Although most surgeons will not be intubating patients in the office, roughly 7% of patients are considered a difficult intubation, which can be relevant in emergency settings [25].

Table 6.5 Adapted from Klinger K, Infosino A (2018) Airway Management. In: Basics of Anesthesia, 7th ed. Elsevier, Philadelphia, PA, pp 239–272

Airway examination component	Nonreassuring findings
Length of upper incisors	Relatively long
Relationship of maxillary and mandibular incisors during normal jaw closure	Prominent "overbite" (maxillary incisors anterior to mandibular incisors)
Relationship of maxillary and mandibular incisors during voluntary protrusion of mandible	Patient cannot bring mandibular incisors anterior to (in front of) maxillary incisors
Interincisor distance	Less than 3 cm
Visibility of uvula (Mallampati score)	Not visible when tongue is protruded with patient in sitting position (e.g., Mallampati class ≥2)
Shape of palate	Highly arched or very narrow
Compliance of mandibular space	Stiff, indurated, occupied by mass, or nonresilient
Thyromental distance	Less than three ordinary finger breadths
Length of neck	Short
Thickness of neck	Thick
Range of motion of head and neck	Patient cannot touch tip of chin to chest or cannot extend neck

Table 6.6 Adapted from El-Orbany M, Woehlck HJ (2009) Difficult Mask Ventilation. Anesthesia & Analgesia 109:1870–1880

Predicted difficult mask ventilation
Increased body mass index
History of snoring or sleep apnea
Presence of beard
Lack of teeth
Age >55 years
Mallampati III or IV
Limited mandibular protrusion
Male gender
Airway mass or tumor

Venous Access

Assess peripheral venous anatomy and document likely access points for the day of anesthesia. Inquire about history of failed intravenous cannulation or need for advanced techniques such as ultrasound guidance or other technologies such as vein finders. Examples of patients that may have difficult access are IV drug users, advanced age, obese, dehydrated, or diabetic patients. If intravenous access is predicted to be difficult based on physical examination, but the patient is otherwise a candidate for office anesthesia, ultrasound guidance may be indicated.

Preanesthesia Counseling

Patient Education

Patient expectations for anesthesia should be set at the initial appointment to prevent confusion and frustration on the day of surgery. Patients may fear not knowing what to expect with the sedation and feel that they do not have control. The anticipated anesthetic plan should be reviewed with the patient from start to finish. As most oral and maxillofacial surgeons will use moderate to deep sedation in the office, the patient should be instructed that they will not have memory of the procedure, but they likely will remain conscious enough to respond to simple commands or tactile stimulation. Psychological readiness for office sedation should be assessed and anesthetic plans adjusted accordingly.

Preanesthesia Instructions

At the consultation appointment, the patient should receive both verbal and written instructions on how to prepare for the day of anesthesia. The patient should be counseled on the most up-to-date fasting recommendations to decrease incidence of pulmonary aspiration of gastric contents as depicted in Table 6.7 [26]. The patient is expected to arrive on the day of anesthesia with a responsible escort that will be spending the day caring for the patient. The escort should be instructed to remain in the office for the duration of anesthesia and recovery. The patient should be instructed to dress comfortably, wear shoes that will not easily fall off while walking, and to not wear nail polish as this affects the pulse oximeter.

Medications

Medications that should be stopped or continued should be reviewed and adjusted on a case-by-case basis. Beta-blockers should generally be continued in the perianesthesia period as they have been shown to be cardioprotective [27]. Although widely debated, for the purposes of the oral and maxillofacial surgeon, ACE inhibitors (ACE-I) and angiotensin receptor blockers (ARBs) should be continued as the risk of rebound hypertension with discontinuing likely outweighs the hypotension observed with continuing [27]. Diuretics, with the exception of thiazide diuretics for hypertension, should be discontinued [19]. Insulin-dependent diabetic patients should discontinue short-acting insulin on morning of surgery and use 1/2 to 1/3 of basal dose of insulin. Generally, oral hypoglycemic medications are held on the morning of surgery to prevent hypoglycemia [19]. Generally, antidepressants, antipsychotics, and anxiolytics are continued on the day of anesthesia [19].

Table 6.7 ASA fasting recommendations (2016)

Ingested food or liquid	Minimum fasting time before surgery (h)
Clear liquids	2
Breast Milk	4
Infant formula	6
Nonhuman milk	6
Light meal	6
Fried or fatty foods, meat	8

Adapted from (2017) Practice Guidelines for Preoperative Fasting and the Use of Pharmacologic Agents to Reduce the Risk of Pulmonary Aspiration. Anesthesiology 126:376–393

Preparation: Day of Anesthesia

Preanesthesia Checklist

Table 6.8 is a checklist that reviews common causes of delayed or postponed anesthetics. Review this list with the patient early on the day of anesthesia to ensure compliance with preanesthesia instructions and identify other obstacles to a safe anesthesia experience.

Venipuncture

One of the first interactions with the patient on the day of anesthesia is the placement of the peripheral intravenous catheter, an area of intense anxiety in many patients. Providing efficient placement with minimal discomfort is a chance to earn the patient's trust.

Venipuncture Anatomy

Choice of vein for elective anesthesia in the maxillofacial surgery office typically is in the dorsum of hand, ventral forearm, or antecubital fossa [28]. Dorsal hand veins are superficial, distant from other anatomically important structures, but tend to be smaller than proximal veins and mobile due to superficial location [28]. The ventral forearm includes larger caliber veins, less mobility, but can be challenging due to deeper location [28]. The antecubital fossa has several large caliber veins that are readily accessible and minimally mobile, but caution should be taken on the medial aspect to avoid nearby important anatomic structures [28].

Venipuncture Technique

Basic setup for placement of the peripheral IV should be simple and done the same way each time, an example is depicted in Fig. 6.2.

Prior to starting the IV, the tubing should be run entirely with fluids to eliminate all air bubbles, which have potential to be hazardous to the patient. The drip chamber should be filled about halfway with fluids to reduce the risk of turbulence

Table 6.8 Day of anesthesia checklist

Day of anesthesia checklist
The patient is NPO according to current ASA guidelines
The patient is present with responsible adult escort
The patient has a responsible adult to care for the patient until fully recovered from anesthesia
The patient has taken home medications as recommended at previous appointment
Informed consent obtained with written confirmation
Vital signs obtained and within normal limits for the patient
Recent illness with focused reevaluation for respiratory tract sensitivity including upper respiratory infection, bronchitis, pneumonia, asthma exacerbation, etc.

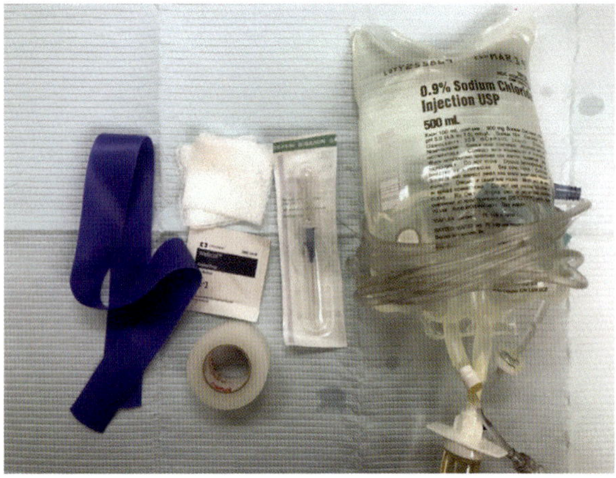

Fig. 6.2 Basic peripheral IV setup

and air bubble formation. The patient is positioned comfortably and the tourniquet is applied to the upper arm tight enough to prevent venous flow but still allows for arterial flow (radial pulse maintained). The tourniquet should be applied in such a way that it can be simply removed with one hand after the catheter is inserted. The arm is allowed to hang below the level of the heart while venous blood pools and the patient can be asked to open and close a fist, which redistributes blood from the musculature into the veins [29]. Venodilation can be encouraged by light tapping of tissue overlying vein or application of warm towel [29]. Nitrous oxide-oxygen can be used to promote venodilation and provide analgesia during venipuncture. Skin is cleaned with 70% isopropyl alcohol or other equivalent solution over IV insertion site and allowed time to dry completely. If desired, injection of local anesthetic (Lidocaine 1% or 2%) with 27-gauge needle to form a wheal may be used to minimize discomfort at the time of intravenous cannulation as depicted in Fig. 6.3. A cream such as EMLA® (Eutectic mixture of local anesthetic) can be applied over IV insertion site for the indicated time period to achieve similar effect [29]. This technique is generally reserved for larger gauge catheters (at least 18 gauge), but this is based on surgeon preference. A 20 or 22 gauge catheter is generally sufficient for use in the office [29].

Traction is applied with nondominant hand distal to injection site to pin the vein in place and prevent movement during venipuncture. Hold the nondominant hand in such a way that the proper angulation of the angiocatheter can be maintained. The needle is advanced with bevel up at 15–30° angle from the skin until through the skin layer and into the vein as shown in Fig. 6.4 [29]. After the vein is penetrated, the angulation of the needle is decreased to parallel that of the vein.

When the needle enters the vein, blood will appear in the clear chamber, known as "flash." When the flash appears, advance the needle another 2–3 mm while remaining parallel to vein to ensure that the plastic catheter is also within the vein as seen in Fig. 6.5.

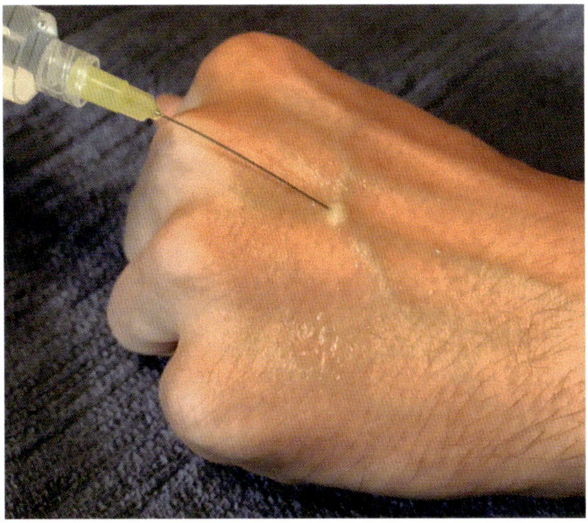

Fig. 6.3 Injection of local anesthetic into subcutaneous tissue to alleviate pain during peripheral IV insertion

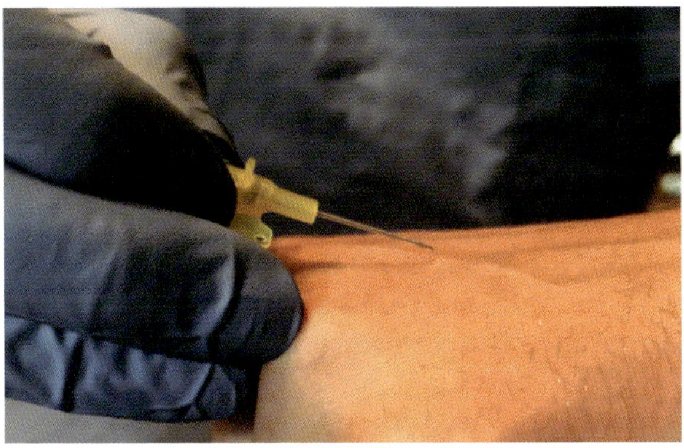

Fig. 6.4 Angulation of angiocatheter as it passes through skin

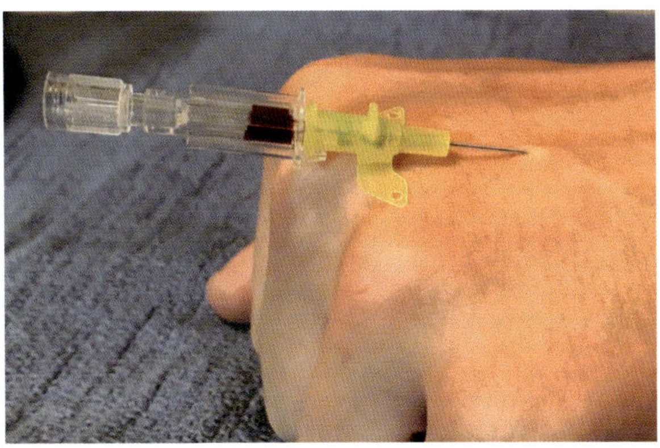

Fig. 6.5 Blood return into chamber as needle enters the vein, known as "flash"

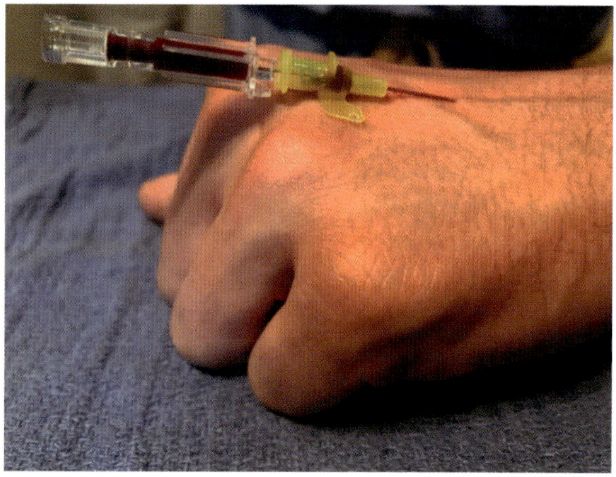

Fig. 6.6 Blood return into the plastic catheter is observed when needle is withdrawn and the catheter is within the lumen of the vein

While holding the plastic catheter stationary, the needle is then withdrawn 2–3 mm. If the catheter is indeed within the vein, blood will be seen entering the catheter as the needle is withdrawn as shown in Fig. 6.6.

The catheter can now be advanced to the hub, the tourniquet is immediately released, and the catheter is secured with adhesive tape. The catheter is then flushed with saline or connected to IV tubing and observed to ensure surrounding tissues are not infiltrating with fluids. Infiltration is a sign that the tip of the catheter is outside of the vein. If infiltrated, the catheter must be removed and a new one started at a more proximal location on the same limb, or any location on opposing limb.

Emergency Drug and Equipment Checklist

A well-organized compilation of emergency drugs and equipment should be stored in an easily accessible location and stocked regularly [30]. Medications are to be arranged in a simplistic fashion to avoid confusion in the case of an office anesthesia emergency [30]. Example contents of each medication compartment should include generic and proprietary name of drug, dosage, and quick instructions for use in emergency setting. Table 6.9 demonstrates recommended drugs and equipment, but only drugs that the practitioner is trained to administer should be stocked [30].

Intraoperative Management

Levels of Sedation

According to the American Society of Anesthesiologists, there is a spectrum of depths of sedation ranging from anxiolysis to general anesthesia as described in Table 6.10 [31]. This model depicts the levels of sedation with clear-cut parameters, but in reality it is a continuum, and a patient may drift between levels [31]. For this reason, it is important that the anesthetist be prepared to "rescue" the patient from a deeper plane of anesthesia than intended, as response to medications is unpredictable [31].

Table 6.9 Recommended equipment and medications for office anesthesia

Basic equipment setup
Oxygen source
Yankauer suction
Intravenous access—tourniquet, alcohol wipe, angiocatheter, adhesive tape, IV tubing, IV fluids
Sterile water—for reconstitution of medications
Intraoperative monitoring
Stethoscope (precordial recommended)
Blood pressure cuff
Pulse oximeter
Capnograph
Electrocardiogram
Temperature probe
Glucometer
Respiratory/cardiac equipment
Nasopharyngeal and oropharyngeal airway adjuncts
Bag-valve-mask or positive pressure ventilation system
Supraglottic laryngeal mask airways (LMA)
Laryngoscope and blades (or video laryngoscope)
Endotracheal tubes
McGill forceps
Instruments for surgical airway (cricothyrotomy)
Automatic external defibrillator (AED)
Medications
Epinephrine
Atropine
Glycopyrrolate
Nitroglycerine
Phenylephrine
Ephedrine
Lidocaine
Verapamil
Magnesium sulfate
Adenosine
Naloxone
Flumazenil
Esmolol
Labetolol
Hydralazine
Succinylcholine
Dantrolene OR Ryanodex

Intramuscular Anesthesia

Intramuscular Sedation Overview

The intramuscular route of anesthesia administration provides opportunities for sedation in special populations that cannot tolerate oral or intravenous sedation. For example, the uncooperative child, special needs child or adult, or the patient where intravenous access is not feasible [32]. This technique is praised for its relatively fast onset of action (10–15 min) by bypassing the gastrointestinal tract, patient cooperation is not required, and reabsorption is more predictable than with oral administration [32]. There are risks more specifically associated with IM technique,

Table 6.10 Excerpted from "Continuum of Depth of Sedation: Definition of General Anesthesia and Levels of Sedation/Analgesia," 2014 of the American Society of Anesthesiologists. A copy of the full text can be obtained from ASA, 1061 American Lane Schaumburg, IL 60173-4973 or online at www.asahq.org [31]

Levels of sedation
Minimal sedation (anxiolysis) is a drug-induced state during which patients respond normally to verbal commands. Although cognitive function and physical coordination may be impaired, airway reflexes and ventilatory and cardiovascular functions are unaffected
Moderate sedation/analgesia (conscious sedation) is a drug-induced depression of consciousness during which patients respond purposefully to verbal commands, either alone or accompanied by light tactile stimulation. No interventions are required to maintain a patent airway, and spontaneous ventilation is adequate. Cardiovascular function is usually maintained
Deep sedation/analgesia is a drug-induced depression of consciousness during which patients cannot be easily aroused but respond purposefully following repeated or painful stimulation. The ability to independently maintain ventilatory function may be impaired. Patients may require assistance in maintaining a patent airway, and spontaneous ventilation may be inadequate. Cardiovascular function is usually maintained
General anesthesia is a drug-induced loss of consciousness during which patients are not arousable, even by painful stimulation. The ability to maintain ventilatory function is often impaired. Patients often require assistance in maintaining a patent airway, and positive pressure ventilation may be required because of depressed spontaneous ventilation or drug-induced depression of neuromuscular function. Cardiovascular function may be impaired

including intra-arterial injection, nerve damage, inability to titrate drugs, needle breakage, and possible needle-stick injury [32].

Intramuscular Injection Sites

There are four anatomic locations that are generally utilized for intramuscular injection of drugs, including deltoid area, gluteal area, ventrogluteal area, and vastus lateralis [32]. The deltoid area is a common location in the adult as it is easily accessible, extremely vascular, and can accommodate up to 4 mL of fluid [32]. Injection in the deltoid area should be administered between the upper and lower areas of the muscle to avoid damaging the radial nerve. The vastus lateralis is the lateral aspect of the thigh and can be used in patients of all ages, easily accessible in most cases, moderate vascularity, few nearby anatomic structures, and can accommodate up to 15 mL of fluid [32]. Injections in the gluteal area should be done in the upper outer quadrant to avoid injuring nearby nerves and arteries. Access for gluteal injection requires the patient to lay face down with arm and legs hanging off the table to allow for relaxation of the muscle; therefore this injection is not commonly used [32]. The gluteal area is able to accommodate 4–8 mL of fluid and is minimally vascular [32]

Intramuscular Injection Technique

The site chosen for injection must be adequately exposed and anatomic landmarks identified [32]. Apply antiseptic such as isopropyl alcohol and allow sufficient time to dry. Squeeze the soft tissue with nondominant hand to keep taut while holding the syringe in the dominant hand in a dart-like fashion [32]. Quickly introduce the needle to the depth of the muscle then release the soft tissue with nondominant hand

[32]. Aspirate to ensure that needle is not intra-arterial, turn syringe quarter turn, and re-aspirate to ensure needle tip was not against vessel wall [32]. If conditions permit, inject drug slowly to reduce discomfort. Remove the needle slowly, apply gauze, and hold firm pressure [32]. Gently massage muscle to encourage increased blood flow [32].

Commonly Used Intravenous Drugs

Opioids

Opioids are often used during office-based anesthesia due to potent and short-acting analgesia by acting on pain pathways. Opioids also induce a euphoric state and provide an antitussive effect, both of which are beneficial during sedation [18]. Opioids act synergistically with propofol and other anesthetics allowing for decreased effective amounts of each and improved hemodynamic stability [18]. The side effect with greatest clinical impact is dose-dependent respiratory depression and decreased responsiveness to carbon dioxide [18]. Respiratory depression can be exacerbated by factors such as older age, use of other CNS depressants, renal impairment, and decreased hepatic blood flow [18]. Another serious but less common side effect is chest wall or glottis rigidity that can be caused by rapid administration of the drug [21]. Gastrointestinal manifestations may occur with opioid use including postoperative nausea and vomiting, decreased gastric emptying, and ileus [18, 33]. Opioids may cause bradycardia due to increased vagal activity or decreased sympathetic tone [18]. The negative effects of opioids can be reversed by naloxone, which is a pure opioid antagonist.

Benzodiazepines

Benzodiazepines are used for office sedation due to the amnestic, anxiolytic, and sedative properties [34]. The patient will have no memory of intraoperative events, even with a lighter plane of anesthesia, due to the anterograde amnestic effects. Caution used when administering to obese patients or patients with OSA as benzodiazepines relax airway musculature, which may cause upper airway obstruction and decrease response to carbon dioxide. Benzodiazepines act synergistically with propofol and opioids and increase risk of upper airway obstruction and apnea when used together. Oversedation may be observed in patients with renal or hepatic impairment due to decreased clearance and active metabolites [3]. The effects of benzodiazepines can be completely reversed using flumazenil, which is a competitive benzodiazepine antagonist [34].

Propofol

Propofol is an induction agent that causes hypnosis and sedation by effects on the GABA receptor and inhibition of NMDA receptor [34]. This drug is often used for its fast on and fast off properties, allowing quick recovery and discharges. Another benefit that propofol provides for office sedations is its antiemetic properties in doses as small as 10 mg [34, 35]. Bronchodilatory effects make propofol a favorable drug to use with patients with asthma or COPD [34]. Propofol causes vasodilation, which results in a decreased mean arterial pressure with minimal change in heart rate [34]. Apnea may result from administration of propofol in a dose-dependent manner. Propofol can cause burning pain on injection, which can be alleviated by first injecting lidocaine. Although propofol contains egg lecithin and soybean oil, its use has not been shown to be contraindicated in patients with egg, soy, or peanut allergy [36].

Ketamine

Ketamine is a sedative and potent analgesic drug that produces a dissociative anesthesia by acting as an antagonist of the NMDA receptor. The analgesic effects allow for pain control during sedation in patients with opioid tolerance or chronic pain [34]. The use of ketamine reduces the required dosage of postoperative opioids [13]. Most protective reflexes are maintained with ketamine unlike other anesthetics, and it even causes bronchodilation. Ketamine is a sympathomimetic drug; therefore, it causes an increase in arterial blood pressure, heart rate, cardiac output, and myocardial oxygen consumption [34]. Despite many desirable properties of ketamine, the anesthetist must be aware of many side effects of the drug. The sympathomimetic side effects may be harmful to a patient with existing ischemic heart disease. Emergence reactions such as vivid dreams, confusion, and fear occur in around 10–30% of patients, and therefore this drug should be avoided in patients with psychiatric disorders and history of delirium [34]. Ketamine increases intraocular pressure and should not be used on patients with open eye injuries or other eye disorders [34]. Patients are routinely pretreated with an anticholinergic such as glycopyrrolate since ketamine causes salivation and lacrimation [34]. The use of benzodiazepines with ketamine can blunt the sympathomimetic and psychomimetic effects [34].

Dexmedetomidine

Dexmedetomidine is an alpha-2-adrenergic agonist that acts on the brain and spinal cord to produce sedative, hypnotic, anxiolytic, and analgesic effects [34]. This drug is similar in structure to the antihypertensive drug Clonidine, but much more specific to the alpha-2 receptor [34]. The difference between Dexmedetomidine and other sedative drugs like propofol and benzodiazepines is that it does not act on the GABA pathway, but instead, sedation is via endogenous sleep promoting pathways [34]. For this reason, patients treated with dexmedetomidine tend to have smooth wake ups and are easily arousable [34, 37]. Dexmedetomidine can be an advantageous drug for office sedation as it has very little effect on the respiratory system and preserved response to CO_2 [34]. Dexmedetomidine acts as a sympatholytic drug resulting in a decrease in mean arterial pressure, heart rate, and cardiac output. Changes in blood pressure appear to be related to drug concentrations in the blood; hypertension with greater concentration and hypotension with lower concentration [37, 38]. Dexmedetomidine is used less frequently for office sedation due to prolonged recovery and discharges. There is currently no reversal drug that is approved for use in humans [37].

IV Fluids

IV fluids can be divided into two distinct categories: crystalloids and colloids. Colloids are principally used to expand the plasma volume in the case of resuscitation and are not routinely utilized in the oral and maxillofacial surgery office. Crystalloids on the other hand are used routinely to compensate for relative fluid deficit from NPO status, decrease PONV, and maintain patency of the peripheral IV [39]. Only a few types of IV fluids are necessary to review, as patients selected for office sedation will likely have stable hemodynamics.

Normal saline (0.9% NaCl) is a slightly hypertonic crystalloid that contains equal parts of sodium and chlorine in sterile water [40]. Balanced salt solutions such as Lactated Ringer and Plasma-Lyte are crystalloids that contain similar physiologic electrolyte profile (Na, K, Mg, Ca) as plasma with added buffers to prevent metabolic disturbances [40]. The isotonic nature of these fluids allows for a longer intravascular time, which can counter the vasodilatory properties of many anesthetics [21]. Dextrose 5% in water (D5W) is a hypotonic crystalloid that is often combined with normal or half normal saline as it is rapidly metabolized into free water that leaves the intravascular space [21, 39].

With few exceptions, any of the mentioned IV fluids will be appropriate for office sedation due to the relatively short durations of surgery and the health of the patients selected.

Intraoperative Safety

Patient Monitoring

Patient monitoring alerts the anesthetist to changes in physiologic status before it may be clinically apparent. There are minimum requirements for monitoring during office anesthesia that are set by AAOMS parameters of care. Each component, whether measured continuously or intermittently, should be documented in 5-min intervals on the anesthetic record. Requirements for continuous monitoring include continuous pulse-oximetry, capnography, and electrocardiography. Blood pressure should be measured at least every 5 min. Auscultation, visual inspection of ventilation, and level of sedation should be monitored as indicated clinically [8]. Although temperature measurement is not required, it should be immediately available any time a triggering agent for malignant hyperthermia is administered [8].

Anesthesia Team Model

Oral and maxillofacial surgeons have a long track record of safe office-based anesthesia, centered on the anesthesia team model [41]. This model consists of the surgeon as the operator-anesthetist, one trained assistant to observe and monitor patient, and one trained assistant to directly assist the surgeon [41]. The assistants should be trained in recognizing office anesthesia emergencies and assisting the surgeon with management. The anesthesia team is expected to regularly rehearse anesthesia emergencies to ensure that each team member understands their role and can be effective in the case of a real emergency [41].

Airway Protection

Increased levels of sedation may relax the tongue and pharyngeal musculature enough to cause airway obstruction with resulting hypoxia. If a simple chin lift and jaw thrust are unsuccessful, an airway adjunct such as oropharyngeal or nasopharyngeal airway may be inserted. Oral airways should be avoided if the patient is only mildly sedated and has maintained gag reflex as this may trigger vomiting and aspiration or laryngospasm [42]. Nasopharyngeal airways tend to be better tolerated than oral airways especially in lighter sedation but have potential to cause trauma to the mucosa resulting in bleeding in the nasopharynx [42]. If the plane of anesthesia is unintentionally deepened resulting in general anesthesia, airway reflexes and spontaneous breathing may be lost. In this case, the patient may require assistance with breathing that can be accomplished with a supraglottic laryngeal mask airway (LMA) and manual bag ventilation. The appropriate size of airway adjunct or LMA should be determined and pulled prior to initiating anesthesia to allow for rapid insertion if needed.

Intraoperative Emergencies

Laryngospasm

Laryngospasm is a spasm of the vocal cords usually caused by irritation from blood or secretions, light anesthesia, or removal of endotracheal tube during extubation [43]. Signs of laryngospasm include inspiratory stridor, paradoxical chest movement, nasal flaring, diminished or absent breath sounds, and hypoxemia [44]. Although most prevalent in the pediatric population, other risk factors include upper respiratory infection, asthma, smokers, and acid reflux. Treatment consists of stimulus removal, jaw thrust, and 100% oxygen administered via continuous positive airway pressure (CPAP) with facemask [43, 44]. If laryngospasm continues, the level of sedation can be deepened with propofol (0.5–1 mg/kg). Lastly, muscle relaxation with succinylcholine (0.1–1 mg/kg IV or 4 mg/kg IM) can be administered to break the spasm [43]. Studies have demonstrated breaking of laryngospasm by placing firm pressure bilaterally on the "laryngospasm notch," located behind the ear, posterior to the ascending ramus and anterior to mastoid process [44]. This causes a pain-induced autonomic reflex that relaxes the vocal cords [44].

Bronchospasm

Bronchospasm is a constriction of bronchial smooth muscle often in patients with reactive airways such as asthma caused by local irritation and medications [45]. Signs of bronchospasm include wheezing, prolonged expiratory phase, and lack of chest fall [45]. Treatment consists of removal of irritants, administration of medications, and 100% oxygen via facemask [45]. Beta-2 adrenergic agonists (8–10 puffs) via metered-dose inhaler are first line during bronchospasm due to rapid onset [45].

Prevention of bronchospasm occurs by patient selection and an optimal anesthetic plan. Patients with well-controlled asthma with few exacerbations may still be good candidates for office anesthesia [45]. Anticholinergics can be used prophylactically to decrease secretions and airway reactivity [45].

Anaphylaxis

Anaphylaxis is a severe, life-threatening, generalized or systemic hypersensitivity reaction that can be caused by medications or other allergens [46]. Signs include rash, angioedema, hypotension, cough, and airway obstruction [46]. Early recognition of anaphylaxis is critical as shock and airway obstruction may progress quickly. Treatment involves maintaining hemodynamic stability by administering fluids and increasing vascular tone, generally epinephrine in boluses of 50 mcg [46]. Certain patient populations are affected by anaphylaxis differently. Patients with asthma are more likely to have a bronchospasm [46]. Patients with cardiac disease are less likely to tolerate hemodynamic changes and may lead to refractory shock [46]. Patients treated with beta-blockers are not able to mount a tachycardic response, and likely will develop shock at a faster rate [46].

Malignant Hyperthermia

Malignant hyperthermia is a rare, but life-threatening, genetic disorder of hypermetabolism caused by a defect in a skeletal muscle calcium channel [47]. It is important to ask if the patient or any family members have had a history of malignant hyperthermia. This is rarely seen in the oral and maxillofacial surgery office, as the main triggers are inhaled anesthetics (not nitrous oxide) and succinylcholine [47]. Signs include elevated end-tidal CO_2, hyperthermia, muscle rigidity, and tachycardia, among other laboratory findings [47]. The treatment of malignant hyperthermia is dantrolene, a drug that binds to the defective receptor and prevents excess calcium release [44]. The dosage of dantrolene is an initial bolus of 2.5 mg/kg, then again every 10–15 min until signs resolve [47]. A newer medication called Ryanodex is an alternative to dantrolene and is simpler to reconstitute and is more shelf stable [47]. If possible, the patient should be cooled using ice packs or cooled IV fluid [47].

Postanesthesia Management

Recovery From Office Anesthesia

Definition of Recovery

Recovery from anesthesia is a gradual process that comprises three distinct stages [48]. The early stage of recovery occurs from the time administration of anesthesia is completed until all protective reflexes and motor control is reestablished [48, 49]. The intermediate stage of recovery demonstrates readiness for transport out of the surgical facility and to home under the care of a responsible adult [48, 49]. The late stage of recovery occurs at home and may take place several hours to days after receiving anesthesia when the patient is fully recovered from the anesthetic [48, 49].

Monitoring

According to the ASA, signs and systems that should be monitored in the recovery unit include respiratory function, cardiovascular function, neuromuscular function, mental status, temperature, pain, nausea and vomiting, fluid assessment, urine output, and bleeding or drainage [50]. Although encouraged in the recovery room, a requirement to void and take in oral fluids is not a criterion to postpone discharge, unless indicated on a case-by-case basis [50, 51]. Forced oral fluid intake increases the likelihood of PONV, especially in patients that have received opioids [51]. Risk factors for postoperative urinary retention include male sex, older age, increased duration of surgery, and increased IV fluids [51]. Patients with low risk for urinary retention should be given instructions on how to obtain help if they are unable void within 6–8 h after anesthesia [51].

Discharge Planning

Surgeons performing office anesthesia should adopt a scoring system that predicts criteria for safe discharges [49]. There are many systems that have been created and the surgeon should choose one that fits best in their individual practice. The ideal system should be easy to remember and practical for the type of office sedation conducted [51]. One example is the Modified Aldrete's scoring system as depicted in Table 6.11, which measures consciousness, physical activity, circulation, respiration, and oxygen saturation and requires score of ≥9 prior to predicted safe discharge to home [48]. There is no minimum time required prior to discharge, but the surgeon should be confident that the patient is stable from a central nervous system and cardiorespiratory standpoint [50].

Table 6.11 Modified Aldrete's scoring system

Modified Aldrete score	
Level of consciousness	
Fully awake	2
Arousable with verbal cue	1
Nonresponsive	0
Physical activity (voluntary movement)	
Moves four extremities	2
Moves two extremities	1
Moves no extremities	0
Circulation/hemodynamic stability	
Blood pressure within 20 mmHg of preoperative level	2
Blood pressure within 20–50 mmHg of preoperative level	1
Blood pressure greater than 50 mmHg of preoperative level	0
Respiration/respiratory stability	
Able to breathe deeply and cough freely	2
Shortness of breath, shallow or limited breathing	1
Apneic	0
Oxygen saturation status	
SaO_2 maintained above 92% on room air	2
Needs supplemental oxygen to maintain SaO_2 >90%	1
SaO_2 <90% even with oxygen supplementation	0

Postanesthesia Complications

Postoperative Nausea and Vomiting

Postoperative nausea and vomiting (PONV) is an unfortunate adverse effect of anesthesia and surgery affecting up to 20–40% of the general population and up to 80% of high-risk patients [52]. Post-discharge nausea and vomiting (PDNV) occurs after discharge at home and occurs in roughly 33% of the population [48]. Patient-dependent risk factors include female, age less than 50, history of PONV or motion sickness, and nonsmokers [52]. Patient-independent risk factors include increased duration of anesthesia or surgery and use of opioids or nitrous oxide [52]. Two methods exist to overcome this reaction, PONV prophylaxis and treatment. Anti-nausea drugs are not without side effects, so choice to use prophylactically should be on a case-by-case basis for high-risk patients. Although there is no single drug proven to be superior, a multimodal approach is recommended to target different receptor groups [52]. In the office, recommendations to decrease PONV include: prophylactically treat moderate and high-risk groups with multimodal therapy 20–30 min before anticipated end-of-surgery [53], minimize opioids and nitrous oxide, hydrate with IV fluids, and control pain [48, 52]. Small doses of intraoperative propofol have been shown to decrease PONV [54]. If PONV does occur, treatment should be with a different antiemetic than the drug used for prophylaxis [53].

Pain Control

Analgesia in the postoperative setting is important as continued pain can cause PONV, patient dissatisfaction, and delayed discharges [49]. A multimodal approach to pain control should be utilized including long acting local anesthesia, acetaminophen, NSAIDS, and opiates [49]. Targeting multiple receptors will allow for opioid-sparing pain control, which limits the negative effects of opioids [49]. Although a multimodal approach is preferred, severe breakthrough pain may require use of opioids [48]. Adequate pain control will allow the patient to be discharged to home earlier and resume normal daily activities including ambulating and taking PO [54]. NSAIDS may increase postoperative bleeding due to disruption of platelet aggregation and should be used with caution in patients with kidney impairment or gastric ulcers.

Oversedation

Office sedation with opioids and benzodiazepines can lead to oversedation if too much drug is used or if the patient is more sensitive to the drug. Oversedation can cause respiratory depression or delayed recovery from anesthesia [50]. The decision to reverse anesthetic drugs should not be routine practice, but reserved for select cases in which it is for the patient's safety. Naloxone is an opioid antagonist that can reverse the respiratory depression or glottic rigidity that is possible with opioids [50]. Flumazenil is a benzodiazepine antagonist that can reverse the sedation effects of benzodiazepines [50]. Following use of reversal drugs, the patient should be observed for an extended time as the half-life of reversal drugs may be shorter than that of the anesthetics [50].

Discharge and Home Care

Postanesthesia Instructions

As mentioned earlier in this chapter, the discussion about postanesthesia care begins in the preoperative stage [48]. Preferably, this conversation occurs with the patient and the responsible adult that will be caring for the patient during recovery. Postoperative medications including analgesics, antibiotics, and other medications should be reviewed with the patient and escort to ensure safe and proper usage. The patient should be given instructions about who to contact in the case of emergency, whether it is the surgeon's office or local emergency department. Follow-up should be scheduled to ensure proper healing from surgery and full recovery from anesthesia.

Conclusion

Safe and effective office anesthesia begins with careful patient selection and protocols that aim to prevent complications. Patients with OSA, severe cardiorespiratory disease, predicted difficult mask ventilation, or intubation might be better treated in the operating room with a secured airway. A comprehensive knowledge of equipment and drugs is necessary to work efficiently through the inevitable office anesthesia emergency. Drugs utilized during an office sedation should not be cook book, rather, adapted to a specific patient's requirements. Recovery from anesthesia occurs in stages and close observation is required until the patient is deemed stable for discharge based on hemodynamic stability, respiratory stability, and level of consciousness.

References

1. ASA Physical Status Classification System - American Society of Anesthesiologists (ASA). In: American Society of Anesthesiologists. https://www.asahq.org/resources/clinical-information/asa-physical-status-classification-system. Accessed 22 July 2018.
2. Sankar A, Johnson S, Beattie W, Tait G, Wijeysundera D. Reliability of the American Society of Anesthesiologists physical status scale in clinical practice. Br J Anaesth. 2014;113:424–32.
3. deLeon I, Hausman LM. Office-based anesthesia. In: Clinical cases in anesthesia. 4th ed. Philadelphia, PA: Sauders Elsevier; 2014. p. 390–4.
4. Gerlach RM, Sweitzer BJ. Preoperative evaluation and medication. In: Basics of anesthesia. 7th ed. Philadelphia, PA: Elsevier; 2018. p. 189–212.
5. Chung F, Subramanyam R, Liao P, Sasaki E, Shapiro C, Sun Y. High STOP-bang score indicates a high probability of obstructive sleep apnoea. Survey Anesthesiol. 2012;56:312.
6. Chung F, Yegneswaran B, Liao P, et al. STOP questionnaire: a tool to screen patients for obstructive sleep apnea. Anesthesiology. 2008;108:812–21.
7. Joshi GP, Ankichetty SP, Gan TJ, Chung F. Society for ambulatory anesthesia consensus statement on preoperative selection of adult patients with obstructive sleep apnea scheduled for ambulatory surgery. Anesth Anal. 2012;115:1060–8.

8. Sims PG, Kates CH, Moyer DJ, Rollert MK, Todd DW. Anesthesia in outpatient facilities. J Oral Maxillofac Surg. 2012;70:e31–49.
9. Kristensen MS. Airway management and morbid obesity. Eur J Anaesthesiol. 2010;27:923–7.
10. Finucane B, Tsui B, Santora A. Principles of airway management. 4th ed. New York: Springer; 2010.
11. (2017) Patient Assessment. AAOMS Parameters of Care: Clinical Practice Guidelines for Oral and Maxillofacial Surgery.
12. Freeman WK, Gibbons RJ. Perioperative cardiovascular assessment of patients undergoing noncardiac surgery. Mayo Clin Proc. 2009;84:79–90.
13. Koepke EJ, Manning EL, Miller TE, Ganesh A, Williams DGA, Manning MW. The rising tide of opioid use and abuse: the role of the anesthesiologist. Perioper Med. 2018; https://doi.org/10.1186/s13741-018-0097-4.
14. Public Affairs What is the U.S. Opioid Epidemic? In: HHS.gov. https://www.hhs.gov/opioids/about-the-epidemic/index.html. Accessed 17 July 2018.
15. May JA, White HC, Leonard-White A, Warltier DC, Pagel PS. The patient recovering from alcohol or drug addiction: special issues for the anesthesiologist. Survey Anesthesiol. 2002;46:39–40.
16. Mitra S, Sinatra RS. Perioperative management of acute pain in the opioid-dependent patient. Anesthesiology. 2004;101:212–27.
17. Yi P, Pryzbylkowski P. 2015. Opioid induced hyperalgesia | Pain Medicine | Oxford Academic. In: OUP Academic. https://academic.oup.com/painmedicine/article/16/suppl_1/S32/2472483. Accessed 17 July 2018.
18. Vuyk J, Sitsen E, Reekers M. Opioid analgesics. In: Miller's anesthesia. 8th ed. Philadelphia, PA: Sauders Elsevier; 2015. p. 821–63.
19. Wijeysundera DN, Sweitzer B-J. Preoperative evaluation. In: Miller's anesthesia. 8th ed. Philadelphia, PA: Saunders Elsevier; 2015. p. 1085–155.
20. Rodrigo C. The effects of cigarette smoking and anesthesia. Anesth Prog. 2000;47:143–50.
21. Treasure T, Bennett J. Office-based anesthesia. Oral Maxillofac Surg Clin North Am. 2007;19:45–57.
22. Reece-Stremtan S, Campos M, Kokajko L, et al. ABM clinical protocol #15: analgesia and anesthesia for the breastfeeding mother, revised 2017. Breastfeed Med. 2017;12:500–6.
23. Benjamin C, Renyu L, Elizabeth V, Onyi O. Breastfeeding after anesthesia: a review for anesthesia providers regarding the transfer of medications into breast milk. Transl Perioper Pain Med. 2015; https://doi.org/10.31480/2330-4871/023.
24. Apfelbaum JL, Hagberg CA, Caplan RA, et al. Practice Guidelines for Management of the Difficult Airway: An Updated Report by the American Society of Anesthesiologists Task Force on Management of the Difficult Airway. Anesthesiology. 2013; https://doi.org/10.1097/ALN.0b013e31827773b2. http://anesthesiology.pubs.asahq.org/article.aspx?articleid=1918684. Accessed 17 July 2018.
25. Klinger K, Infosino A. Airway management. In: Basics of anesthesia. 7th ed. Philadelphia, PA: Elsevier; 2018. p. 239–72.
26. (2017) Practice Guidelines for Preoperative Fasting and the Use of Pharmacologic Agents to Reduce the Risk of Pulmonary Aspiration. Anesthesiology 126:376–393.
27. Mets B. To stop or not? Anesth Anal. 2015;120:1413–9.
28. Malamed SF. Anatomy for venipuncture. In: Sedation. 6th ed. St. Louis, MO: Elsevier; 2018. p. 298–307.
29. Malamed SF. Venipuncture technique. In: Sedation. 6th ed. St. Louis, MO: Elsevier; 2018. p. 308–18.
30. Malamed SF. Emergency drugs and equipment. In: Sedation. 6th ed. St. Louis, MO: Elsevier; 2018. p. 442–55.
31. Continuum of Depth of Sedation: Definition of General Anesthesia and Levels of Sedation/Analgesia - American Society of Anesthesiologists (ASA). In: American Society of Anesthesiologists. http://www.asahq.org/quality-and-practice-management/standards-guidelines-and-related-resources/continuum-of-depth-of-sedation-definition-of-general-anesthesia-and-levels-of-sedation-analgesia. Accessed 27 July 2018.

32. Malamed SF. Intramuscular sedation. In: Sedation. 6th ed. St. Louis, MO: Elsevier; 2018. p. 134–63.
33. Egan TD, Newberry C. Opioids. In: Basics of anesthesia. 7th ed. Philadelphia, PA: Elsevier; 2018. p. 123–38.
34. Vuyk J, Sitsen E, Reekers M. Intravenous anesthetics. In: Miller's anesthesia. 8th ed. Philadelphia, PA: Sauders Elsevier; 2015. p. 821–63.
35. Mertens MJ, Olofsen E, Engbers FHM, Burm AGL, Bovill JG, Vuyk J. Propofol reduces perioperative remifentanil requirements in a synergistic manner. Anesthesiology. 2003;99:347–59.
36. Asserhøj L, Mosbech H, Krøigaard M, Garvey L. No evidence for contraindications to the use of propofol in adults allergic to egg, soy or peanut † †This Article is accompanied by Editorial Aev401. Br J Anaesth. 2016;116:77–82.
37. Weerink MAS, Struys MMRF, Hannivoort LN, Barends CRM, Absalom AR, Colin P. Clinical pharmacokinetics and pharmacodynamics of dexmedetomidine. Clin Pharmacokinet. 2017;56:893–913.
38. Keating GM. Dexmedetomidine: a review of its use for sedation in the intensive care setting. Drugs. 2015;75:1119–30.
39. Butterfield KJ, Bennett JD, Dembo JB. Outpatient anesthesia. In: Peterson's principles of oral and maxillofacial surgery. 3rd ed. Shelton, CT: People's Medical Publishing House - USA; 2012. p. 63–93.
40. Frost EAM. Fluid management. In: Basics of anesthesia. 7th ed. Philadelphia, PA: Elsevier; 2018. p. 395–401.
41. Office-Based Anesthesia Provided by the Oral and ... https://www.aaoms.org/docs/govt_affairs/advocacy_white_papers/advocacy_office_based_anesthesia_whitepaper.pdf. Accessed 22 Aug 2018.
42. Roberts K. The nasopharyngeal airway: dispelling myths and establishing the facts. Emerg Med J. 2005;22:394–6.
43. Nicholau D, Haehn M. Postanesthesia recovery. In: Basics of anesthesia. 7th ed. Philadelphia, PA: Elsevier; 2018. p. 675–91.
44. Samol NB, Wittkugel EP. Pediatric laryngospasm. In: Complications in anesthesia. 3rd ed. Philadelphia, PA: Elsevier; 2018. p. 758–62.
45. Woods B, Sladen R. Perioperative considerations for the patient with asthma and bronchospasm. Br J Anaesth. 2009;103:i57–65.
46. Nel L, Eren E. Peri-operative anaphylaxis. Br J Clin Pharmacol. 2011;71:647–58.
47. Rosenberg H, Pollock N, Schiemann A, Bulger T, Stowell K. Malignant hyperthermia: a review. Orphanet J Rare Dis. 2015; https://doi.org/10.1186/s13023-015-0310-1.
48. Dickerson DM, Apfelbaum JL. Outpatient anesthesia. In: Basics of anesthesia. 7th ed. Philadelphia, PA: Elsevier; 2018. p. 634–57.
49. Marshall SI, Chung F. Discharge criteria and complications after ambulatory surgery. Anesth Anal. 1999;88:508–17.
50. Apfelbaum JL, Silverstein JH, Chung FF, et al. Practice guidelines for postanesthetic care. Anesthesiology. 2013;118:291–307.
51. Awad IT, Chung F. Factors affecting recovery and discharge following ambulatory surgery. Can J Anesth. 2006;53:858–72.
52. Cao X, White PF, Ma H. An update on the management of postoperative nausea and vomiting. J Anesth. 2017;31:617–26.
53. 2012 CP1 JAN (2012) How to prevent and manage postoperative nausea and vomiting. In: Pharmaceutical Journal. https://www.pharmaceutical-journal.com/learning/learning-article/how-to-prevent-and-manage-postoperative-nausea-and-vomiting/11096163.article?firstPass=false. Accessed 30 July 2018.
54. White PF, Kehlet H, Neal JM, Schricker T, Carr DB, Carli F. The role of the anesthesiologist in fast-track surgery: from multimodal analgesia to perioperative medical care. Anesth Anal. 2007;104:1380–96.

Informed Consent: Process and Practice in the Context of Office-Based Oral Surgery

7

Eric R. Bernstein

Informed Consent

Informed consent is both an ethical and legal construct that, in the case of office-based oral surgery, is situated within a clinical (as opposed to research) context [1]. This chapter addresses the concepts around informed consent through that lens. With respect to ethics, informed consent is a process—not a form or a signature—that reflects respect for patient autonomy and requires provider beneficence. From a practical and legal perspective, informed consent, while still a process and not merely a signature on a form, is an affirmative step that may reduce provider liability. In either case, the essence of informed consent is "a conversation between physician and patient about a proposed treatment, alternative treatments, nontreatment, and the risks and benefits of each of these options" [2].

The commitment of the medical and dental professions to the principle of informed consent is evident in sect. "Informed Consent" of the ADA Principles of Ethics and Code of Professional Conduct and Chap. 2 of the AMA Code of Medical Ethics.

The ADA Code states that professionals have:

> *...a duty to treat the patient according to the patient's desires, within the bounds of accepted treatment. ... Under this principle, the dentist's primary obligations include involving patients in treatment decisions in a meaningful way, with due consideration being given to the patient's needs, desires and abilities...*[3]

Opinion 2.1.1 of the AMA Code explains that:

> *[i]nformed consent to medical treatment is fundamental in both ethics and law. Patients have the right to receive information and ask questions about recommended treatments so*

E. R. Bernstein (✉)
University of Connecticut School of Dental Medicine, Farmington, CT, USA
e-mail: erbernstein@uchc.edu

E. M. Ferneini, M. T. Goupil (eds.), *Office-Based Maxillofacial Surgical Procedures*, https://doi.org/10.1007/978-3-030-22371-7_7

that they can make well-considered decisions about care. Successful communication in the patient-physician relationship fosters trust and supports shared decision making [4].

The fundamental principles of informed consent do not vary from procedure to procedure or from patient to patient. That said, with the emergence of new and often elective treatment options and the influence of the information age on patient knowledge and expectations, understanding the underpinnings of the process, the "what" and "why" at the root of informed consent, becomes even more critical for today's providers.

The legal origins of modern-day informed consent in healthcare arose out of the common law concepts of trespass and assault. This was explained in the seminal New York Court of Appeals decision, *Schloendorff v. Society of New York Hospitals*. In that opinion, Justice Benjamin Cardozo wrote that "every human being of adult years and sound mind has a right to determine what shall be done with his own body; and a surgeon who performs an operation without his patient's consent, commits an assault, for which he is liable in damages" [5]. All jurisdictions in the United States recognize the obligation for physicians and dentists to obtain informed consent from patients prior to treatment. The legal obligation may arise in statute, case law, under accepted common law doctrine, or a combination of the three, with the specific legal "requirements" varying from state to state.[1]

Broadly, informed consent involves the communication between patients and their care providers about treatments, treatment options, and treatment decisions. The primary goal of the informed consent process is to make sure that patients fully understand the procedures that will be performed (and/or the care that will be provided). A full understanding requires understanding the expected benefits and risks and any alternatives to the proposed procedure that may be available; the opportunity discuss their treatment choice, to ask questions, and to reflect on the decision; and, finally, to provide a clear indication of their ultimate decision free from coercion or pressure [7]. Consent in the light of all of these elements, together, make up informed consent.

Coupled with the increased risks of office-based oral surgical procedures are increased potential for malpractice claims resulting from adverse procedural outcomes and complications. Dym explained that "a well-informed patient is more likely to have more reasonable expectations as to outcome and possible complications" [8] and thus reduces the likelihood of a malpractice claim. While informed consent is and should always be equally important from an ethical perspective, when the risk of legal liability increases, the *legal* importance of appropriate and documented informed consent increases, as well. The legal importance comes from both a legal defense to malpractice claims and, as Dym noted, the reduction of claims in the first place.

[1] In an appendix of the opinion in the Georgia Court of Appeals case Ketchup v. Howard, the Court described informed consent origins in each state [6].

Underlying Theoretical Constructs

There are a variety of theories through which to understand the structures and functions of consent and the consent process. What follows is a brief discussion of several of those lenses: real consent, constructed consent, functionalist consent, and postmodern choice.

Real Consent

One theory, perhaps considered the "gold standard" for understanding the goal of informed consent in healthcare, is known as "real consent." Real consent adopts a positivistic approach to consent which is black and white—either a patient is or is not sufficiently informed, voluntary, and competent to give consent or they are not. This theory takes seriously into account whether the patient was given sufficient information about the proposed treatment or procedure and all appropriate alternatives or not. Moreover, was the consent give voluntarily—that is, completely without coercion—again, with no gray area. Finally, the patient is either competent or not competent to give their consent to treatment. While this approach may be a gold standard of sorts, it is also likely never truly attainable and very difficult to truly measure beyond the information component [9]. It is far less a gold standard in the way that it suggests that the informed consent process would be one-way flow from provider to patient, rather than a dialogic approach.

Constructed Consent

Another theory, constructed consent, is far more reflective of the process aspects that have been discussed earlier in this chapter. Constructed consent relies heavily on the interpersonal aspects of the consent elements, with "numerous social and personal influences [shaping] a recipient's ability [to understand] and [their] choices" [10]. While the focus of constructed consent on process is consistent with the ideal notions of informed consent, there is an extreme variability based on the different social and personal influences between different patients.

Functionalist Consent

Functionalist consent is, ostensibly, the type of consent that boils down to a signature on the form. While we might reject this notion out of hand, too often this is a common approach to consent by providers who, for many different reasons, tend to treat consent as "a simple or tedious formality" [9]. It is true that any consideration of informed consent as a mere formality should be avoided. However, the functionalist approach does also speak to the very pragmatic legal reasons for obtaining informed consent and, in particular, mitigating liability risks.

Postmodern Choice

As discussed later in this chapter, patient autonomy and the ability to make informed choices is complex. Postmodern choice focuses, however, on the patient as a consumer with the ability to pick and choose among options presented to them. On its face, this definitely seems aligned to ethical notions of patient autonomy [11].

It becomes complicated for providers, however, when patients are making bad choices—as discussed later in the chapter with respect to informed refusals and waivers of informed consent, as well as providers' ethical principle of beneficence.

It is evident, when surveying the different theoretical constructs for making real meaning of the informed consent process, that no single theory can stand on its own. This chapter takes elements of each theory, and other approaches to informed consent concepts, and weaves them together to have the most realistic and meaningful discussion of the topic.

Fundamental Elements of Informed Consent

Just as no single theory can adequately frame informed consent, there is no universally accepted structure for the informed consent process. One common framework breaks it down into five basic elements: decisional capacity; information; understanding; voluntarism; and a final decision by the patient [7].

Decisional Capacity

Put simply, patients must have the capacity to understand, deliberate, and communicate about their condition and the proposed treatment, as well as relevant issues related to their condition and that treatment. It is essential that patients can participate in all aspects of the process in a meaningful and complete way. Decisional capacity requires not only the cognitive ability to understand the information provided, but also the legal maturity to make reasonable and independent decisions in light of that information and the way that it interacts with their own values and beliefs.

The complexity and inherent risks of surgical procedures may impact certain aspects of the consent process. A patient with decreased cognitive ability (e.g., a patient with a mild intellectual disability) may have decisional capacity and be capable of understanding tooth cleaning and polishing, but when the proposed procedure involves cosmetic procedures, that same patient may not have the decisional capacity to provide informed consent [12]. Issues may also arise with higher risk procedures that can involve stressors that may result in extreme pressure on the patient that undermines the voluntariness of the consent [13].

Information

Patients need the appropriate knowledge to make informed decisions about the management of dental problems. They must have information about the nature of their problem and the treatment being proposed. Information about the nature of the proposed treatment should include both the risks and benefits of the treatment. In addition, alternative treatment options, if available, must be presented along with their risks and benefits. Finally, patients must also have information on the option of nontreatment. One way to ensure that all appropriate information is discussed is the acronym BARN: B—benefits; A—alternatives; R—risks; and N—no treatment [12].

As the complexity of a procedure increases, the amount of information necessary to allow for informed consent also increases, compared to more routine procedures. The information that must be provided to obtain informed consent for a restorative procedure is less than that necessary for a surgical extraction or implant.

With the massive increase in information available to patients, many will have conducted their own research prior to or throughout the treatment planning and decision-making stages. Such research can be supportive of the patient's understanding of their problem and the treatment options while simultaneously posing a challenge to providers who increasingly face the need to help patients make sense of the inaccurate or incomplete information they find in their own search. In any case, patients should be heard with respect to their own research and providers should take their own response to that information seriously.

Understanding

Information, alone, is not sufficient for a patient to provide informed consent. Patients must comprehend the information for consent to be valid. This requires a dialogue between the provider and the patient to assess and ensure understanding. Through that dialogue, providers help the patient clarify issues, answer questions that have arisen, and verify, through conversation, that the patient, in fact, has an understanding of the relevant information regarding their condition and the treatment plan.

Voluntarism

In order for patients to make their own decisions, their decisions must be voluntary. Neither the provider nor a family member should coerce or manipulate the patient into making a decision around treatment. Nevertheless, should the course chosen by the patient—in the provider's professional opinion—be likely to do more harm than good, the provider's concerns and reasons for those concerns should, indeed, be communicated in an attempt to persuade the patient to reconsider. Failure by the provider to do so is a violation of the ethical principle of beneficence.

When engaging in the consent process for more complex or anxiety inducing oral surgical procedures, additional time must be taken to ensure patients are not making their decisions under duress and that they maintain decisional capacity in the light of the complexity of the procedure.

Final Decision

The final step in obtaining informed consent is to obtain an actual decision from the patient. While the final decision does not necessarily need to be communicated in writing by the patient (e.g., a form may or may not be required to be signed), the decision—and the process leading up to the decision—should always be documented formally in the patient chart by the provider. The greater the risks and complexities of the proposed treatment, the greater the value, however, of capturing the patient's final decision in a writing that is signed by the patient.

Supporting Informed Consent for Surgical Procedures with TRAAM

Timing

Whenever appropriate, based on the nature of circumstances, the consent process for surgical procedures should begin at a separate appointment prior to treatment. This time gap allows patients to fully consider the information provided, without undue or unnecessary pressure (including time constraints).

Revisiting

When treatment does take place at an appointment subsequent to the initiation of the consent process, the initial information and consent (if already offered) should be revisited and affirmed at the appointment or appointments where treatment will take place.

Alternatives

Fully informing the consent process requires disclosure of sedation options, information about the surgical treatment and proposed technique along with alternative treatments and techniques, and a full discussion of the benefits and risks of those sedations, treatments, and techniques.

Appropriateness

Whatever information is provided should be appropriately adapted to the individual patient's age, general health literacy, and learning ability. Moreover, the provider should check frequently for understanding, even considering techniques like teach-back, where the patient is asked to explain the proposed treatment to the provider [14].

Multi-modality

Not every patient will learn the same way—and providers will often be unaware of a patient's best learning modality. In addition to verbal discussions, information should be provided in written or other formats that support the information shared verbally (see, e.g., discussion on technologically supported informed consent discussed later in this chapter).

It is not until an entire, sufficient process is completed that a final decision by a patient can be considered informed consent.

Additional Aspects of Informed Consent

The fundamental elements of informed consent have nuanced aspects when the process is put into practice.

Treatment Planning

With respect to "information," practitioners should ensure that the proposed treatment plan is clear to the patient. Regarding the "final decision," the patient must then authorize the treatment plan.

Waiver of Informed Consent

Patients have both the right to be informed prior to consenting to treatment and the right to refuse treatment, with limited exceptions. Two circumstances may arise that place the practitioner in a difficult situation with respect to those patient rights. Rights are inherently waivable—think, for example, of the right to free speech which does not require speech but protects the right to it. Individuals may, then, choose not to exercise a right. If a patient says, "I don't need any more information and I don't care what the risks are, Doc…I am going to do whatever you suggest," it places the practitioner in a tricky position. While it has been long held that patients may decline the information while retaining the right to decide to undergo treatment [15], it should be carefully documented when a patient does so and it is prudent to inform the patient that they have the right to know the risks, benefits, and alternatives before making a decision.

"Informed Refusal"

The other challenge to informed consent arises when a patient decides to refuse treatment while declining to be informed. A theory of "informed refusal" has been articulated in some instances, which would require patients to have the same information required to consent to treatment before declining. However, similarly, to declining information and giving consent, one can decline information and decline treatment—for example, "No matter what you say, Doc, I will not have surgery." In such instances, it is still important for the waiver and the refusal to be documented and prudent for the dentist to clearly inform the patient that they have a right to the information before deciding against treatment [16].

It is also worth noting that informed consent, as a process that may span multiple visits (see TRAAM above), may involve multiple conversations over an extended period of time. This is particularly true as the circumstances and/or treatment options change. Take the extraction of a third molar as an example. A patient may indicate that they will not consent to the prophylactic removal of the third molar or molars and decline to hear the benefits of such removal. Over time and at subsequent visits, the surgeon may revisit the discussion and the patient may decide to hear more information. If the condition of the patient changes over time—such as the emergence of evidence of disease in the third molars—the revisited conversation now becomes obligatory, not optional [17]. In either case, the continued conversations and the patient's responses should be documented appropriately.

Informing, but Less Than Informed Consent

There are circumstances where a full informed consent process may not be necessary or contextually appropriate—often with respect to some isolated element of an entire treatment plan or procedure.[2] In these cases, some level of informing may still be called for. This is not to suggest that something "less than informed consent" is

[2] This should be distinguished from emergency circumstances, such as unconsciousness, where treatment is provided explicitly *without consent* and where providers have a defense against a claim of assault through their duty to care and the exigent life-saving patient necessity [18].

ever a reasonable substitute when informed consent is appropriate and/or required. It is never appropriate to inform, but less than the level of informed consent, merely for convenience [19]. A specific example relevant to the context of office-based surgery involves medical imaging that exposes patients to radiation. Basic, health literacy information regarding exposure to radiation from imaging is arguably sufficient and appropriate, as opposed to a full informed consent process. Nievelstein and Frush suggested that "high-quality (electronic) brochures and information for patients… can help to appropriately weigh the risks and benefits of radiologic procedures and avoid causing patients undue anxiety about medical radiation exposure" [20].

Informed Consent Is Not an Assumption of the Risk

When consent forms are signed, concluding a full and informed consent process, providers are often left wondering why, if a known risk of a procedure occurs, the patient hasn't agreed to take on that risk. Indeed, in common law and under the Federal Rules of Civil Procedure, there is a defense against liability for negligence known as the assumption of the risk. However, with respect to the medical sciences, in almost every case where a doctor is sued later, "the assumption of risk defense is unavailable to [doctors] who have shared decision-making with patients" [21].

The Assumption of the Risk Defense

In its simplest form, the assumption of the risk defense arises when an individual gives express "consent to relieve [someone] of an obligation to exercise care for [their] protection and agrees to take [the] chances as to injury from a known or possible risk." The defense effectively relieves a defendant from an otherwise existing duty to exercise care and eliminates any duty to protect that individual [22]. Due to the complexity of health sciences and the special relationship between a doctor and patient, patients have the right "to be protected from [their] own decisions" and "to rely totally on the [doctor's] medical expertise" [21]. American courts follow a traditionalist view that the power differential between doctor and patient prevents providers from "relieving themselves of liability on the grounds of a patient's agreement to assume the risk of malpractice" [23].

Limited Exceptions

While the prevailing view is that patients cannot "sign away" the right to make a malpractice claim and that consent to treatment does not constitute an assumption of the risks associated with that treatment, like virtually any legal construct, there are case-specific exceptions. This is true, in the most limited sense, with respect to the applicability of the assumption of the risk defense in a healthcare malpractice context. The specific types of cases where providers have been able to successfully defend against a malpractice or negligence claim using the assumption of the risk doctrine have generally been limited to patients who agree to "an experimental… procedure where the standards of care have not yet been fully developed or consents to treatment modalities known to be outside of the medical mainstream" [24]. Even in such cases, however, the courts have held a very high standard of informed consent, requiring evidence that the patient knew of, understood, and expressly consented to the particular risks "of refusing conventional treatment" [25].

Beneficence

Another question that often arises is whether the general exclusion of the assumption of the risk defense contradicts the ethical demand for patient autonomy. It is generally accepted that, based on the ethical principal of beneficence, patients "cannot pre-emptively excuse their doctor from any harm they may suffer from what they convince the doctor to do" [26]. Part of the doctor's duty of care requires the assessment of the reasonability of what the patient is requesting of the doctor and a refusal to comply if such a request is inherently threatening to the patient's safety or well-being. Even with informed consent, the provider cannot merely "rubber stamp" a bad patient decision under the guise that the decision was informed. The issue of "informed refusal" addressed this in more detail above.

Special Issues Regarding Informed Consent and Oral Surgical Procedures

While the underlying elements of the informed consent process are the same (capacity, information, understanding, voluntarism, and decision) from case to case, there are certain nuanced aspects or related topics that merit additional discussion in the context of surgical and/or office-based procedures. Of particular interest and considered here are the ways that informed consent intersects with elective procedures, office-based anesthesia, opioids and postoperative pain management, and pediatric patients. Finally, it is also worth considering the ways that technology may impact the substance and delivery of information with respect to informed consent.

Informed Consent and Elective Procedures

With a drastic increase in mass media advertising of specific treatment options and the sociocultural focus on esthetics, patients increasingly seek "the instant gratification of the esthetic treatments they have heard about from others and have seen on television advertisements and the Internet." Technological advances (as discussed later in this chapter) have made such treatments that were once so cost-prohibitive to only be afforded by a select few, much more widely accessible. This has fostered "a practice model of commercialism previously unseen in dentistry" [27]. While these types of treatments are patient driven and often economically advantageous to the practitioner, they are elective procedures and may even have little or no therapeutic benefit. Elective procedures raise certain issues with respect to informed consent. In the esthetics-driven commercialism seen ever more frequently in dentistry, there are issues related to therapeutic value that must be considered in the informed consent process. For those conditions that are elective, but with clear therapeutic value, they often arise from preference-sensitive conditions. Preference-sensitive conditions also call for some specific consideration during the consent process.

Elective Procedures, Generally

How elective surgery is defined varies greatly. The definition ranges from procedures that are considered optional to procedures that are considered necessary, but not urgent. In its simplest form, elective surgery can be defined as "pre-planned surgery as opposed to urgent or emergent surgery." The approach to informed consent for all elective procedures, then, necessarily varies as patients must be able to include considerations around the need (or lack of need) as well as the "benefit-harm balance" for the timing and/or delay of the procedure given the specific circumstances [28]. It becomes the responsibility of the provider to ensure that the patient has this information to inform their decision-making.

In addition to different patient information demands in the context of elective procedures, the provider must also consider the need and the impact of timing and/or delay on their original and continuing recommended course of treatment. Circumstances may arise that change whether a particular course of treatment remains the preferred or recommended course and the provider is obliged to update the informed consent if their recommendation has or may change or the benefit-harm balance has changed.

The most likely recommended change to an elective procedure is the scheduling. For example, "elective oral surgery procedures should be deferred in patients with acute exacerbations of respiratory disease" [29]. In a case like that, the patient would be explained the reason delay is recommended, as well as the impact that the delay may have on the intended outcomes and any other new information necessary to re-inform their decision. There are, however, both provider and patient forces that threaten informed decision-making about rescheduling elective procedures.

Patients, for example, may have already "made psychological and logistical provisions for the procedure on a particular day" or may be afraid they cannot reschedule in a timely manner and/or with their preferred provider [30]. In such cases, it is incumbent upon the provider to ensure that the patient understands the newly emerged risks. Logistical concerns or provider scheduling fears from the patient may threaten the voluntariness of the consent. Providers may also threaten the previously informed consent when deferral may be clinically indicated, but the provider opposes rescheduling. Providers may be less likely to properly inform the patient about changes to the benefit-harm balance for fear of lost income, encumbrances of their schedule, and/or the loss of a case to a colleague [30]. In either case, it is the provider who bears the primary responsibility for re-informing the consent and ensuring that the patient is able to make a decision in light of the new circumstances.

Preference-Sensitive Conditions

Elective procedures frequently treat what are known as preference-sensitive conditions. Preference-sensitive conditions are those conditions where the practice guidelines may be less declarative on which treatment course is most appropriate. These are also cases where the decision to delay surgical intervention or to attempt nonsurgical options prior to surgery are very reasonable choices that the provider would, given the context, not be compelled to try to dissuade in order to prevent harm to the patient. In 2007, Washington state passed a law that allowed for a shared decision-making (SDM) model, ostensibly in lieu of traditional informed consent [31]. Preference-sensitive conditions, given the less declarative nature, must rely on an even more patient-centered informed decision-making process. Even in the absence of specific authorizing legislation (as in the case of Washington state), preference-sensitive conditions are a fertile ground for shared decision-making between patients and providers [32].

Therapeutic Value and Aesthetic Surgery

All elective surgeries are not necessarily synonymous with needs-driven interventions. When an elective procedure is not a needs-driven intervention, the decisions associated with the procedure are not based on need. This can have a significant impact on decision-making and informed consent [28]. In the case of cosmetic dentistry and aesthetic surgery, "there is a strong ethical imperative to assure that [shared decision-making] is embedded in the clinical process...the values and preferences of the patient should dictate the treatment choices and together with the provider" and only then should "a pathway for treatment [be] agreed upon" [32]. Moreover, the provider should take extra care when advancing a proposed treatment plan that includes even potentially unnecessary elective surgery [27].

Where it is the patient who is bringing the apparently unnecessary treatment to the provider, it is particularly important for providers to understand patient motivations when they seek treatments that, on their face, seem to lack any therapeutic value [33]. Once the provider understands the patient's motivations, if the unnecessary elective procedure remains at odds with their own ethical standards, they should not "succumb to the entreaties of a patient and embark on [such] a treatment plan." Instead, just as they would in the informed consent process, the provider should "have a discussion with the patient, explain [their] position and offer to refer the patient elsewhere to pursue the desired treatment" [27].

Informed Consent and Anesthesia

Surgery procedures may use a variety of forms of anesthesia, across the continuum of sedation. Because sedation is a continuum, individual patients may respond differently to different types of sedation approaches. Patients may become more deeply sedated than intended and need rescue or patients may not be as sedated as expected and feel more pain than desired. These are the types of issues that should be addressed in the part of the informed consent process covering anesthesia plans [34].

What further complicates informed consent where it comes to anesthesia is that a main purpose of anesthesia in oral surgery is to manage fear and anxiety "satisfactorily during the perioperative period to permit safe and effective completion of the surgical procedure" [34]. Appropriately informed consent does not require the disclosure and discussion of every conceivable risk or complication. It therefore becomes especially important with anesthesia to "determine patients' attitudes, concerns, and expectations regarding being informed of the specific risks associated with the administration of anesthesia" in guiding decisions around the extent of the information provided about anesthesia and anesthesia choices [35]. The balance with informed consent around anesthesia comes with controlling the anxiety that the anesthesia and information around anesthesia may, itself, cause in the patient.

Informed Consent and Opioids

Postoperative management of pain is an important aspect of patient care. In the 1990s, there was recognition that pain was not being managed adequately. This led to, among other things, efforts to increase the use of opioids for acute pain management. Those decades-old policy changes led to a massive spike in opioid abuse and, in the 2010s, a public health crisis around their improper use. Certainly, there are still appropriate uses of opioids, especially for acute, postoperative pain management [36]. However, for both public health reasons and for individual patient care outcomes, much greater care should be taken when prescribing opioids for any reason and alternatives should always be considered.

Given the increased scrutiny on opioid prescribing patterns and the massive increases in risks of opioid use disorders (OUDs), it makes sense to take explicit steps in the informed consent process when including opioids as part of a recommended treatment plan. The societal and public health implications of the "opioid epidemic" need not be part of the informed consent discussions, unless such issues are raised by the patient, themselves. Individual patient risks, however, should be explicitly discussed and patients informed of the potential for the development of tolerances and/or opioid dependence that may arise even from acute use. In addition, the risks associated with opioid overdose should be explicitly discussed and weighed against the analgesic benefits. Just like all other aspects of informed consent, potentially effective alternatives, including acetaminophen or nonsteroidal anti-inflammatory drugs (NSAIDs) or a specific regimen that structures postsurgical opioid analgesia to a combination of acetaminophen and/or NSAIDs [37].

Informed Consent and the Pediatric Patient

Even if a patient lacks the legal capacity to consent, where a parent, guardian, or other legal proxy provides the legal consent for the procedure, the patient may still have sufficient levels of understanding to be included in some or all of the discussions about the procedure. In such circumstances, it is both good ethical practice and important to confirm that the patient is ready to proceed. That said, there are ways that minor children can be involved in clinical decision-making and reasons to do so. McCabe discusses five goals for involving children in that process: patient

Table 7.1 US states with some form of legal recognition of the mature minor doctrine

Alabama	Kansas	Oregon
Alaska	Louisiana	Pennsylvania
Arkansas	Maine	S. Carolina
Delaware	Massachusetts	Tennessee
Idaho	Montana	W. Virginia
Illinois	Nevada	

autonomy; doctor-patient-parent communication; improved cooperation with treatment; provide a sense of self-control; and respect and develop children's capacity [38]. Just as with any patient, the way in which a child should be involved in the informed consent process should take into consideration the specific needs, abilities, maturity, and health literacy of the specific child.

There is also a legal doctrine, known as the "mature minor doctrine," that may give (sometimes limited) legal decision-making capacity to the child themselves, to provide informed consent. In the table below, the states listed have some form of recognition of the mature minor (Table 7.1).

Coleman and Rosoff provide an excellent discussion of the sources of legal authority for the mature minor doctrine in each state [39]. However, no two states have the exact same treatment of mature minors, making it even more important to get competent legal advice to address any questions about minors providing their own informed consent.

Technology and Informed Consent

Technology impacts informed consent in at least two types of ways. First, new technologies open the door to new treatment techniques, materials, and tools for use in procedures. In that respect, they become a *subject* of the information provided about treatment options. Second, the way that information is provided to patients and the way that patient understanding can be assessed can impact the informed consent *process*, itself.

New Treatments

New instruments and new techniques, many of which are the result of massive technological advances, have "allowed extraction techniques and outpatient oral and maxillofacial surgery to evolve" [40]. Indeed, beyond techniques and procedures, even the delivery, management and monitoring of office-based anesthesia agents and their use have been impacted by technology [41]. These advancements and technological evolutions have potential to benefit surgeons and patients. However, with these new technologies and advancements come new responsibilities for the provider, especially as it relates to informed consent. Under the ADA Principles of Ethics and Code of Professional Conduct, for example, it is clear that "just because it can be done does not mean it necessarily should be" [27]. Providers need to be certain that they do not allow an eagerness to pursue the newest treatment advance (from the provider themselves or brought to them by patient request) to cloud the way that consent is informed. This means that providers must still fully explain the treatment plan they consider to be optimal (whether recommending the newest technology or not, as well as an explanation of the likely short- and long-term outcomes, alternatives and risks with all procedure options, with particular focus on any specific treatment preferences the patient brought to the attention of the provider. When a very new procedure or tool or material is to be used, it is especially important to inform patients of the breadth or dearth of evidence that supports that new technology.

Patient Decision Aids

An emerging use of technology to support more informed patient consent is the development of patient decision aids (PDAs). While some PDAs do not leverage technology (e.g., decision grids), the most common PDAs include multimedia rich content or online resources [42]. It is particularly noteworthy that the effectiveness of PDAs has a strong evidence base. Patients presenting with impacted third molars who were shown an informational video regarding third molars and treatment options prior to meeting with the treating doctor to continue the informed consent process had significantly greater recall of the information provided throughout the process than those who only met with the provider and did not view the video [43]. In other studies, patients who "received a decision aid…as compared with usual care, had greater knowledge of the evidence, felt more clear about what mattered to them, had more accurate expectations about the risks and benefits, and participated more in the decision-making process" [44].

As discussed above, multi-modalities (the "M" in TRAAM) should be used in presenting patients' information to meet the needs of different types of learners and to help ensure all patients make real meaning of the information being provided. Different modalities include the traditional verbal discussions, written documentation explaining the treatment options, but also include video and interactive multimedia wherever possible. As more general information is shared via video and multimedia online, patients may be increasingly reliant upon those types of mediums to garner understanding of new topics, making the integration of technology into the informed consent process even more important. Studies have shown that patients presented with preoperative information in multimedia formats have better recollection of the information they were provided [45].

Assessing Patient Understanding

Finally, providers can utilize new technology to help assess patient understanding of the information provided them. This is a direct corollary to the use of technology to provide information. The idea of teach-backs was discussed earlier as a way of assessing patient understanding. Similarly, interactive multimedia presentations can allow patients to demonstrate their understanding and identify specific gaps that may need to be revisited.

Concluding Remarks

Despite its critical importance in providing high-quality, safe healthcare that is patient-centered, the informed consent process in practice is very often insufficient. This is a high-risk inadequacy on many levels, as failure to obtain appropriately informed consent is not only an ethical conflict because it compromises patient autonomy, but it places patient safety at risk and could constitute negligence or even battery from a legal perspective. It may be frustrating to practitioners that adequate informed consent is nebulous and not able to be concretely defined. It has been said that "one cannot know with certainty whether a consent is valid until a lawsuit has been filed and resolved" [46]. This vagueness, however, can be best mitigated by ensuring that informed consent always includes consideration of patient capacity, provides sufficient and accurate information, that patient understanding is checked, and that the consent is given voluntarily. Moreover, with respect to surgical procedures in particular, the TRAAM model is also integrated, considering the TIMING of information provided, REVISITING the consent, discussing ALTERNATIVES, ensuring APPROPRIATENESS of information, and utilizing MULTI-MODALITIES when providing information.

Ultimately, the best case for patients and providers—legally, ethically, and with respect to outcomes—is a provider who knows and understands the elements of informed consent and commits to making a good faith effort to engage patients in a meaningful and ongoing process.

References

1. Berg JW, Appelbaum PS, Lidz CW, Parker LS. Informed consent: legal theory and clinical practice. Oxford: Oxford University Press; 2001.
2. Whitney SN, McGuire AL, McCullough LB. A typology of shared decision making, informed consent, and simple consent. Ann Intern Med. 2004;140(1):54–9.
3. American Dental Association. Principles of ethics and code of professional conduct. With official advisory opinions revised to January 2005. Hawaii Dent J. 2007;38(1):9.
4. American Medical Association. Code of Medical Ethics Opinion 2.1.1 - Informed Consent 2017.
5. Schloendorff v. Society of New York Hospital (211 N.Y. 125). NY: Court of Appeals; 1914.
6. Ketchup v. Howard (543 S.E.2d 371). Georgia: Court of Appeals; 2000.
7. Mukherjee A, Livinski AA, Millum J, Chamut S, Boroumand S, Iafolla TJ, et al. Informed consent in dental care and research for the older adult population: a systematic review. J Am Dent Assoc. 2017;148(4):211–20.
8. Dym H. Risk management in the dental office. Dent Clin North Am. 2012;56(1):113–20. https://doi.org/10.1016/j.cden.2011.07.001.
9. Alderson P, Goodey C. Theories of consent. BMJ. 1998;317(7168):1313–5.
10. Wolf A. The emergence and implementation of the advance informed agreement procedure. Governing global biodiversity. Abingdon: Routledge; 2017. p. 127–44.
11. Benedict JL. The ethics of consent. a revised consent model for the transplantation of face and upper limbs: covenant consent, International library of ethics, law, and the new medicine, vol. 73. New York: Springer; 2017.

12. Bernstein ER, Lazzarini Z. Medicolegal and ethical considerations in oral surgery by the general dentist. In: Ferneini EM, Goupil MT, editors. Evidence-Based oral srgery: a clinical guide for the general dental practitioner. New York: Springer; 2019.
13. Roberts LW. Informed consent and the capacity for voluntarism. Am J Psychiatry. 2002;159(5):705–12.
14. Tamura-Lis W. Teach-back for quality education and patient safety. Urol Nurs. 2013;33(6):267–73.
15. Meisel A. The exceptions to the informed consent doctrine: striking a balance between competing values in medical decisionmaking. Wis L Rev. 1979;1979:413–88.
16. Ridley DT. Informed consent, informed refusal, informed choice – what is it that makes a patient's medical treatment decisions informed. Med Law. 2001;20(2):205–14.
17. Gray DG, Franklin JL, Nicholls MK, Eaton KA, Barrett AW. Compliance of referral and hospital documentation with National Institute of Health and Care Excellence guidelines for the extraction of third molars: a comparative analysis of two NHS Trusts. Br J Oral Maxillofac Surg. 2017;55(6):575–9.
18. Lynch J. Consent to treatment. Oxford: Radcliffe Pub; 2011.
19. Cole CA. Implied consent and nursing practice: ethical or convenient? Nurs Ethics. 2012;19(4):550–7.
20. Nievelstein RAJ, Frush DP. Should we obtain informed consent for examinations that expose patients to radiation? Am J Roentgenol. 2012;199(3):664–9. https://doi.org/10.2214/AJR.11.8319.
21. Dobson T. Medical malpractice in the birthplace: resolving the physician-patient conflict through informed consent, standard of care, and assumption of risk. Nebraska Law Rev. 1986;65(4):655–85.
22. American Law Institute. § 496A - assumption of risk. Restatement (Second) of Torts. St. Paul, MN: American Law Institute Publishers; 1965.
23. Sawicki NN. Choosing medical malpractice. Wash Law Rev. 2018;93(2):891–966.
24. Brady v. Urbas (631 Pa. 329). Pennsylvania: Supreme Court of Pennsylvania; 2015.
25. Schneider v. Revici (817 F.2d 987). F.2d: 2nd Circuit Court of Appeals; 1987.
26. Assumption of the Risk. Physician's Weekly 2017 May 23, 2017.
27. Leffler WG, et al. J Am Dent Assoc. 2008;139(11):1546–7. https://doi.org/10.14219/jada.archive.2008.0086.
28. Bernal-Delgado E, Ridao-López M, Garcia-Armesto S. Medical practice variations in elective surgery. In: Medical Practice Variations. New York: Springer; 2016. p. 53–78.
29. Renton T, Woolcombe S, Taylor T, Hill CM. Oral surgery: part 1 introduction and the management of the medically compromised patient. BDJ. 2013;215:213. https://doi.org/10.1038/sj.bdj.2013.830.
30. Nurok M, Czeisler CA, Lehmann LS. Sleep deprivation, elective surgical procedures, and informed consent. N Engl J Med. 2010;363(27):2577–9. https://doi.org/10.1056/NEJMp1007901.
31. Spatz ES, Krumholz H, Moulton BW. The new era of informed consent: getting to a reasonable-patient standard through shared decision making. JAMA. 2016; https://doi.org/10.1001/jama.2016.3070.
32. Moulton B, Birkeland S. Shared decision-making and liability in aesthetic surgery. Aesthet Surg J. 2016;36(8):NP254–NP5. https://doi.org/10.1093/asj/sjw067.
33. Bruckner A, Zentner A, Klages U. Dental aesthetics, self-awareness, and oral health-related quality of life in young adults. Eur J Orthod. 2004;26(5):507–14. https://doi.org/10.1093/ejo/26.5.507.
34. Rollert MK, Busaidy K, Krishnan D, Van Heukelom E. Anesthesia in outpatient facilities. J Oral Maxillofac Surg. 2017;75(8, Supplement):e34–49. https://doi.org/10.1016/j.joms.2017.04.032.
35. Burkle C, Mann C, Steege J, Stokke J, Jacob A, Pasternak J. Patient fear of anesthesia complications according to surgical type: potential impact on informed consent for anesthesia. Acta Anaesthesiol Scand. 2014;58(10):1249–57.

36. Dineen KK, DuBois JM. Between a rock and a hard place: can physicians prescribe opioids to treat pain adequately while avoiding legal sanction? Am J Law Med. 2016;42(1):7–52.
37. Morris BJ, Mir HR. The opioid epidemic: impact on orthopaedic surgery. J Am Acad Orthop Surg. 2015;23(5):267–71. https://doi.org/10.5435/jaaos-d-14-00163.
38. McCabe MA. Involving children and adolescents in medical decision making: developmental and clinical considerations. J Pediatr Psychol. 1996;21(4):505–16. https://doi.org/10.1093/jpepsy/21.4.505.
39. Coleman DL, Rosoff PM. The legal authority of mature minors to consent to general medical treatment. Pediatrics. 2013;131(4):786. https://doi.org/10.1542/peds.2012-2470.
40. Weiss A, Stern A, Dym H. Technological advances in extraction techniques and outpatient oral surgery. Dent Clin. 2011;55(3):501–13. https://doi.org/10.1016/j.cden.2011.02.008.
41. Robert RC, Liu S, Patel C, Gonzalez ML. Advancements in office-based anesthesia in oral and maxillofacial surgery. Atlas Oral Maxillofac Surg Clin. 2013;21(2):139–65. https://doi.org/10.1016/j.cxom.2013.05.007.
42. Boss EF, Mehta N, Nagarajan N, Links A, Benke JR, Berger Z, et al. Shared decision making and choice for elective surgical care: a systematic review. Otolaryngol Head Neck Surg. 2016;154(3):405–20. https://doi.org/10.1177/0194599815620558.
43. Olsen BT, Sherwood CJ, Carrico CK, Priest JH, Laskin DM. Patient recall of information on a third molar informed consent video. J Oral Maxillofac Surg. 2017;75(12):2507–11. https://doi.org/10.1016/j.joms.2017.06.006.
44. Gillies K, Cotton SC, Brehaut JC, Politi MC, Skea Z. Decision aids for people considering taking part in clinical trials. Cochrane Database Syst Rev. 2015:(11). https://doi.org/10.1002/14651858.CD009736.pub2.
45. Michalski A, Stopa M, Miśkowiak B. Use of multimedia technology in the doctor-patient relationship for obtaining patient informed consent. Med Sci Monit. 2016;22:3994–9. https://doi.org/10.12659/MSM.894147.
46. Moore v. The Regents of the University of California et al. (271 Cal. Rptr. 146). California: Supreme Court; 1990.

Part II

Dentoalveolar Procedures

Differential Diagnosis and Biopsy Techniques

8

Steven Halepas, Michael T. Goupil, and Christine Niekrash

Gathering Information

Medical History

The first step when treating a patient is to gather pertinent and relevant information. The fundamentals of the medical assessment explained in Chap. 1 apply to patients with unknown lesions. It is necessary to gather both a current and past medical history since lesions of the oral cavity may be presentations of systemic diseases. An accurate medical assessment can also change the definitive treatment decisions. Certain medications may produce mucosal alterations as known side effects. Patients also may develop hypersensitivity reactions to medications that may present themselves in the perioral area. A review of systems may also help discover any undiagnosed medical conditions that could be manifesting as the lesion(s) in question. A good medical assessment includes a detailed social history. Habits such as alcohol or tobacco products are vital information when diagnosing pathologic conditions. Asking questions regarding routines, holding objects in the mouth, oral hygiene products, trauma, and diet can be equally as important.

S. Halepas (✉)
Department of Oral and Maxillofacial Surgery, New York Presbyterian Hospital, Columbia University Medical Center, New York, NY, USA

M. T. Goupil
University of Connecticut School of Dental Medicine, Farmington, CT, USA
e-mail: mtgoupil@comcast.net

C. Niekrash
Frank H Netter MD School of Medicine, Quinnipiac University, Hamden, CT, USA
e-mail: Christine.Niekrash@quinnipiac.edu

E. M. Ferneini, M. T. Goupil (eds.), *Office-Based Maxillofacial Surgical Procedures*, https://doi.org/10.1007/978-3-030-22371-7_8

History of the Lesion

There is a saying in medicine that the diagnosis is in the patient's story. Many lesions in the oral cavity and perioral region can be diagnosed with a good clinical history and examination. Therefore, it is important to ask the right questions. A focused history should be obtained with the chronological events related to the pathologic condition of concern. When was the condition first noticed? Was it noticed by the patient or by a healthcare provider? How long has the lesion been there? What is the rate of growth? Growth rate is a fundamental question because a lesion that has been there for years without progressing is more likely to be congenital or benign while a rapidly growing lesion is more likely to be malignant. Have there been any changes in the texture or appearance of the lesion? An example of this is an ulcer that previously presented as a vesicle. Are there any associated symptoms? What makes it better or worse? What treatments has the patient tried, if any? Is the patient aware of any event that could have caused this, such as trauma or recent dental procedures?

Focused Exam

When conducting an examination, the practitioner needs to remember that all information obtained in the clinical examination must be fully documented in the patient's chart. The written description should be so comprehensive that any reader would be able to mentally visualize the pathologic condition present at that time (see Table 8.1). In addition, taking a photograph to be placed in the patient's chart is an excellent form of documenting. This same information should be conveyed to the pathologist when the biopsy specimen is submitted.

The location of the lesion in question is very important, and the clinician must be as specific as possible when describing its location. White lesions on the floor of the mouth may be of greater significance than along the occlusal line of the buccal mucosa. Multifocal and/or bilateral lesions may be more suggestive of an autoimmune process or a variation from normal. The location is also an important factor in considering whether to biopsy the lesion or not. Lesions close to vital structures or in areas of limited accessibility may be better referred to a specialist. The location determines which tissue is contributing to the lesion. If one ascertains the type of tissue involved, such as keratinized vs. unkeratinized epithelium, this can provide additional information when developing a differential diagnosis.

The size of the lesion should be measured. Many of the instruments in the office have a basic ruler imprinted on them. A periodontal probe should be readily available as well and can be used to measure lesions. Next, the practitioner should assess the color and texture. Is the lesion flat or raised? Rough or smooth? If nodular, is it firm, doughy, or soft? Is the color distinct from the surrounding tissue? Or is it diffuse and indistinct? Is it movable or tightly bound down? Is it painful?

Great care must be taken when palpating the lesion. One should assess if the lesion can be removed when wiped with a sterile gauze, specifically in the case of white lesions. Once the texture and color have been identified assess the borders.

Table 8.1 Descriptive pathologic terms usefully in describing pathologic conditions of the oral cavity

Term	Definition
Bulla	A blister, fluid containing lesion of skin or mucosa
Crust	Dried serum on the surface of the skin or mucosa
Cyst	Pathological cavity lined by epithelium
Dysplasia	Changes in architecture—regarded as potentially malignant
Erosion	A superficial ulceration (loss of epithelium)
Fluctuant	Fluid-filled
Hyperkeratosis	An abundance of the keratinized layer of epithelium
Hyperplasia	An increase in the number of normal cells
Hypertrophy	An increase in size of cells
Indurated	Hard, firm, fixed mass
Keratosis	An increased number and size of the keratinized layer of epithelium
Leukoplakia	Slowly developing thickened white patches that are firmly attached to the skin or mucosa
Macule	A well-demarcated, non-elevated, non-depressed area of color that is different from the surrounding tissue
Nodule	A large elevated solid palpable mass of the skin or mucosa (greater than 1 cm in diameter)
Papule	A large elevated solid palpable mass of the skin or mucosa (less than 1 cm in diameter)
Pedunculated	Mass attached to adjacent structure by a stalk
Plaque	Flat or slightly raised superficial lesion, 2 cm or greater in diameter
Pustule	A small, cloudy, elevated pus containing vesicle of the skin or mucosa
Scale	A thin flat, superficial flake of the keratinized epithelium
Sessile	Broach based raised mass
Stomatitis	A generalized inflammatory condition of the oral mucosa
Telangiectasia	Surface vascular markings
Ulcer	A crater-like, well-demarcated break in the epithelium and dermis
Vesicle	A small fluid-filled blister

Are the edges distinct and well demarcated or are they diffuse? Changes in the surrounding tissue can also provide information. An example of this is if the body is attempting to "wall off" this pathologic condition. If it is a bony lesion, assess if teeth are being moved or eroded? For bony lesions, appropriate radiographs should be obtained and reviewed to see if they provide any additional information. Are neighboring lymph nodes enlarged or tender?

Differential Diagnosis

Before performing a biopsy, the clinician should develop a working differential diagnosis using a systematic and orderly standard protocol. It is often best to approach this task by considering potential diagnoses within specific diagnosis groups. Pathologic conditions essentially fall into one of these six categories:

1. Congenital/developmental
2. Reactive/inflammatory

3. Infection
4. Immune mediated (local/systemic)
5. Neoplastic
6. Oral manifestations of systemic diseases

The clinician should use these subgroups to populate a rank ordered list of possible diagnoses for the pathologic condition. Using the history and clinical exam to compile all available information, a differential diagnosis is developed from most likely to least likely with all possible conditions included. In certain instances, a diagnosis can be made from history and clinical exam alone. In other instances, a biopsy maybe warranted. The biopsy results will be used to confirm one of the diagnoses within the differential.

The differential diagnosis is important to determine whether the pathologic condition contains a vesicular bullous lesion or an immune response. Special stains or immunofluorescence studies may be required when processing the biopsied tissue. In the case of infectious processes culturing and sensitivity studies may be required. In these situations, extra samples and/or special handling of the biopsy specimens is required. Transport in formalin solution is contraindicated in these situations.

A verbal and written consent must be obtained before any biopsy is performed.

Biopsy Principles

Several decisions are required in determining the need for a biopsy. The term "biopsy" is a procedure to remove a piece of tissue or group of cells from a living organism for the purpose of being analyzed in a laboratory. The first question is—Is a biopsy required in order for the clinician to confidently diagnose the pathologic condition in question? Often the area of concern may be a normal anatomical variation, or the history and clinical exam may be so characteristic or pathognomonic that the diagnosis is obvious and does not warrant additional investigation. Even in these cases, a biopsy maybe required to satisfy the patients concerns, or to provide confirmation to a third-party payer.

After the decision has been made to obtain a biopsy then the next determination is to decide what type of biopsy to perform. There are two different kinds of biopsy—excisional or incisional. An excisional biopsy involves the removal of the entire area of concern, and in an incisional biopsy a representative sample is obtained. Both incisional and excisional biopsies should include adjacent normal tissue. The goal is to obtain a representative sample suitable for the pathologist to interpret.

Excisional Biopsy

An excisional biopsy in most cases should be reserved for well-circumscribed lesions less than 1 cm in diameter and not closely associated with significant anatomical structures. Local anesthesia should be obtained with nerve blocks whenever possible. If a nerve block is not possible, then local anesthesia should be directed at peripheral structures and not injected directly into the lesion in question. Injecting directly into the area can distort tissue and make pathological examination and an accurate diagnosis more difficult. The standard incision for an excisional biopsy is an ellipse (Fig. 8.1). The goal is to have the length 3× longer than the width, allowing for better closure. The elliptical incision allows for tension-free closure. The incision is "V" shaped, meaning widest at the superficial layer going to a point at the base of the lesion. It is important to keep a border of normal tissue in all directions around the lesion (Fig. 8.2). The buffer zone of excised normal tissue can be as little as 2–3 mm for benign conditions to at least a centimeter or more in malignant conditions. Surgeons often place suture tags in one aspect of the specimen to help orient the pathologist to the lesion's anatomical position.

In cases of well-demarcated lesions such as a mucocele utilization of a Chalazion clamp is very useful. The Chalazion clamp is situated around the lesion causing firm pressure and hemostasis to the surrounding tissue (Fig. 8.3). This clamp allows easier manipulation when the surgeon removes the lesion with a scalpel blade.

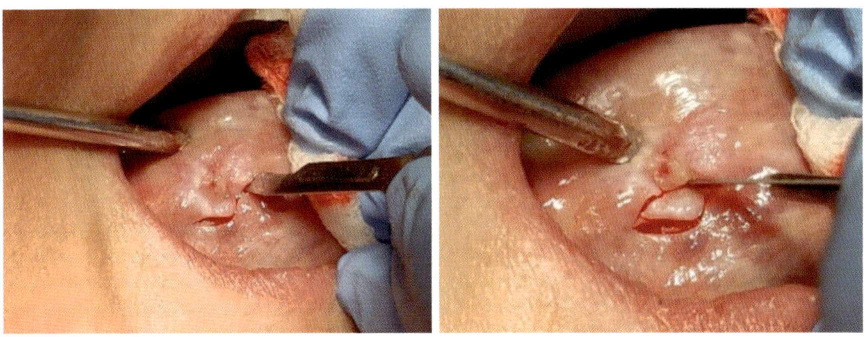

Fig. 8.1 Excisional biopsy using an elliptical incision

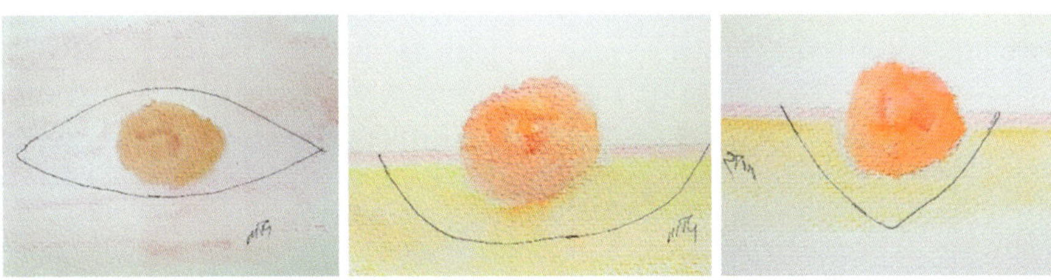

Fig. 8.2 Excisional biopsy. Length is approximately three times the width and includes normal tissue all around the lesion

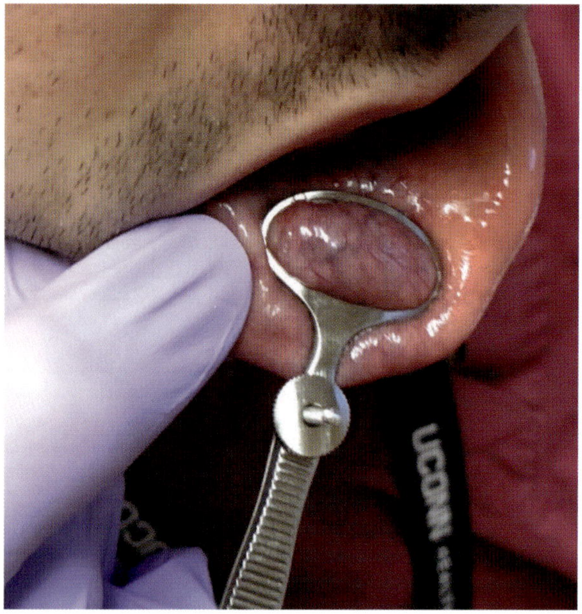

Fig. 8.3 A Chalazion clamp in place to assist in the biopsy

Incisional Biopsy

Incisional biopsies can be broken down into several different subcategories. An incisional biopsy should not be performed for vascular lesions. An aspiration biopsy may be useful in determining if a lesion is vascular to minimize risk of hemorrhage, especially in intraosseous radiolucencies [1, 2]. A fine needle aspirate (FNA) is a type of incisional biopsy that utilizes a 16- to 18-gauge needle on a syringe with the goal of aspirating cells from a nodule. This is usually performed for deep-seated nodules and is not often utilized in oral surgery. FNA is particularly useful in lesions of the neck that are otherwise inaccessible without surgical intervention.

A brush biopsy is another type of incisional biopsy because it only removes a portion of the area of interest. The brush biopsy is used to obtain cells from the surface of a lesion. The biopsy is performed by placing the brush on the lesion in question and rotating with firm pressure about 5–10 times [3]. Anesthesia is generally not required, and the procedure is usually well tolerated by patients. Although the brush biopsy is convenient, its value has been questioned in the literature [4–7]. However, a brush biopsy can be a useful screening tool. Generally, the cytology report is categorized into (1) negative, i.e., no abnormalities, (2) positive, i.e., cellular evidence of dysplastic changes, or (3) atypical, i.e., abnormal epithelial changes [8]. If the brush biopsy is in the second or third category, a more invasive biopsy, such as an incisional biopsy, is performed to determine a more definitive diagnosis.

As stated earlier incisional biopsies are indicated for larger lesions, especially when more than one representable sample is required. The basic principles are the same as with the excisional biopsy. The surgeon should utilize anesthesia with blocks whenever possible or inject in the periphery of the pathologic condition. An elliptical incision is utilized to allow the best closure and the sample should include the interface between normal and abnormal tissue (Fig. 8.4). When multiple samples are taken it is important to be specific as to where each specimen came from anatomically and one tissue sample is submitted per specimen bottle. When lesions are large, multiple site biopsy allows for better diagnosis [9].

A punch biopsy can be either an incisional or excision biopsy depending on the size of the punch and the size of the lesion. A punch biopsy is a relatively easy technique for most providers. A punch biopsy utilizes a circular cutting blade to make a circular incision around the lesion. The diameter of the punch is generally fairly small, 2–5 mm (Fig. 8.5), and therefore it is not difficult to obtain primary closure. With careful handling of the soft tissue, the punch biopsy is placed over the lesion and turned in a clockwise/counter clockwise twisting fashion with slight pressure. The lesion can then be gently lifted with a tissue forceps, and the remaining

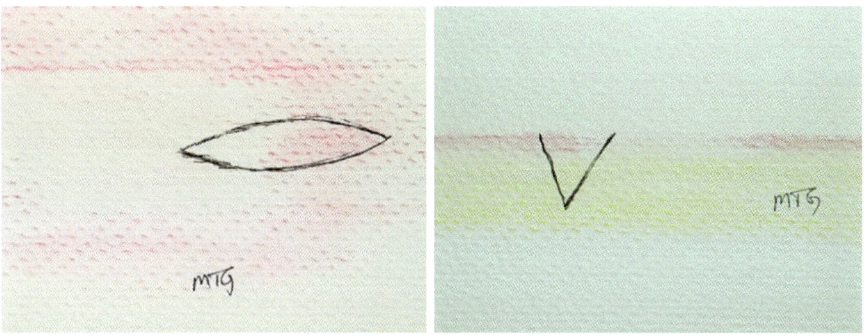

Fig. 8.4 Incisional biopsy of diffuse white lesion that includes both abnormal and normal tissue

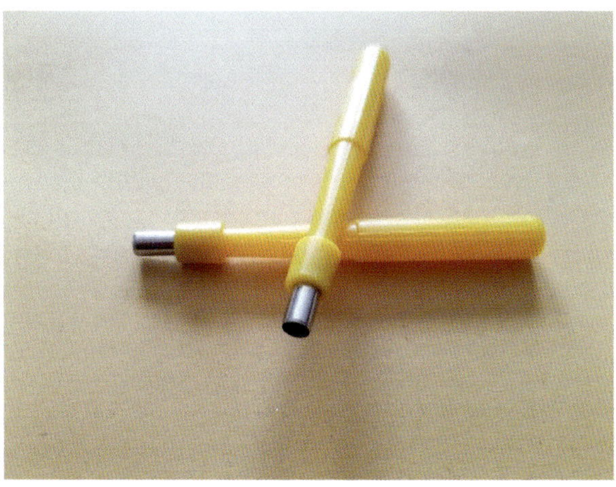

Fig. 8.5 Biopsy punches come in a variety of diameters

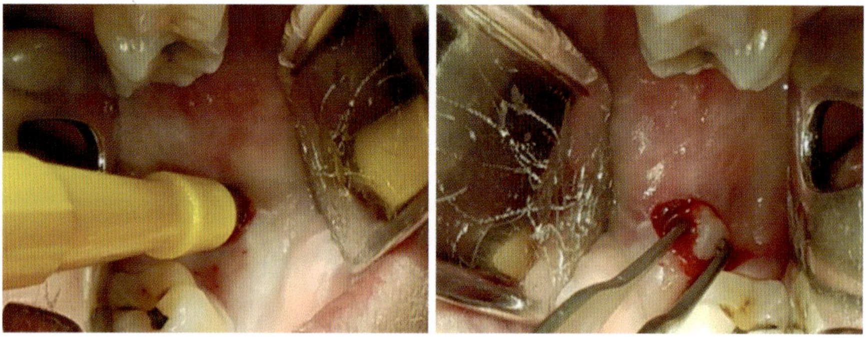

Fig. 8.6 Incision is made by rotating the circular bladed punch instrument to the desired depth. The specimen is gently lifted and the base is sharply incised for removal with a scalpel blade

connecting tissue gently separated from under the lesion with a #15 scalpel blade (Fig. 8.6). It is important to use sharp instruments and avoid distorting the lesion.

Special Considerations

Special considerations need to be taken with bone biopsies. As mentioned previously, when dealing with a radiolucent lesion, the lesion should be aspirated first to ensure that the lesion is not vascular in nature [10]. It is recommended that a radiograph is taken postoperatively to ensure that a representative specimen has indeed been obtained. Copies of both the preoperative and postoperative radiographs should be submitted with the specimen to the pathologist. Histologically many boney lesions can be similar, and the radiograph is necessary to make a more definitive diagnosis. Because many bone biopsies need to undergo decalcification, the pathologic report can be delayed from the standard 2–3 days for soft tissue specimens to 10–14+ days.

Wound Stabilization

After the biopsy is performed proper hemostasis needs to be achieved. During biopsy procedures, the use of suction should be minimized to lessen the risk of losing the specimen. Using 2 × 2 gauze with firm pressure will allow control of hemostasis during the procedure as well as after. Often excision of a larger biopsy specimen results in the need for sutures. Biopsies taken from keratinized surfaces such as the hard palate or gingiva generally are not sutured and heal by secondary intention. Biopsies performed on nonattached mucosa, however, often require closure by suturing. When choosing a suture, it is best to use materials that are nonreactive such as black silk. When a biopsy takes place in an area of limited accessibility one can use a slowly resorbing material such as Vicryl® to avoid the need to remove the sutures later.

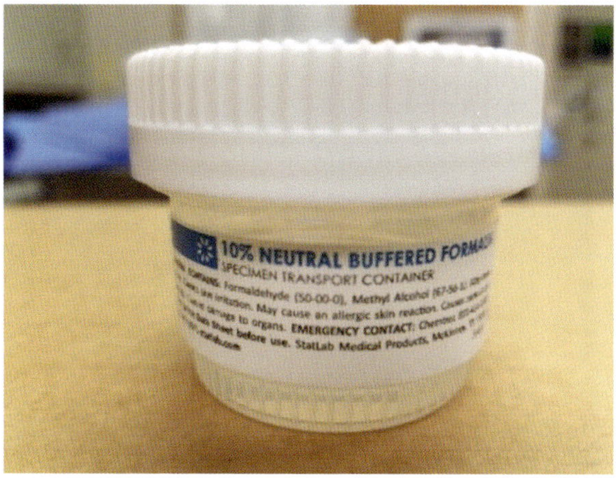

Fig. 8.7 Biopsy specimens are transported to the laboratory in 10% buffered formalin. One specimen per container with labeling as to patient and location source. Appropriate hazard labels required especially when specimens are sent through the mail

Specimen Submission

The specimen must next be sent to the pathologist for interpretation. The pathologist should be provided with a complete summary of the history, the clinical description, and the differential diagnosis [at least the best guess] [11]. A copy of a representative clinical photo should also be sent if photos had been obtained. Biopsy specimens are generally transported in a 10% buffered formalin [12] (see Fig. 8.7).

When the differential diagnosis includes a vesicular-bullous lesion and/or an autoimmune process, it is imperative that at least two biopsy specimens are submitted. This can easily be accomplished by obtaining one larger specimen and dividing it into two representative pieces. One specimen should be placed in the standard 10% buffered formalin solution and will undergo the standard H&E examination. A second specimen should be sent in saline gauze for quick freezing. This will allow the second specimen to be used for specialized immune-fluorescent studies.

When mailing tissue specimens, it is important to use an approved biohazard labeled container with appropriate outer labeling (Fig. 8.8). Whenever possible, samples should be mailed to an oral maxillofacial pathologist as opposed to a general pathologist due to their increased familiarity with the pathologic conditions of the oral cavity and perioral structures. Highly competent general pathologists may be less familiar with odontogenic pathologic conditions which may lead to an incorrect diagnosis.

Follow-up

If the biopsy results are benign then the provider can resume routine, follow-ups and periodic monitoring. If the biopsy results are positive for malignancy, proper referral is needed to a healthcare provider specializing in head/neck malignancies. It is important for the clinician to keep a close follow-up to these types of patients.

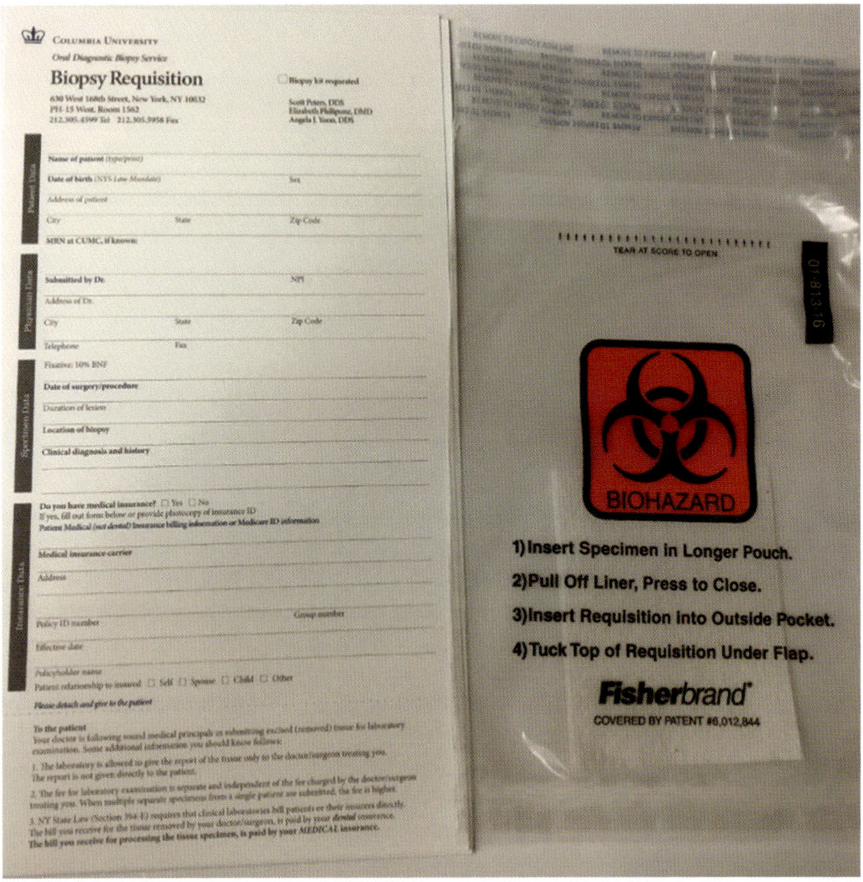

Fig. 8.8 Biopsy laboratory request form and biohazard label

References

1. August M, Faquin WC, Ferraro NF, Kaban LB. Fine-needle aspiration biopsy of intraosseous jaw lesions. J Oral Maxillofac Surg. 1999;57:1282–6. discussion 1287
2. Larsen PE, Peterson LJ. A systematic approach to management of high-flow vascular malformations of the mandible. J Oral Maxillofac Surg. 1993;51:62–9.
3. Sciubba JJ. Improving detection of precancerous and cancerous oral lesions. Computer-assisted analysis of the oral brush biopsy. U.S. Collaborative OralCDx Study Group. J Am Dent Assoc. 1999;130:1445–57.
4. Bhoopathi V, Kabani S, Mascarenhas AK. Low positive predictive value of the oral brush biopsy in detecting dysplastic oral lesions. Cancer. 2009;115:1036–40.
5. Eisen D, Frist S. Efficacy of the brush biopsy. J Oral Maxillofac Surg. 2003;61:1237.
6. Rick GM. Oral brush biopsy: the problem of false positives. Oral Surg Oral Med Oral Pathol Oral Radiol Endod. 2003;96:252.
7. Slater LJ. Brush biopsy: false negative results. J Oral Maxillofac Surg. 2004;62:764.

8. Hupp JR, Ellis E, Tucker MR. Contemporary oral and maxillofacial surgery. St. Louis, MO: Mosby; 2014.
9. Chen S, Forman M, Sadow PM, August M. The diagnostic accuracy of incisional biopsy in the oral cavity. J Oral Maxillofac Surg. 2016;74:959–64.
10. Najjar TA, Gaston GW. Biopsy technique for fibro-osseous and osteolytic lesions of the jaws. Oral Surg Oral Med Oral Pathol. 1977;44:177–82.
11. COOKE BE. Biopsy procedures. Oral Surg Oral Med Oral Pathol. 1958;11:750–61.
12. STOOPACK JC. Biopsy techniques in oral surgery. Oral Surg Oral Med Oral Pathol. 1952;5:1034–46.

Frenectomy

9

Michael T. Goupil, Tyler J. Thomas, and Stephan Goupil

Definitions

Depending on the healthcare provider, different names may be used for this membrane fold that restricts movement. The terms frenum (frena, pl) and frenulum (frenula, pl) can be used interchangeably.

The surgical correction is termed a frenotomy, which releases the frenum through a single incision, or a frenectomy, which removes the frenum through multiple incisions. The corresponding terms would be frenulotomy and frenulectomy. To confuse the issue more frequently, a clinician will state they have performed a frenectomy when, in actuality, they have performed a frenotomy.

The term ankyloglossia refers to an abnormal restriction of the tongue secondary to an abnormally placed lingual frenum. This condition is frequently referred to as "tongue-tie(d)."

Surgical Indications

There are two indications for the release of frena in the oral cavity—functional and cosmetic. The cosmetic concern is usually related to the maxillary labial frenum, especially when the frenum extends between the maxillary permanent central incisors and results in a diastema (Fig. 9.1).

M. T. Goupil (✉)
University of Connecticut School of Dental Medicine, Farmington, CT, USA
e-mail: mtgoupil@comcast.net

T. J. Thomas
Indiana Restorative Dentistry, Carmel, IN, USA

S. Goupil
Emerson Family Medicine at Emerson Hospital, Concord, MA, USA
e-mail: sgoupil@emersonhosp.org

E. M. Ferneini, M. T. Goupil (eds.), *Office-Based Maxillofacial Surgical Procedures*, https://doi.org/10.1007/978-3-030-22371-7_9

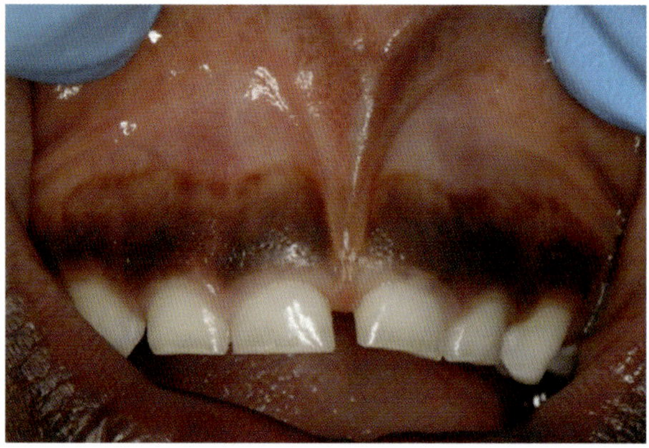

Fig. 9.1 Diastema related to a maxillary labial frenum. (Photo courtesy of Ronald Albert, DMD)

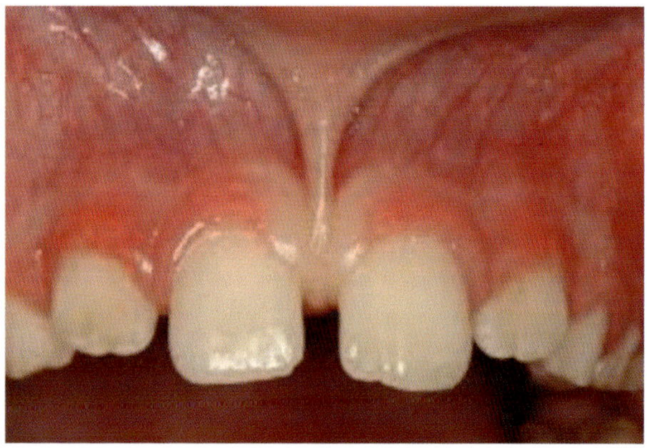

Fig. 9.2 Note blanching of the mucosa between the central incisors

When a frenum extends between the incisors it should be surgically corrected before orthodontic closure of the diastema can be accomplished. As part of the orthodontic exam, the upper lip is retracted in an upward and forward direction in order to place tension on the frenum. Blanching of the mucosa between the maxillary central incisors is an indication that the frenum extends between the incisors and may insert into the incisive papilla on the palate (Fig. 9.2). This band of frenal tissue needs to be removed so that the diastema can be closed orthodontically. When the frenum is surgically corrected early, there is a potential that the diastema may close naturally through the eruption process of the other maxillary permanent anterior teeth. However, closure of the diastema is more predictable with a frenectomy and orthodontics than a frenectomy alone [1].

There are functional reasons for the surgical correction of oral frena (Fig. 9.3). As mentioned above, one of the most common reasons is due to ankyloglossia or tongue-tie. Ankyloglossia's reported prevalence is approximately 5% of newborns with a 3:1 male predilection. A variety of concerns have been raised including breast-feeding problems for both the infant and the mother, swallowing difficulties,

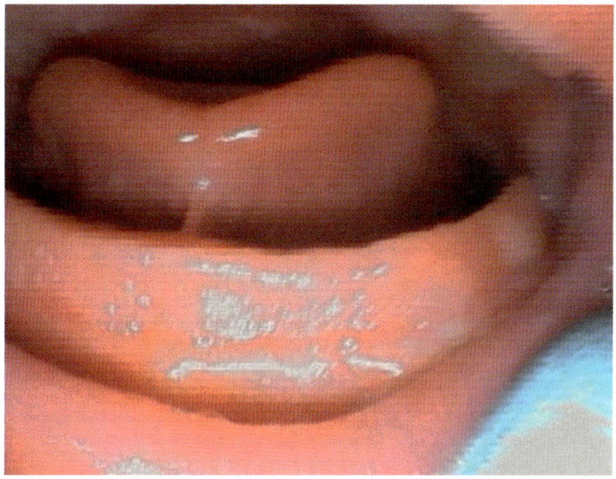

Fig. 9.3 Ankyloglossia causing feeding problems. (Photo courtesy of Ronald Albert, DMD)

speech problems, and altered posture [2, 3]. The first documented case of a breast-feeding problem corrected with a frenum surgery occurred in 1601 on the infant Dauphin of France [4].

Although the majority of breast-feeding issues can be corrected by consultation with a lactation specialist, surgical correction of the frenum may still be required. This also holds true for bottle-fed infants. Maternal nipple pain secondary to ankyloglossia may also be improved with a lingual frenum release [5].

Currently there is no substantial support for prophylactic frenectomy to prevent speech problems [6]. Consultation with a speech pathologist (therapist) should be considered when contemplating a lingual frenectomy for speech issues especially in adults and older children where speech habits and tongue positions are already well established.

Another potential functional indication for frenectomy surgery would be in the fabrication of a removable dental prosthesis for a partially or totally edentulous individual. The lingual and labial frena are composed of extremely delicate non-keratinized tissue. This tissue can be easily traumatized and may become irritated from the constant rubbing of the frena against the hard, non-flexible surface of an overextended prosthesis. Not only will an overextension traumatize the tissue, but it may also dislodge the prosthesis. This is especially true when dealing with a patient with an atrophic alveolar ridge where the frenum attaches high on the ridge (Fig. 9.4). The removable prosthesis may also be dislodged secondary to a tight or high frenum during speech or eating.

To accommodate a frenum without any surgical modification, a large notch may need to be cut in the labial flange of a maxillary denture or lingual flange of a mandibular denture in order to reduce irritation. This may result in a cosmetic problem in a patient with a high smile line. In addition, these adjustments in the notch may be considered a cleavage point resulting in an increased risk of fracture of the denture [7]. A vestibulopathy type frenum procedure can eliminate this concern and may also improve denture stability (Fig. 9.5).

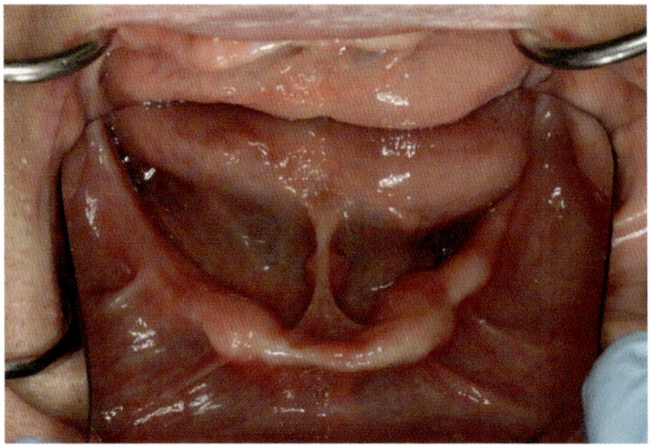

Fig. 9.4 Lingual frenum adversely effects mandibular denture stability. Photo courtesy of Tyler Thomas, DMD, MS

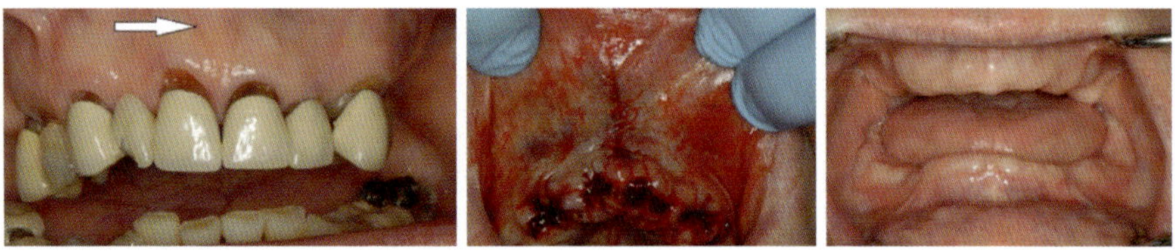

Fig. 9.5 Localized maxillary labial frenum removal vestibulopathy along with extractions in preparation for a maxillary denture. (Photo courtesy of Tyler Thomas, DMD, MS)

Surgical Options

Regardless of the indication for surgical intervention there are two options—release of the immobile part (--otomy) or removal of the frenum (--ectomy). The two modalities usually employed to perform the surgical procedure are laser or sharp incision with a scalpel/scissors. The surgical modality is usually clinician preference.

Surgical Techniques

Anesthesia—In adults and most cooperative children frenum surgery can usually be accomplished as an in-office procedure with local infiltration anesthesia. In the case of neonates where the lingual frenum can be easily freed with a snip of the scissors, no anesthesia is required. For more complex procedures or where the patient cannot fully cooperate (neonates and young children), then general anesthesia may be required.

Surgical options range from a simple release of the frenum (frenotomy) to removal of a portion of the frenum (frenectomy) to more complex procedures such as a Z-plasty or localized vestibulopathy. The choice of the surgical technique is based on the problem the frenum is causing, the end result desired, and the experience of the operator.

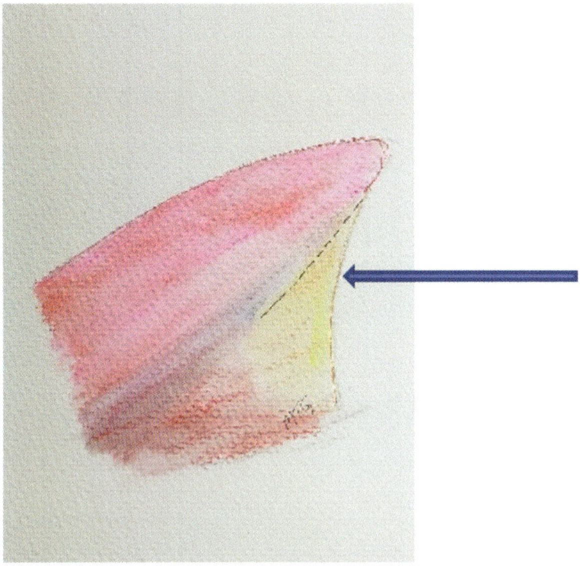

Fig. 9.6 Frenum is released from ventral surface of tongue with scissors, scalpel, or laser

Lingual Frenotomy is probably the most common procedure performed to release the lingual frenum. In the case of neonates with breast-feeding issues this should be performed within the first couple of weeks of age [4]. The frenum is freed from the ventral surface of the tongue using either sharp scissors or a scalpel blade (Fig. 9.6). Since the frenum is midline, the lingual neurovascular elements are easily avoided. The surgery should not extend into the floor of the mouth to avoid the submandibular ducts. Since the frenum is essentially avascular, bleeding should not be an issue.

In the case of older children and adults where the procedure is being performed as part of a speech correction program or to improve comfort/stability of a dental prosthesis, a similar technique can be utilized. Some providers may utilize laser surgery which has an advantage of cauterizing small blood vessels in the area. Regardless of the technique as long as the incision is placed in the avascular frenum bleeding is usually not an issue. Sutures are usually not required and may present more as an irritant and pain stimulus.

Lingual Frenectomy by definition requires removal of tissue. A frenectomy can be easily performed by grasping the frenum with a hemostat between the ventral surface of the tongue and the floor of the mouth. The frenum is then cut along the surface of each side of the hemostat and the "frenum" is then removed (Fig. 9.7). This may result in a larger open surgical would, and partial closure may be required. When suturing the surgical site, the operator must be cognizant of adjacent vital structures such as the lingual neurovasculature and the submandibular ducts. Bleeding should not be an issue.

Maxillary Labial Frenotomy is very useful for patients that have issues with their maxillary denture. In the case of a narrow frenum the upper lip is pulled superiorly and the frenum is released by sharply incising the frenum at its junction with

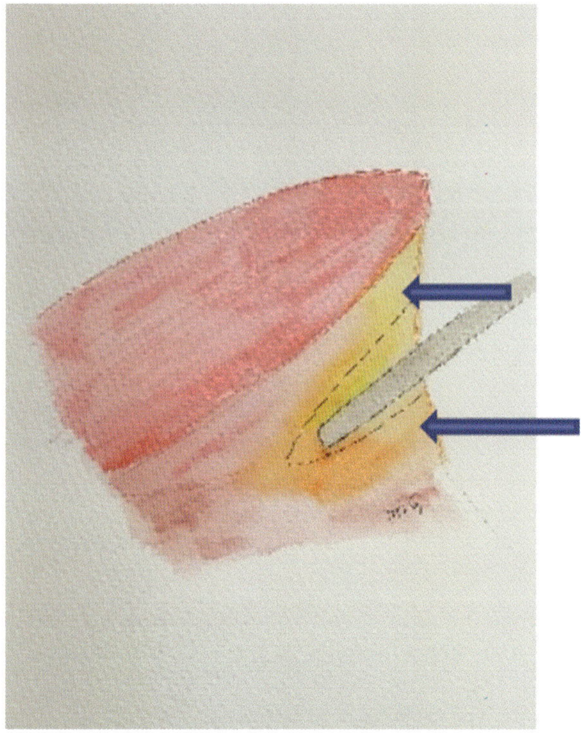

Fig. 9.7 Frenum is grasped with a hemostat and an incision is made on the superior and inferior aspect of the hemostat

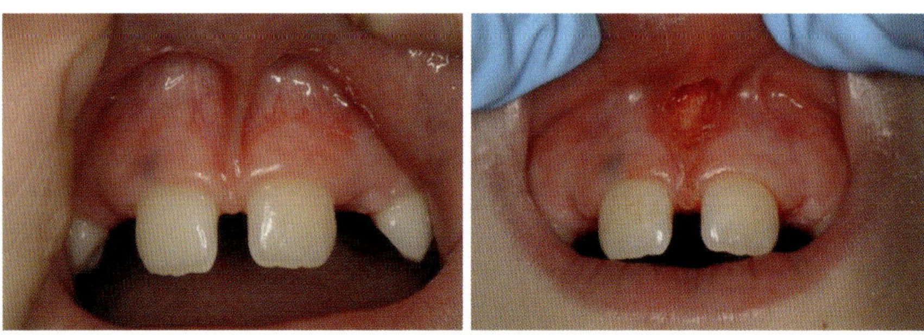

Fig. 9.8 Maxillary labial frenum release utilizing a laser. (Photo courtesy of Ronald Albert, DMD)

the maxillary ridge. This is easily accomplished with a scalpel blade, but a laser or electrocautery may also be utilized. There is minimal bleeding and suturing is usually not required (Fig. 9.8).

For broad-frena a “V”-shaped incision is made extending submucosally but not through the periosteum (Fig. 9.9). This “V” flap is then released in a superior direction along a supraperiosteal plane. This flap is then repositioned superiorly and sutured to the periosteum at the superior extent of the labial vestibule (Fig. 9.10).

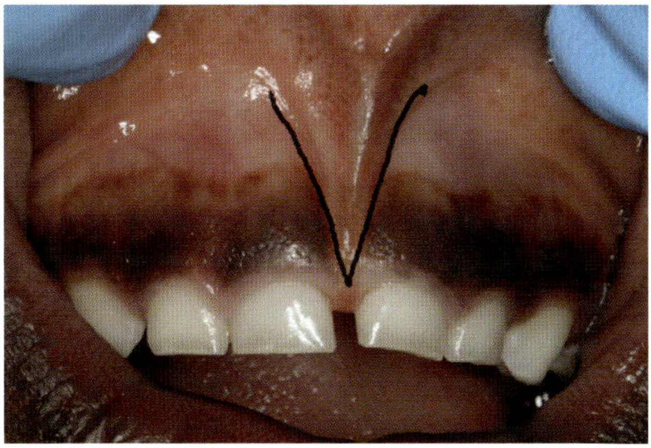

Fig. 9.9 Incision for "V" type frenotomy

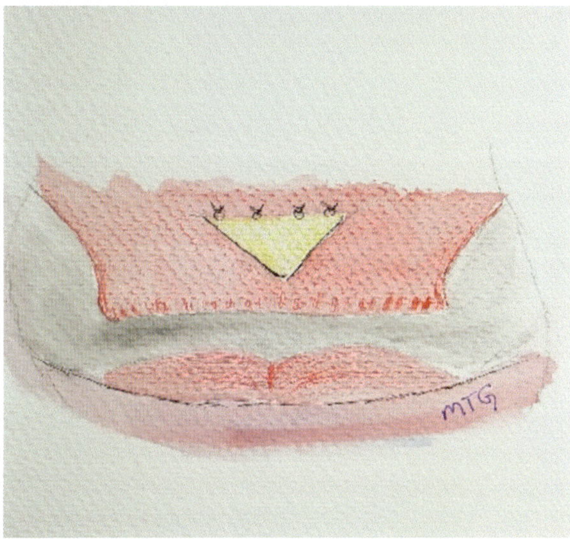

Fig. 9.10 Partial thickness flap is repositioned superiorly

This results in removal of the frenum as well as a localized vestibuloplasty. The surgical site is then allowed to undergo secondary epithelialization. A variation of this procedure would be to undermine the mucosa laterally and to close the wound primarily in a "V" to "Y" fashion.

Another option available that allows primary wound closure is to perform a Z-plasty (Fig. 9.11). This technique realigns the frenum from a vertical to a horizontal alignment (Fig. 9.12). The flaps are developed supraperiosteally. With generous undermining a localized vestibuloplasty is also accomplished.

By performing a localized vestibuloplasty, the labial notch is removed from the denture and the denture flange can be extended superiorly with an end-result of better retention. The labial flange of the maxillary denture should be modified at the time of surgery by using a soft reline material. The patient can leave the office with the denture in place.

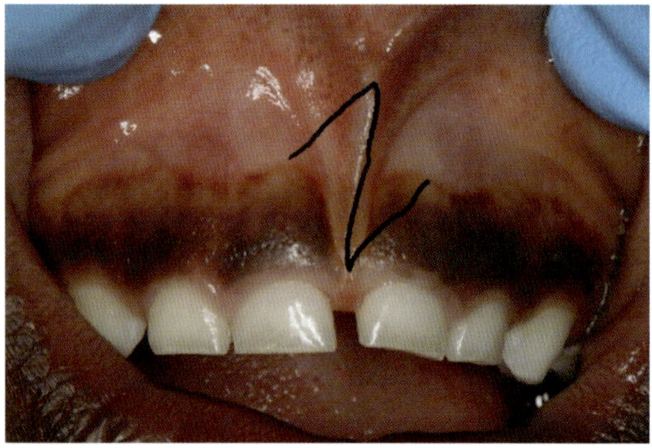

Fig. 9.11 Incision for Z-plasty

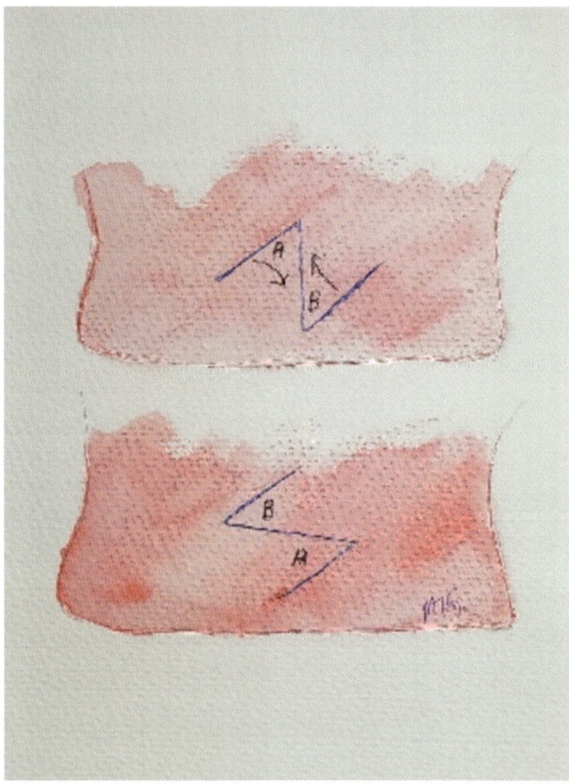

Fig. 9.12 Flaps repositioned from vertical to horizontal alignment

Maxillary Labial Frenectomy can be accomplished in a similar fashion as described for the lingual frenum. The frenum is grasped with a hemostat. The frenum is then sharply incised on each side of the hemostat. The resulting surgical wound can easily be closed primarily.

When the frenectomy is performed as part maxillary incisor diastema closure then additional tissue needs to be removed from between the incisors back to the incisive papilla on the palate. This tissue can be removed with either a sharp scalpel dissection or a laser. If insufficient tissue is removed, there is the potential the diastema will return once the orthodontic apparatus has been removed.

Postoperative Considerations

There is minimal bleeding or pain following frenal surgery procedures. Obviously, when the surgery becomes more complex as in the case of a Z-plasty, there may be more discomfort. Bleeding is more likely to occur with lingual frenum surgery. This complication is rare when the surgery is confined to the midline. When the surgery deviates from the midline, vital structures are more likely to be encountered.

Summary

For the most part, surgical procedures on the oral frenum are relatively simple. Most corrections can usually be accomplished using a simple release of the frenum or a frenotomy, with healing through secondary epithelialization. In most cases sutures are not required. A lingual frenum release in a neonate usually does not require any anesthesia and is accomplished with a sharp pair of scissors. Services of a speech pathologist may be required if speech patterns are already set. Closure of maxillary incisor diastemas usually requires the removal of the frenum extending between the teeth. Retention of removable dental prosthesis may be enhanced by both lingual and labial frenal surgery.

The postoperative course is generally uneventful with minimal pain that can usually be controlled with non-prescription pain medication. Complications are rare. Because of the low complication rate lingual frenum release may be considered for the potential correction of speech issues.

References

1. Suter VGA, Heinzman AE, Grossen J, Sculean A, Burnstein MM. Does the maxillary midline diastema close after frenectomy? Quintessence Int. 2014;45(1):57–66.
2. Baker AR, Carr MM. Surgical treatment of ankyloglossia. Oper Tech Otolaryngol. 2015;26(1):28–32.
3. Olivi G, Signore A, Olivi M, Genovese MD. Lingual frenectomy: Functional evaluation and new therapeutical approach. Eur J Paediatr Dent. 2012;13(2):101–6.
4. Steehler MK, Harley EH. A retrospective review of frenectomy in neonates and infants with feeding difficulties. Int J Pediatr Otorhinolaryngol. 2012;76:1236–40.
5. O'Callahan C, Macary S, Clmente S. The effects of office-based frenectomy for anterior and posterior ankyloglossia on breastfeeding. Int J Pediatr Otorhinolaryngol. 2013;77:827–32.

6. Brookes A, Bowley DM. Tongue tie: the evidence for frenectomy. Early Hum Dev. 2014;90:765–8.
7. Al Jabbari YS. Frenectomy for improvement of a problematic conventional maxillary complete denture in an elderly patient: A case report. J Adv Prosthodont. 2011;3:236–9.

Gingival Augmentation Surgery for Specific Mucogingival Problems

10

Frank C. Nichols, A. Michael Brown, Clarence L. Trummel, and James E. Kennedy

Introduction

Gingival augmentation surgery has been advocated for more than a half century to correct specific deficiencies in gingival tissues. The types of gingival augmentation procedures used today are based on biological principles applicable to all surgical interventions involving pedicle or free graft surgical approaches. The purpose of this chapter is to discuss the use of gingival augmentation surgery to manage three clinical problems affecting natural teeth and dental implants, specifically, gingival recession, the lack of an adequate zone of attached gingiva, and attachment of a frenum which compromises the function of the marginal tissue. Where appropriate, the preferred surgical approach and graft material will be identified. Emphasis will be given to the healing characteristics of the surgical wound as reinforcement of the type of surgical procedure selected. It is not the intent of this chapter to discuss the etiology, pathogenesis, or prevention of mucogingival problems. This chapter will also not address nonsurgical approaches or maintenance of mucogingival problems, nor will this chapter address considerations related to adjunctive procedures for correcting mucogingival problems, e.g., orthodontic tooth repositioning or odontoplasty.

Today, most practitioners utilize the free connective tissue graft (subepithelial connective tissue graft) procedures to provide root coverage where gingival deficiencies are esthetically problematic for the patient [1–7]. Donor tissue for free connective grafts is typically harvested from the palate (autograft) but may also utilize xenograft materials (such as Mucoderm) or allograft materials (such as Alloderm from human cadavers) [8]. The alternate donor tissue products reduce the surgical

F. C. Nichols (✉) · A. M. Brown · C. L. Trummel · J. E. Kennedy
Division of Periodontology, University of Connecticut School of Dental Medicine, Farmington, CT, USA
e-mail: nichols@uchc.edu; mibrown@uchc.edu; jayhawk1960@comcast.net; kennedy@uchc.edu

E. M. Ferneini, M. T. Goupil (eds.), *Office-Based Maxillofacial Surgical Procedures*, https://doi.org/10.1007/978-3-030-22371-7_10

time because harvesting palatal tissue is not required which reduces the likelihood for postsurgical morbidity at the donor site (severe bleeding) [9]. The use of alternative sources of connective tissue is particularly helpful with gingival recession that extends over several teeth and where harvesting a very large graft from the palate is not possible.

This chapter will also review the use of gingival augmentation procedures for the purpose of establishing an adequate zone of keratinized gingival tissue where other dental problems may exist such as a minimal depth of the vestibule or a specific mucogingival problem that has contributed to dental disease such as caries. For these specific mucogingival defect problems, the free gingival graft (epithelialized gingival graft) procedure has particular advantages in treating problem sites. When performed properly, the free gingival graft provides a predictable zone of immovable keratinized gingiva. This chapter describes the use of this procedure for managing dental problems associated with mucogingival deficiencies or problem areas.

The presurgical considerations for gingival augmentation surgery include the patient's age, tooth root prominence, orthodontic treatment options, the restorative treatment plan, the patient's compliance with home care instructions, and esthetic requirements. If the patient is primarily concerned about esthetic issues regarding a mucogingival deficiency, a free connective graft procedure is the preferred approach to manage a gingival deficiency (gingival recession) that is an esthetic concern. However, increasing vestibular depth [10], problematic frenum attachments or continued progression of recession can often be managed with a free gingival graft procedure with excellent treatment results [11]. The following cases provide examples of how these procedures can provide a satisfactory solution to specific issues with mucogingival deficiencies.

Types of Gingival Augmentation Procedures

Gingival augmentation procedures include the procedures listed in Table 10.1. Many of the pedicle graft procedures are not performed routinely today and are not considered to be mainstream gingival augmentation procedures. Of the procedures listed, this chapter will concentrate on free gingival graft, frenectomy/frenotomy procedures, and laterally positioned flaps. The specific examples described in this chapter are not intended to address only a deficiency of gingival tissue but rather to address specific dental problems associated with the mucogingival deficiencies.

Table 10.1 Classification of gingival augmentation surgical procedures

- Pedicle grafts
  - Laterally positioned flap
  - Rotated pedicle flap
  - Double pedicle flaps
  - Coronally positioned flap
- Free gingival graft
- Frenectomy/Frenotomy
- Free connective tissue graft

Currently, pedicle grafts are rarely used for treating mucogingival defects. However, as described later in this chapter, a laterally positioned pedicle flap can be used to manage keratinized tissue deficiencies in cases where the implant procedure includes the surgical uncovering of an implant or implants. The pedicle grafts retain attachment of the gingiva to the body whereas free grafts release the grafted tissue from the body so that positioning at a distant recipient site can occur. Free gingival grafts primarily augment gingiva at sites were minimal keratinized gingival tissue is present but are not intended to provide substantial coverage of denuded root surfaces.

The Free Gingival Graft Procedure to Augment Gingiva and Increase Vestibular Depth

Figure 10.1 shows the steps involved with the free gingival graft procedure. The free gingival graft survives initially by plasmatic support from the recipient site because the connective tissue side of the graft contacts the recipient bed, thereby providing vascular support for the overlying graft to survive. When placed directly

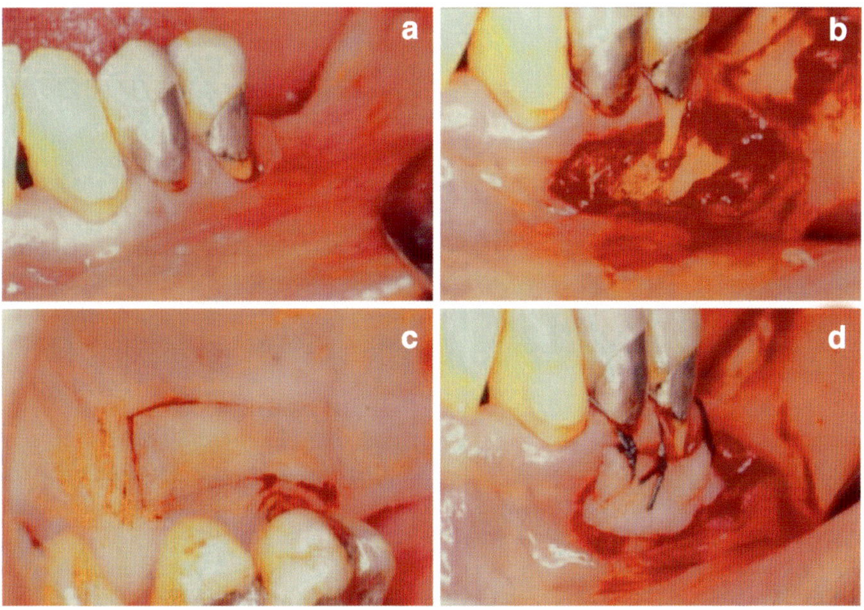

Fig. 10.1 Free gingival graft procedure. (**a**) Preoperative location of the free gingival margin shows a minimal zone of keratinized gingiva on the facial aspect of #21 and no keratinized gingiva on the facial aspect of #20. (**b**) Preparation of the graft recipient site. (**c**) Preparation of the donor site. (**d**) Placement of the free gingival graft on the recipient site. (**e**) Appearance of the donor site after the graft is removed from the palate. (**f**) Healing of the donor site after 1 week. Note the striations of epithelium extending from the edge of the donor excision site. (**g**) Appearance of the site before performing the graft procedure and the appearance of the site after 6 months of healing (**h**). Photographs courtesy of Dr. James Bussiere

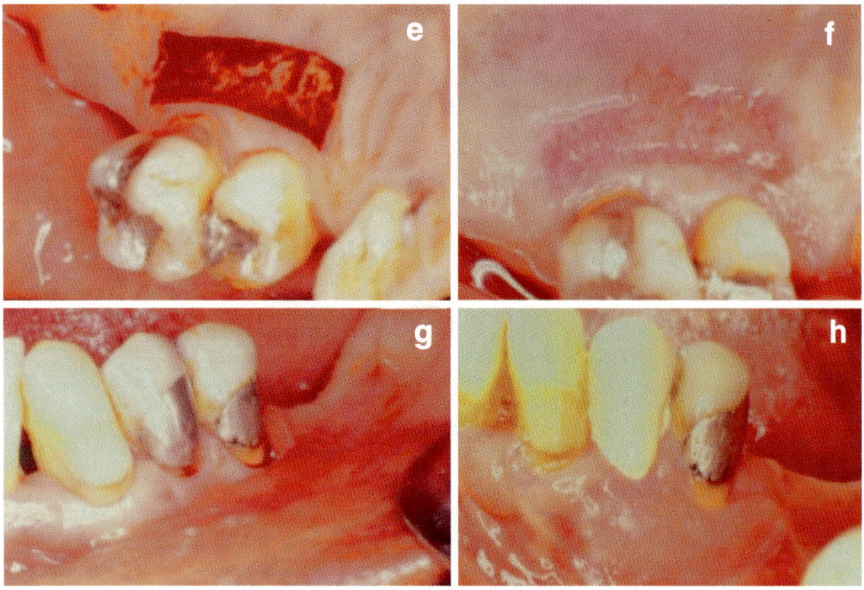

Fig. 10.1 (continued)

over an exposed root surface, the free gingival graft will likely not survive due to lack of vascular support to the graft from the tooth root. When the graft is placed on the recipient site, it is also important to ensure that the graft sits on a bed of immovable connective tissue. Preparation of the recipient site involves a beveled incision coronal to the mucogingival junction so that the bed separates the moveable oral mucosa from the underlying alveolar bone (Fig 10.1b). Only a thin layer of immovable connective tissue remains on the exposed alveolar bone. The tissue elements remaining on the alveolar bone are usually minimal in thickness or as an alternative, a fenestration through soft tissue to the alveolar bone is also acceptable. The recipient site must be extended mesially and distally to accommodate for secondary contraction (shrinkage) of the graft during healing (see below). Vertical incisions are made at the mesial and distal extent of the recipient bed. Care must be taken to avoid excising nerves or other critical structures in the area. The dimensions of the graft to be taken from the palate are determined by measuring the height and width of the recipient site and increasing these dimensions by 10–20%. The freed graft will shrink by about 10–20% in size when it is released from the palate (primary contraction). The graft size is outlined on the palatal donor site by making an incision to approximately the depth of the bevel of the Bard Parker blade (Fig. 10.1c). The graft is then released by using the scalpel to excise the tissue parallel with surface of the palate. Bleeding should be well controlled within a normal clotting time. If a particular area shows excessive bleeding, a stricture suture in the palatal soft tissue can be placed to control a local area of excessive bleeding. The graft is then placed on the recipient site with the epithelial surface of the graft contacting the cheek and not the alveolar bone. Once the graft is positioned on the recipient site, a good way to test that the graft is resting on an immovable recipient site is to pull the cheek or lip mesially and distally in order to verify visually that the graft does not move. If movement of the graft is observed, the recipient site should be extended, or the graft trimmed in order to ensure that the graft rests on an immovable recipient bed. The graft is then attached coronally to the keratinized gingiva using suspensory sutures (Fig. 10.1d). Typically, a periodontal dressing (Coe-Pak dressing) is placed over the graft in order to maintain contact between the graft and the underlying recipient tissue. The dressing and sutures are removed in 7–10 days.

Revascularization of the connective tissue portion of the free gingival graft occurs from 30 h to 6 days after graft placement. The overlying graft epithelium will slough but will regenerate as the graft matures with additional healing. The graft will also shrink even more with the healing and maturation at the recipient site and is termed secondary contraction. Secondary contraction can be up to 50% of the graft size depending on the thickness of the graft. Thicker grafts tend to shrink less with healing and are generally much lighter in color than the surrounding keratinized tissue after healing. If an esthetic problem exists for the patient because it is too light in color after graft healing, the thickness of the healed graft can be reduced by dermabrasion using a high-speed handpiece and diamond bur. A better way to avoid the very light color of a healed gingival graft is to resect the graft with a minimal connective tissue layer. A guide for incision depth for excising an epithelialized graft is the width of the bevel on a #15 Bard Parker blade. The outline of the graft is made to the depth of the bevel and this depth is maintained during the surgical harvesting of the graft. Another helpful tip is to excise the graft to a depth where the side of the Bard Parker blade is barely visible through the keratinized tissue of the palate as the graft is released. A uniformly thin free gingival graft heals with a color approximately matching the usual gingival tissue coloration of the facial gingiva (Fig. 10.1h). Note the increased vestibular depth evident after healing of the graft. Increasing the depth of the vestibule allows better access for cleaning of the recession areas on the facial aspects of the bicuspid teeth and also provides greater depth for a denture flange along the lateral aspect of the alveolar process.

For this and all subsequent procedures described in this chapter, postoperative pain management rarely requires the use of opioid analgesics. Generally, use of a nonsteroidal anti-inflammatory (NSAID) medication such as ibuprofen (400–600 mg tid) is usually sufficient to manage postoperative discomfort. As with any NSAID, this medication also provides additional benefit by reducing postoperative inflammation. It is advisable to begin analgesic coverage 1 h prior to the surgical procedure in order to maximize the anti-inflammatory effect of this medication. Although these medications are known to increase bleeding times, use of NSAIDS rarely lead to significant postoperative bleeding unless it is combined with other well-known anticoagulant medications. Acetaminophen is an effective alternative to ibuprofen for those individuals who cannot take NSAID medications. Periodic topical anesthetic application (Benzocaine) to the palate will also help patients who experience significant pain at the graft donor site when oral function occurs, such as eating or speaking. Topical anesthetic application is rarely needed for extended periods.

The Free Gingival Graft Procedure to Manage Aberrant Frenum Attachment

Another example of how a free gingival graft can be used to correct a facial mucogingival problem is shown in Fig. 10.2 [12]. The facial aspect of the mandibular bicuspid is concealed by a buccal frenum; the buccal frenum prevents adequate cleaning of the facial aspect of this tooth. Retraction of the frenum with a periodontal probe revealed that the frenum is covering a class V carious lesion. Treatment of this problem area included excising the frenum followed by preparation of a free gingival graft recipient site (see free gingival graft procedure above). The sutured graft is sutured to an immovable bed of connective tissue verified by manipulating the cheek as described in Fig. 10.1. A Coe-Pack dressing can also be used to provide contact between the graft and the recipient site. After healing of the graft, the facial aspect of the tooth was accessible for oral hygiene measures and the facial class V carious lesion was restored with a composite restoration.

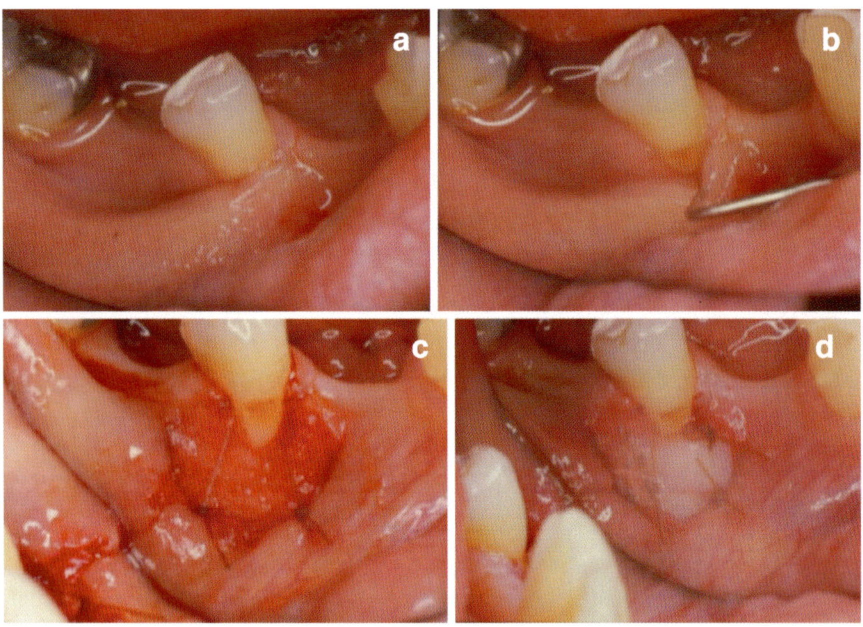

Fig. 10.2 Management of an aberrant frenum attachment with a free gingival graft. (**a**) Preoperative appearance of the buccal frenum attachment facial to #29. (**b**) Retraction of the frenum revealed that the frenum is concealing a facial carious lesion. (**c**) Excision of the frenum and preparation of a free gingival graft recipient site. (**d**) The apical end of the freed oral mucosa is sutured in order to maintain the apical position of the oral mucosa. The class V carious lesion was restored as soon as the facial tissue had matured sufficiently to allow cavity preparation without disrupting the graft attachment

The Free Connective Tissue Graft Procedure

Figure 10.3 provides the surgical steps in performing the free connective tissue graft on the facial aspect of a tooth with severe gingival recession. The primary consideration for survival of the connective tissue graft is to provide vascular support for the graft directly over the exposed root surface. This is accomplished by coronally positioning gingival tissue over the graft or by preparing laterally positioned pedicle flaps from each side of the exposed root surface, as shown

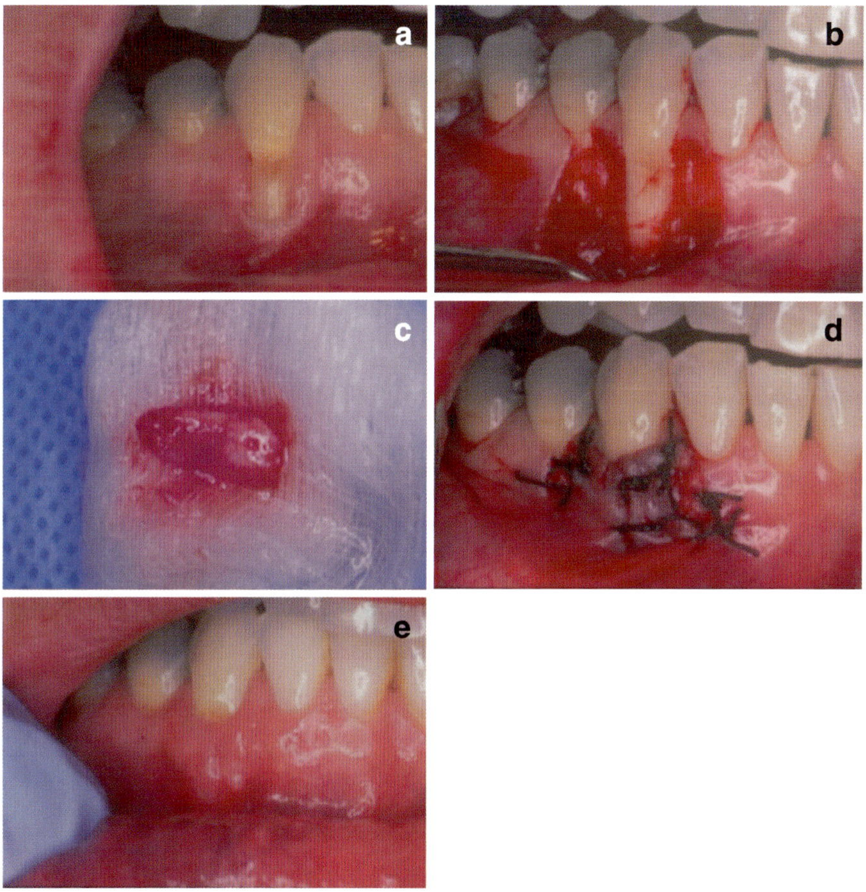

Fig. 10.3 Free connective tissue graft procedure to treat an isolated area of severe gingival recession. (**a**) The preoperative appearance of recession on the facial aspect of #27. (**b**) Preparation of the recipient site using a double pedicle flap procedure. (**c**) The harvested connective tissue graft should be as long as the recipient bed. (**d**) The palatal connective graft is harvested and secured to the recipient site. (**e**) The healed graft demonstrates a zone of keratinized gingiva and substantial root coverage where gingival recession was evident preoperatively. Photographs courtesy of Dr. Nina Hirshman

in Fig. 10.3b. Once the two pedicle flaps are released by dissecting full-thickness flaps using vertical incisions well beyond the mucogingival junction, the flap margins should contact each other on the facial aspect of the exposed root and lay passively in this location. The margins of the pedicle flaps are sutured together with interrupted sutures to achieve primary closure. The joined pedicle flaps provide vascular support to the underlying connective tissue graft when it is placed over the root surface. Therefore, the connective tissue graft will receive plasmatic support and eventual vascular ingrowth from the pedicle flaps during the graft healing. In contrast to the free gingival graft, the free connective tissue graft harvests palatal connective tissue without including the overlying epithelium. This is usually accomplished by making two parallel incisions in the palate approximately 1.5 mm apart followed by releasing the connective tissue at its base. Care must be taken to avoid severing the greater palatine artery during the harvesting of the graft [9]. The connective graft should be as long as the recipient bed (Fig. 10.3c). Once harvested from the palate, the connective graft is placed over the recipient site and secured to the mesial and distal keratinized gingiva at the coronal and lateral margins. The previously joined pedicle flaps are then secured over the connective tissue graft using interrupted and sling sutures as needed (Fig. 10.3d). This procedure is not associated with sloughing of the gingival keratinized epithelium. As shown, healing of free connective graft will provide substantial root coverage (Fig. 10.3e) so long as the interproximal tissue height is adequate as described for the Miller class type I or II defects [13–15]. Although an increase in keratinized tissue width is also evident, this procedure will not increase vestibular depth. In addition, root coverage is more predictable when the facial aspect of a prominent root is reduced by odontoplasty. Figure 10.3 shows that the free connective tissue graft procedure is an effective technique in managing root recession.

Surgical Management of High Frenum Attachment

The frenum release (frenectomy or frenotomy) procedure shown in Fig. 10.2 required the placement of a free gingival graft to provide vestibular extension and prevention of frenum reattachment. By contract, it is not always necessary to place a free gingival graft to maintain vestibular extension. Figure 10.4 shows a frenotomy procedure where the narrow frenum was excised with a scalpel and because the oral mucosa passively retracted from its attachment site, a free gingival graft was not needed at this site. For this procedure to be successful, it is necessary to excise the frenum from labial alveolar bone well apical to the frenum attachment (Fig. 10.4c) so that a triangular area of thin unmovable connective tissue is exposed. An interrupted suture can be placed in the apical extent of the exposed connective tissue bed in order to prevent reattachment of the frenum. The suture bridges the two sides of the excision site so that primary closure of the oral mucosa is achieved from the left and right tissue margins at the base of the exposed connective tissue bed. Release of the labial frenum can provide an improved gingival architecture for cleaning the facial aspects of the mandibular incisors.

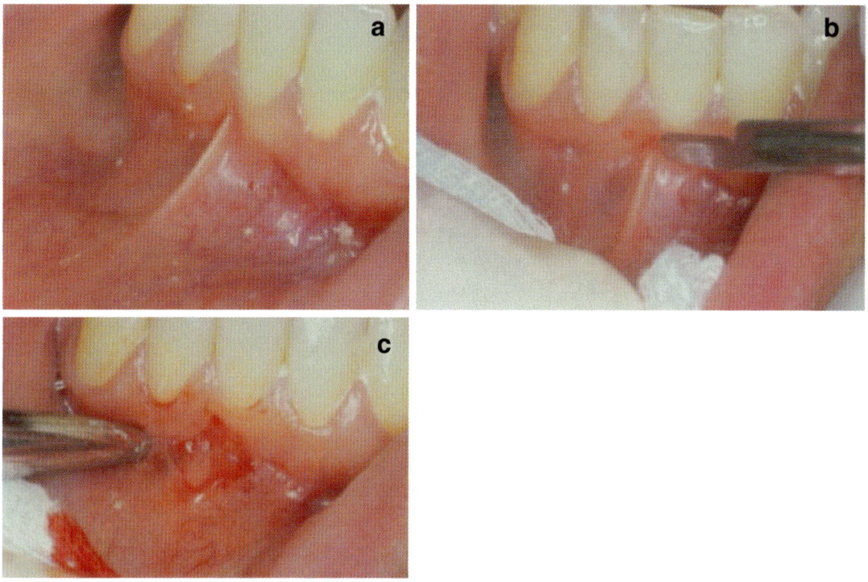

Fig. 10.4 Frenotomy procedure. (**a**) Note the high frenum attachment on the facial aspect of #24 with a minimal zone of keratinized gingiva. (**b** and **c**) Dissection of the labial frenum at its base using a Bard Parker scalpel. Also consider placing a free gingival graft over the exposed connective tissue if vestibular extension is desired or if a coronal positioning of gingiva is planned during a second procedure (see Figs. 10.1 and 10.2 for details)

Creating a Zone of Keratinized Gingiva on the Facial Aspect of Bone Level Implants

The last example shows the management of keratinized gingiva associated with bone level implants [16–19]. Two implants were placed distal to the lower left cuspid and were surgically covered. After osseointegration of the implants, it was noticed that the facial aspect of the mesial implant cover screw was exposed through a gingival fistula at the junction of the keratinized gingiva and oral mucosa. Because of the shallow buccal vestibule and the presence of a fistula to the cover screw, the keratinized gingival tissue was excised horizontally over the closure screws of the implants and two vertical incisions were extended laterally into the buccal vestibule for apical/lateral displacement of the keratinized gingiva much like an apically positioned flap procedure (Fig. 10.5b). The buccal flap was elevated as a pedicle flap and the implant closure screws were removed and replaced with healing abutments (Fig. 10.5c). The buccal flap was then adapted to the buccal alveolar process by using sling sutures around the healing abutments (Fig. 10.5d). Note that the excision of the gingival tissue was initiated lingual to the actual implants in order to ensure preservation of the maximum amount of keratinized gingival tissue on the facial aspect of the implants (Fig. 10.5e). After healing, the implants were restored with splinted crowns and the keratinized gingival tissue on the facial aspect was preserved (Fig. 10.5f).

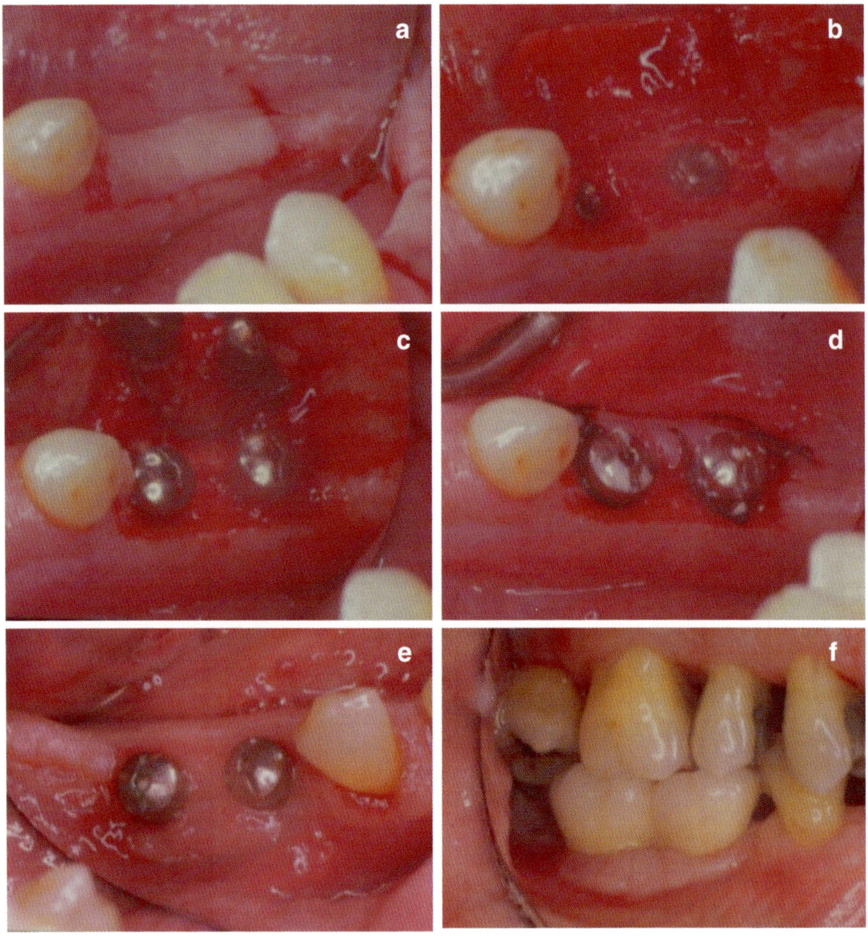

Fig. 10.5 Creating a zone of keratinized gingiva on the facial aspect of submerged implants during surgical uncovering. (**a**) Horizontal gingivectomy and vertical incisions used to reflect the keratinized gingiva covering two posterior implants (**b**) Lateral reflection of the flap that extends beyond the mucogingival junction as with an apically positioned flap. (C) Healing abutments placed on the implants. (**d**) The pedicle flap secured to the healing abutments with sling sutures. (**e**) Healing of the surgical site after 1 week. (**f**) Appearance of the healed keratinized gingiva facial to the restored implants

Summary Comments

These procedures demonstrate the use of free gingival grafts or laterally positioned flaps, or both, to provide not only a zone of keratinized tissue but also to increase vestibular depth. By doing so, the patient's oral hygiene measures are facilitated with better access to the facial aspects of teeth. The surgical principles outlined in this chapter also provide a guide for successful management of grafting procedures and manipulation of gingival tissues to help to preserve the dentition where dental disease persists due to the architecture of the gingiva. Connective tissue grafts are not generally helpful in this regard. Further information about these procedures can be found in the following references.

References

1. Cairo F. Periodontal plastic surgery of gingival recessions at single and multiple teeth. Periodontol 2000. 2017;75(1):296–316. https://doi.org/10.1111/prd.12186. PubMed PMID: 28758301
2. Carnio J, Camargo PM, Pirih PQ. Surgical techniques to increase the apicocoronal dimension of the attached gingiva: a 1-year comparison between the free gingival graft and the modified apically repositioned flap. Int J Periodontics Restorative Dent. 2015;35(4):571–8. https://doi.org/10.11607/prd.2386. PubMed PMID: 26133147
3. Lee YM, Kim JY, Seol YJ, Lee YK, Ku Y, Rhyu IC, Han SB, Choi SM, Chung CP. A 3-year longitudinal evaluation of subpedicle free connective tissue graft for gingival recession coverage. J Periodontol. 2002;73(12):1412–8. https://doi.org/10.1902/jop.2002.73.12.1412. PubMed PMID: 12546090
4. Sedon CL, Breault LG, Covington LL, Bishop BG. The subepithelial connective tissue graft: part II. Histologic healing and clinical root coverage. J Contemp Dent Pract. 2005;6(2):139–50. PubMed PMID: 15915213
5. Sedon CL, Breault LG, Covington LL, Bishop BG. The subepithelial connective tissue graft: part I. Patient selection and surgical techniques. J Contemp Dent Pract. 2005;6(1):146–62. PubMed PMID: 15719086
6. Sonick M. Root coverage: a comparison of techniques: the free gingival graft versus the subepithelial connective tissue graft. Pract Periodontics Aesthet Dent. 1992;4(8):39–48. PubMed PMID: 1286177
7. Wessel JR, Tatakis DN. Patient outcomes following subepithelial connective tissue graft and free gingival graft procedures. J Periodontol. 2008;79(3):425–30. https://doi.org/10.1902/jop.2008.070325. PubMed PMID: 18315424
8. Agarwal C, Tarun Kumar AB, Mehta DS. Comparative evaluation of free gingival graft and AlloDerm((R)) in enhancing the width of attached gingival: a clinical study. Contemp Clin Dent. 2015;6(4):483–8. https://doi.org/10.4103/0976-237X.169838. PubMed PMID: 26681852; PMCID: PMC4678545
9. Tavelli L, Barootchi S, Ravida A, Oh TJ, Wang HL. What is the safety zone for palatal soft tissue graft harvesting based on the locations of the greater palatine artery and foramen? A systematic review. J Oral Maxillofac Surg. 2018. https://doi.org/10.1016/j.joms.2018.10.002. PubMed PMID: 30395825.
10. Schmitt CM, Moest T, Lutz R, Wehrhan F, Neukam FW, Schlegel KA. Long-term outcomes after vestibuloplasty with a porcine collagen matrix (Mucograft((R))) versus the free gingival graft: a comparative prospective clinical trial. Clin Oral Implants Res. 2016;27(11):e125–e33. https://doi.org/10.1111/clr.12575. PubMed PMID: 25720794
11. Park JB. Widening keratinized tissue using modified free gingival graft. J Oral Implantol. 2016;42(1):114–6. https://doi.org/10.1563/aaid-joi-D-13-00353. PubMed PMID: 24968262
12. Hall WB, Lundergan WP. Free gingival grafts. Current indications and techniques. Dent Clin North Am. 1993;37(2):227–42. PubMed PMID: 8477866
13. Tatakis DN, Chambrone L, Allen EP, Langer B, McGuire MK, Richardson CR, Zabalegui I, Zadeh HH. Periodontal soft tissue root coverage procedures: a consensus report from the AAP Regeneration Workshop. J Periodontol. 2015;86(2 Suppl):S52–5. https://doi.org/10.1902/jop.2015.140376. PubMed PMID: 25315018

14. Miller PD Jr. A classification of marginal tissue recession. Int J Periodontics Restorative Dent. 1985;5(2):8–13. PubMed PMID: 3858267
15. Chambrone L, Tatakis DN. Periodontal soft tissue root coverage procedures: a systematic review from the AAP Regeneration Workshop. J Periodontol. 2015;86(2 Suppl):S8–51. https://doi.org/10.1902/jop.2015.130674. PubMed PMID: 25644302
16. Bassetti RG, Stahli A, Bassetti MA, Sculean A. Soft tissue augmentation procedures at second-stage surgery: a systematic review. Clin Oral Investig. 2016;20(7):1369–87. https://doi.org/10.1007/s00784-016-1815-2. PubMed PMID: 27041111
17. Bassetti RG, Stahli A, Bassetti MA, Sculean A. Soft tissue augmentation around osseointegrated and uncovered dental implants: a systematic review. Clin Oral Investig. 2017;21(1):53–70. https://doi.org/10.1007/s00784-016-2007-9. PubMed PMID: 27873018
18. Thoma DS, Naenni N, Figuero E, Hammerle CHF, Schwarz F, Jung RE, Sanz-Sanchez I. Effects of soft tissue augmentation procedures on peri-implant health or disease: A systematic review and meta-analysis. Clin Oral Implants Res. 2018;29(Suppl 15):32–49. https://doi.org/10.1111/clr.13114. PubMed PMID: 29498129
19. Wu Q, Qu Y, Gong P, Wang T, Gong T, Man Y. Evaluation of the efficacy of keratinized mucosa augmentation techniques around dental implants: a systematic review. J Prosthet Dent. 2015;113(5):383–90. https://doi.org/10.1016/j.prosdent.2014.10.001. PubMed PMID: 25681355

Management of Oroantral Communications

11

Kristopher Cooper

Anatomy

The maxillary sinus is the largest of the paranasal sinuses. These facial sinus cavities are empty spaces lined by respiratory type epithelium and thought to play a role in humidification of inspired air, contribution to vocal resonance, reduction in the overall weight of the head, and action as "crumple zones" to protect the brain in the event of facial trauma [1]. The maxillary sinus lies within the maxillary bone inferior to the orbits, and is roughly shaped like a pyramid with the base facing medially and the tip facing laterally toward the zygoma. There is marked variability between the morphology and size of maxillary sinuses among patients, but on average the volume of the adult maxillary sinus is about 15 mL. The sinus develops throughout childhood and usually reaches its maximum size by 18–20 years old [2, 3].

The inferior wall of the maxillary sinus at the posterior maxilla is contiguous with the hard palate medially, with the alveolus supporting posterior tooth roots laterally. Early anatomic studies suggested that out of all teeth, the second maxillary premolar had the closest relationship with the maxillary sinus [4] though more recent CBCT studies have shown that the apices of first and second maxillary molars are more likely to be intimately positioned near the sinus, and the root apices are often located above the level of the sinus floor [5]. Statistically, the palatal root of the first molar invades furthest into this space. The first premolar and the anterior teeth are usually located anterior to the sinus and are much less commonly involved [5].

K. Cooper (✉)
University of Pittsburgh School of Dental Medicine and University of Pittsburgh Medical Center, Pittsburgh, PA, USA
e-mail: Cooperkr@upmc.edu

E. M. Ferneini, M. T. Goupil (eds.), *Office-Based Maxillofacial Surgical Procedures*, https://doi.org/10.1007/978-3-030-22371-7_11

Etiology of Oroantral Communication

The extraction of posterior teeth is the most common etiology leading to the development of oroantral communication (OAC) and is implicated in over 90% of cases. With extraction of posterior teeth, the incidence of oroantral communication has been reported as being between 0.31% and 4.7% [6–10]. Pathologic conditions such as cysts/tumors account for between 4% and 5%, facial trauma about 1.3% [10].

Among dental extractions, data is widely variable regarding which teeth are most commonly implicated in OAC, but most authors agree that 1st/2nd molars are most **common** followed by third molars, then second premolars and finally first premolars [10, 11]. OAC formation as a result of third molar extraction has been extensively studied because of the commonplace nature of this procedure [9, 12–14]. OAC as a result of canine extraction has been reported, but seems to be vanishingly rare [10]. Reports of oronasal communications have been reported with extraction of anterior teeth. These instances are rare and are generally amenable to the same management strategies as oroantral defects of similar size [15].

Traumatic extraction with removal of alveolar bone, tuberosity fracture, or removal of adjacent teeth in the posterior maxilla also increase risk [16]. Lone standing molars are at higher risk because of the pneumatization of the sinuses around them [2, 4]. One major concern for OACs is epithelialization along the oroantral communication leading to oroantral fistula (OAF). Inflammatory changes in the periapical region of the teeth or existing sinusitis can increase the risk of OAC and eventual fistula formation due to the compromised nature of the bone and soft tissue that would normally separate the alveolus from the sinus [16].

Other surgical procedures can also increase the risk of OAC; oroantral or oronasal communication has been reported as a complication from Lefort I osteotomy [17]. OACs/OAFs from posterior dental implant failure or inflammation associated with endodontic materials have been reported. Pathologic conditions such as maxillary cysts and tumors have been implicated [10, 16]. Medication-related osteonecrosis of the jaws (MRONJ) has been reported in the maxilla with consequent development of OAC and OAF [18]. Osteoradionecrosis of the maxilla also has the potential to lead to OA fistula formation [19].

Preoperative Evaluation of OAC Risk

The proximity of maxillary tooth roots to the sinus floor should be carefully evaluated prior to extraction. Patients must be counseled on the risks of extraction and emphasis given to the risk of sinus communication if tooth apices are in close proximity. Various root-sinus classification systems have been described in the literature to help score and quantify OAC risk but haven't gained common use. On panoramic imaging, root apices superimposed or extending into the sinus are suggestive of increased risk of OAC [13]. However, panoramic radiographs have been shown to have poor reliability in predicting the risk of OAC prior to extraction [20, 21]. Consideration can be given to the use of CBCT or medical-grade CT in cases where the surgeon desires to more carefully evaluate the proximity of root apices to the sinus floor.

Traumatic extraction with removal of alveolar bone or extraction of teeth with periapical pathology further increases risk of communication [16, 22]. Regarding age, patients in the 4th decade of life seem to be at highest risk for sinus exposure with dental extraction [7, 19, 23, 24].

The risks of third molar extraction have been studied extensively, and many publications discuss them separately from the risks of extracting other teeth. Mesioangular position or other complete bony impaction, superimposition of roots over sinus, advanced patient age (>35 years), and even the need to make a longer incision are all factors shown to increase the risk of OAC during third molar extraction [9, 12–14, 25].

Immediate Management of OAC

Following extraction, if a communication is suspected but not visualized, providers should avoid curettage or probing of the socket as such manipulation may lead to enlarging a sinus exposure [23]. A *gentle* Valsalva maneuver can be used while looking for fog on a dental mirror that would indicate pathologic air passage from the sinus to the oral cavity. Additionally, a local anesthetic needle can be gently introduced to the root apex. The needle will pass through, and thus identify, a bony communication without causing significant damage to the sinus mucosa. Radiographs should be taken if the provider suspects that a root tip may have been dislodged into the sinus and can also be used to evaluate the size of the bony defect.

Once an oroantral communication is confirmed, it should be managed within 24–48 h to prevent epithelialization and fistula formation [10, 19, 23, 26, 27]. Seven to eight days after creation of the OAC, the epithelial lining of the tract completes organization and an OAF is present and permanent [19, 28]. Many authors contend that closure of bony defects smaller than 2 mm will likely close spontaneously [10, 16, 23, 29] while others have said this of defects smaller than 5 mm in the absence of infection [30, 31]. Most evidence suggests that if OACs >5 mm are left untreated, not only are they unlikely to close spontaneously, but 50% of the patients will likely experience sinusitis after 48 h and 90% after 2 weeks [32]. Unfortunately, there have not been adequate studies to show the likelihood of adequate healing based on OAC size. Thus, it is recommended by the author that OACs be handled in a conservative manner to avoid fistula formation, infection, and the need for future procedures. Surgeons should keep in mind risk factors other than OAC size, understanding that periapical infection associated with the tooth, or existing maxillary sinusitis also increases the likelihood of fistula formation [16, 22, 23, 33].

If an OAC occurs as a result of extraction, recommendations are as follows:

- *All patients* with suspected or diagnosed OAC should receive strict sinus precautions: No nose blowing, sneeze with open mouth, no straws, no smoking, no aggressive spitting for at least 3 weeks. Patients who use CPAP should have pressure of the machine modified for this time, or stop using it if possible (it is important to consult sleep specialist before implementing this).
  - <2 mm bony defect: pack the site with a collagen sponge and oversew with a figure-of-eight suture.
  - 2–5 mm bony defect: place collagen sponge with figure-of-eight sutures and prescribe 1 week oral antibiotics: Amoxicillin/Clavulanate (clindamycin for PCN allergic patients), antihistamines such as loratadine, and decongestants such as topical xylometazoline OR oral pseudoephedrine. Patients should be counseled against using nasal spray decongestants for more than 7 days in a row.
  - >5 mm bony defect: prescribe 1 week ABX, antihistamines, and decongestants plus flap procedure should be used. Options such as the buccal advancement flap and pedicled buccal fat pad graft are discussed in the next section [17, 23, 34].

Surgical Management of the OA Fistula

A patent bony defect between the maxillary sinus and the oral cavity may undergo fistulization, which occurs when Schneiderian cells and oral epithelial cells proliferate and migrate, fusing to one another [22]. OAFs can be classified, based on their location, into alveolo-sinusal, palato-sinusal, and vestibulo-sinusal [35]. A pathologic communication is likely to persist after the epithelial fusion and will require repair.

The following are common symptoms experienced by patients with OAF

- Fluid leaving the nasal cavity while drinking
- Changes in vocal resonance
- Nasal congestion
- Sanguineous or purulent drainage from the nose or mouth
- Chronic pain [22, 36]

Clinical exam may reveal erythema of the mucosa surrounding the fistula on the oral side. Purulence or discharge may be visible. Radiographs may reveal sinusitis or sinus polyposis as a result of maxillary sinusitis. Some fistulae may be well characterized by panoramic tomogram (Fig. 11.8). It may be advisable to obtain a maxillofacial CT scan to evaluate the size of the bony defect and to examine the severity of sinusitis (Fig. 11.1)

When choosing method of treatment, it is important to consider the size of the fistula, its location, and the presence/severity of associated maxillary sinusitis. Larger defects will require specialized procedures like the pedicled buccal fat pad advancement, and many patients exhibiting signs and symptoms of maxillary sinusitis may benefit from combined sinus surgery. Various treatment modalities and their indications are discussed in the following section.

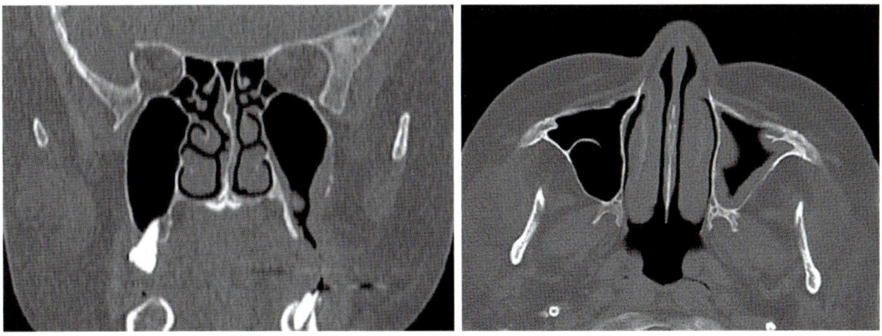

Fig. 11.1 55-year-old female who had a dental extraction in the UL quadrant within the last 6 months. Bony discontinuity of the alveolar bone and left maxillary floor consistent with oroantral fistula (OAF) in the left posterior maxilla. Image on the right shows associated left maxillary sinusitis. *Copyright 2018 Dr Ian Bickle. Image courtesy of Dr Ian Bickle and Radiopaedia.org. Used under license*

Anesthesia Plan and Preoperative Preparation

Many local flaps can be completed under local anesthesia or in-office sedation with local anesthesia. However, the combination of sinus surgery with flap repair of the fistula is best approached under general anesthesia. Nasotracheal intubation in the nare opposite the side of the defect is desirable. If this is not possible, an oral tube taped on the opposite side of the defect can be used [36].

It is recommended to prescribe antibiotics, antihistamines, and nasal decongestants as needed to treat active sinusitis preoperatively. Additionally, the fistulous tract to the sinus should be thoroughly irrigated. Preoperative impressions can be taken, from which a clasp-retained acrylic stent can be fabricated which will be worn for 2 weeks post op and protect the site from trauma postoperatively and prevent pressure differences across the site that could compromise healing [22, 36, 37].

Functional Endoscopic Sinus Surgery

Many OAFs have a component of maxillary sinusitis that, in many cases, should be evaluated and treated with a separate procedure. Leaving severe sinusitis untreated will put the OAF repair at risk of failure [22]. Maxillary sinusitis in this setting used to be surgically treated using a Caldwell-Luc procedure, during which the maxillary sinus is entered orally through the anterolateral sinus wall, the mucosa in the sinus is dissected, and an inferior antrostomy is performed through the lateral nasal wall to allow for drainage into the nasal cavity. Nowadays, functional endoscopic sinus surgery (FESS) has largely replaced the Caldwell-Luc procedure as a very effective and less invasive alternative. FESS was introduced in the 1980s, and involves introduction of a nasal endoscope, uncinectomy followed by a maxillary antrostomy to allow for drainage of the maxillary sinus, which allows for surgical removal of any obstruction to drainage, lavage and debridement of purulence and any significantly diseased mucosa [38–42].

Common Techniques for Repair

Local Buccal Flaps: Rehrmann and Moczair

The buccal advancement flap, initially described by Rehrmann [43] in 1936 and often referred to as a Rehrmann flap, is a common surgical technique available for repair of OAFs and closure of OACs. This technique is most useful for OAFs/OACs positioned at the alveolar crest or more buccal–palatal defects will require too much advancement and other techniques should be considered.

- For the Rehrmann technique, a trapezoidal flap is created by making 2 divergent full-thickness incisions extending into the vestibule away from the defect to be repaired.
- The flap is raised atraumatically, being sure to maintain it at full thickness and remove the periosteum cleanly from the maxilla (Fig. 11.2).
- A #15 blade should be used to excise the tissue from the fistula tract w/ 3 mm margin of healthy tissue [29]. Using a small dental curette or rongeur, any necrotic bone or remaining epithelial tissue within the tract should be removed.
- Using a fresh #15 blade, the periosteum of the raised flap can be scored horizontally which will allow for advancement of the flap toward the palate (dashed lines in Fig. 11.2)
- The flap should be advanced across the oroantral defect and sutured to intact palatal mucosa using horizontal mattress sutures [19, 22, 23, 35].

Another option, known as a sliding trapezoidal flap or Moczair flap, can be utilized when maintaining vestibular depth is of special concern. This procedure

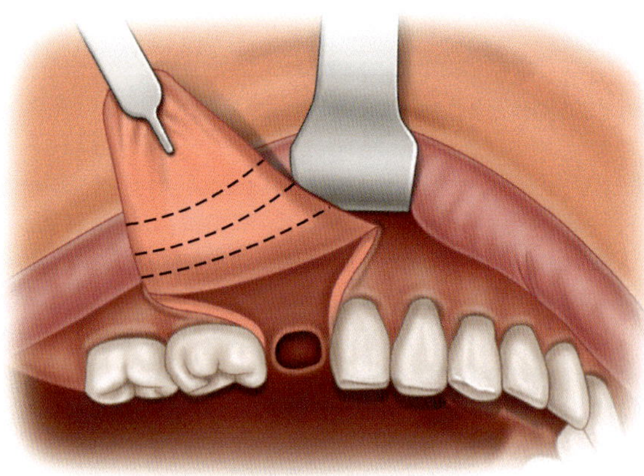

Fig. 11.2 A depiction of the buccal advancement (Rehrmann) flap. The underside of the flap is scored horizontally, through periosteum only, to allow advancement across the OA defect

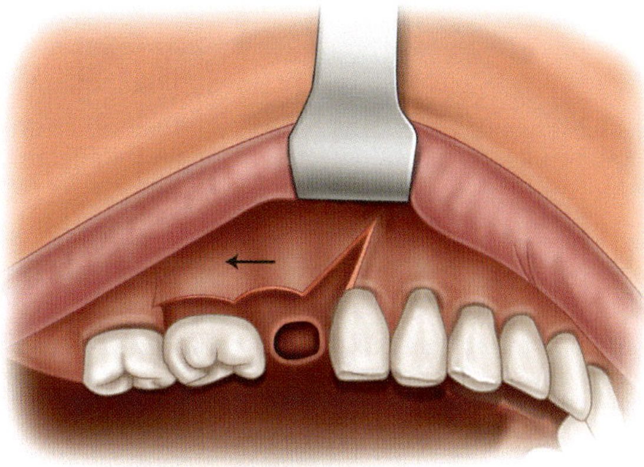

Fig. 11.3 The Moczair flap is shifted laterally (distally in this depiction) which prevents loss of vestibular depth as can be seen in the Rehrmann technique. The papilla from the adjacent tooth should be positioned and sutured over the defect. This technique is more often used in edentulous segments of maxilla (not shown)

is especially useful in edentulous maxillary segments. Its primary advantage is that it does not cause a significant reduction in depth of vestibule if properly performed.

- Trapezoidal flap is created and raised in a similar manner as the Rehrmann flap.
- Instead of advancing over the defect, it is shifted mesially or distally by 1 papilla, so that the papilla from an adjacent tooth covers the defect [44] (Fig. 11.3).

Drawbacks and complications include pain, bleeding, infection, and the risk of flap failure.

Importantly, the buccal advancement flap (Rehrmann) can reduce the depth of the vestibule presenting a problem for patients who use a denture. Some older studies suggest, though, that vestibular height is regained with time [6, 43, 45]. Others have suggested that this risk is significant in up to 50% of patients and can be permanent [44]. Patients should be counseled that a vestibuloplasty might be required in the future if the Rehrmann flap is used. The Moczair flap, because it is shifted laterally, leaves an area to heal by secondary intention, which can lead to more pain and potential for scar tissue formation [44].

Palatal Flaps

The soft tissue overlying the hard palate can be a useful donor site in the setting of oroantral defects. Many surgeons prefer this method because the palatal tissue is thicker and less prone to failure, and because the vestibular depth is left unchanged. These flaps can be used for larger defects when compared with buccal flaps, due to the thickness of palatal tissue [23]. One common method utilizes a finger type flap that is posteriorly based to allow for inflow from the greater palatine artery. The flap should be designed to allow enough length for adequate rotation, and enough width to cover the oroantral defect [23, 35, 46].

- Excise the epithelial tissue from the OAF with 3 mm margin and debride any necrotic bone with small curette or rongeur.
- After marking the flap outline, complete full-thickness incision along its outer edge. Bleeding vessels can be controlled with electrical cautery.
- The full-thickness flap is raised and rotated over the defect. Great care must be taken to ensure that the flap continues to get good blood flow from the greater palatine artery. An area of bony hard palate will be left exposed.
- Inadequate capillary refill might indicate a "kinking" effect of the vessels from turning the flap too sharply, which could lead to flap ischemic necrosis. The surgeon should ensure that the flap is pink and well perfused with adequate capillary refill prior securing it in place with interrupted nonresorbable sutures [23, 35, 46] (Fig. 11.4).

Modifications to this technique such as tunneling the flap under palatal mucosa [47] or basing the flap anteriorly for repair of tuberosity defects [48] have been described but are less common. The palatal flap can also be completed in a split-thickness manner, using the underlying connective tissue to cover the fistula and the superficial mucosal later to cover the donor site, thus avoiding leaving exposed bone in the mouth [24]. Finally, another modification is the palatal island flap in which an island of mucosa and submucosa is incised and lifted while still maintaining its connection with the neurovascular pedicle. This allows for greater rotation and mobility of the flap [49].

Disadvantages to this technique include pain associated with the denuded palatal donor site, which is exposed and left to heal by secondary intention. It can be covered using a stent, or an artificial dermis can be sutured in place [22]. Surface irregularities of the palate can also be seen after healing is complete. Finally, as mentioned above, the risk of flap necrosis is significant if the finger flap is turned too sharply [35].

Buccal Fat Pad

The pedicled buccal fat flap has been one of the most commonly used strategies for repair of OAF. It was described in 1977 by Egyedi and can be used in OA defects

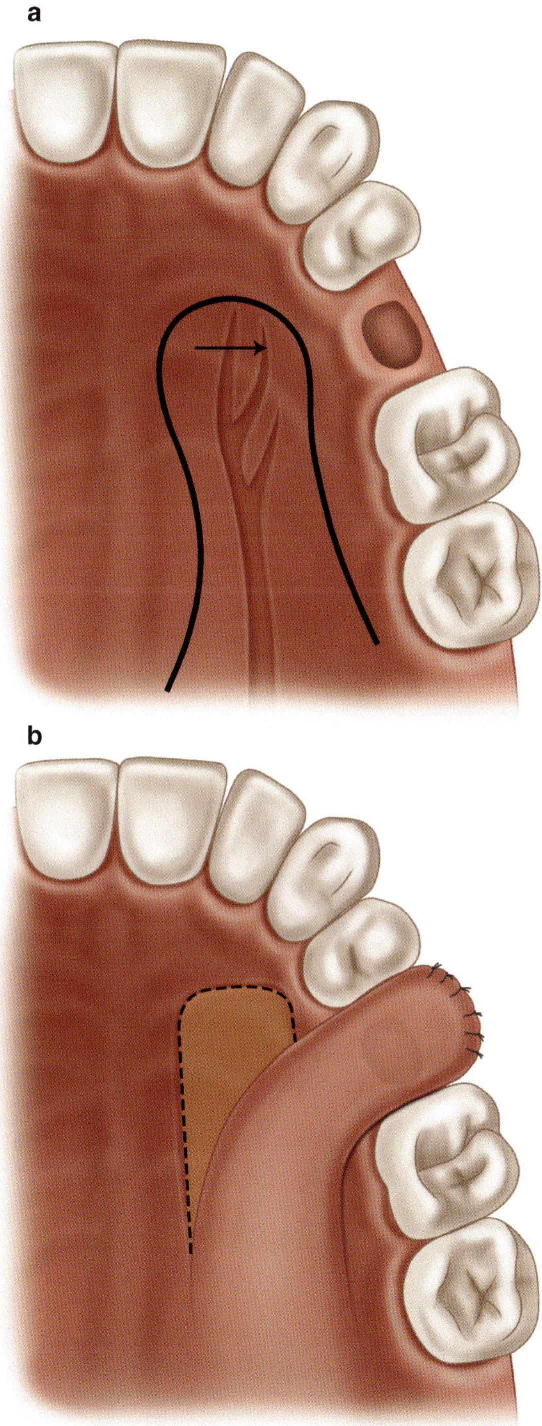

Fig. 11.4 Full-thickness palatal finger flap containing greater palatine vessels and nerves. This flap can be used for premolar and first molar OAFs but cannot usually be turned more posteriorly without risking ischemic necrosis

of up to 4 cm [50]. Some surgeons have shown that it can be used with success in even larger palatal defects of 5 × 6 cm [51]. Because of its versatility, the buccal fat pad has been commonly used in the setting of OAFs and has been used successfully in cases where a buccal advancement flap fails [52]. Studies comparing the pedicled buccal fat flap to the Rehrmann buccal flap have shown that both methods can be used with great success, though the Rehrmann flap must be used on smaller defects, can reduce vestibular depth, and cannot usually be used on palatal defects. However, more post op pain and swelling was noted in the pedicled buccal fat pad group, along with a temporary decrease in maximum interincisal opening [53].

The buccal fat pad lies behind the zygomatic arch and consists of four named processes: buccal, pterygoid, superficial, and deep temporal. The size and shape of the buccal fat pad is similar among individuals regardless of body habitus. Blood flow is supplied by branches of the maxillary, facial, and superficial temporal arteries [54, 55] (Fig. 11.5). Many surgeons are familiar with its location because it can be a clinical nuisance if it is encountered incidentally and herniates into the surgical field.

Pedicled buccal fat graft:

- Excise the epithelial tissue and any necrotic bone around the fistula w/ 3 mm margin of healthy epithelium.
- Design a trapezoidal buccal flap with divergent vertical incisions. Raise flap full thickness from alveolus and lateral wall of maxilla in a manner similar to the

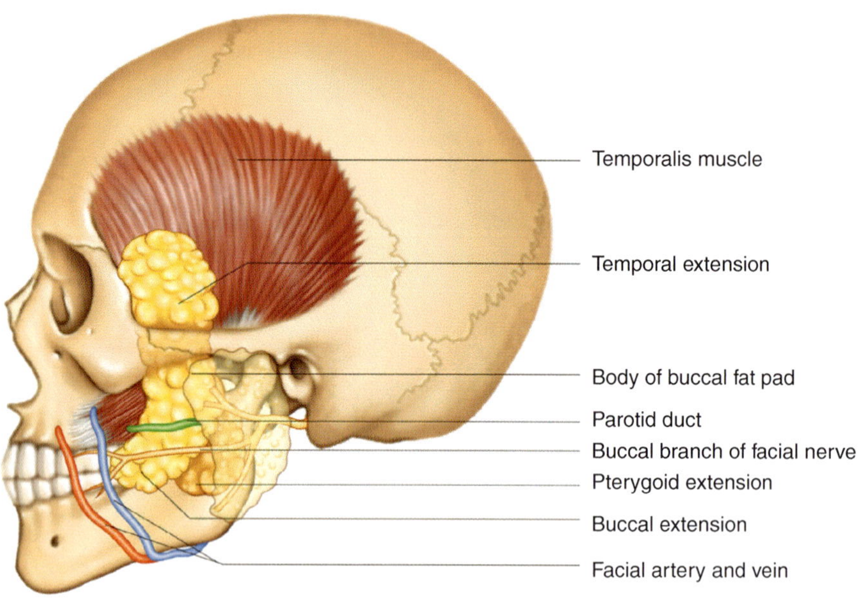

Fig. 11.5 Anatomic depiction of the buccal fat pad. *Image reprinted with permission, courtesy of Kim SG, Kim MK, Han W. The use of the buccal fat pad flap for oral reconstruction. Maxillofacial Plastic and Reconstructive Surgery. (2017) 39:5*

Rehrmann flap. Flap should be raised high into the posterior maxilla in the 1st/2nd molar area.
- 1 cm horizontal incision is made through the periosteum at the height of the posterior aspect of the trapezoidal flap.
- Blunt dissection carried out with a curved or straight Kelly until the capsule of the buccal fat is visualized. #15 blade is used to incise the capsule and expose fat.
- The buccal fat pad, which has a characteristic pale yellow appearance, is delivered into the oral cavity and guided to overlay the defect.
- Using 4-0 braided resorbable suture (such as Vicryl) or 4-0 nonresorbable suture such as nylon, the fat is secured to the palatal mucosa.
- The flap can be secured back into its original position, which usually leaves a significant portion of buccal fat exposed in the oral cavity (Fig. 11.6), which is acceptable. In some cases, a tension-free primary closure over the fat might be possible (Fig. 11.13).
- There is no need to use a surgical splint or dressing for these procedures if buccal fat is exposed [29, 52–54, 56].

Following the procedure, prescribe 7 days of antibiotics (Augmentin, clindamycin), decongestants, and antihistamines. Patients must follow a soft diet and strict sinus precautions for a minimum of 3 weeks. Buccal fat that is exposed has been

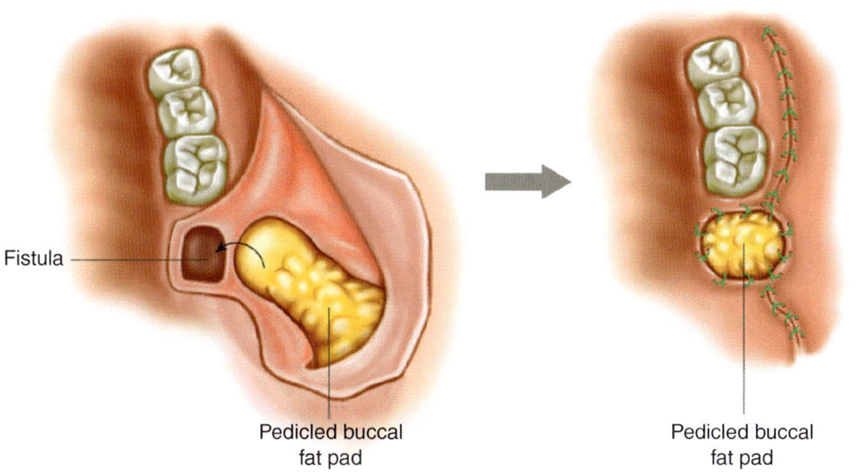

Fig. 11.6 Depiction of flap design and use of buccal fat for repair of an oroantral fistula. Note: the buccal fat remains exposed to the oral cavity immediately postoperatively and will epithelialize in 2–3 weeks. *Image reprinted with permission, courtesy of Kim SG, Kim MK, Han W. The use of the buccal fat pad flap for oral reconstruction. Maxillofacial Plastic and Reconstructive Surgery. (2017) 39:5*

shown to epithelialize in 2–3 weeks at which time the patient should be examined in the office [29, 54].

The following case, Figs. 11.7, 11.8, 11.9, 11.10, 11.11, 11.12, and 11.13, illustrates the use of the pedicled buccal fat graft for repair of an oroantral fistula (OAF). This is a 53-year-old male with history of oral squamous cell carcinoma and head/neck radiation presenting for extraction of remaining grossly carious dentition and repair of an oroantral fistula located at site of tooth #2 that was previously extracted by another provider.

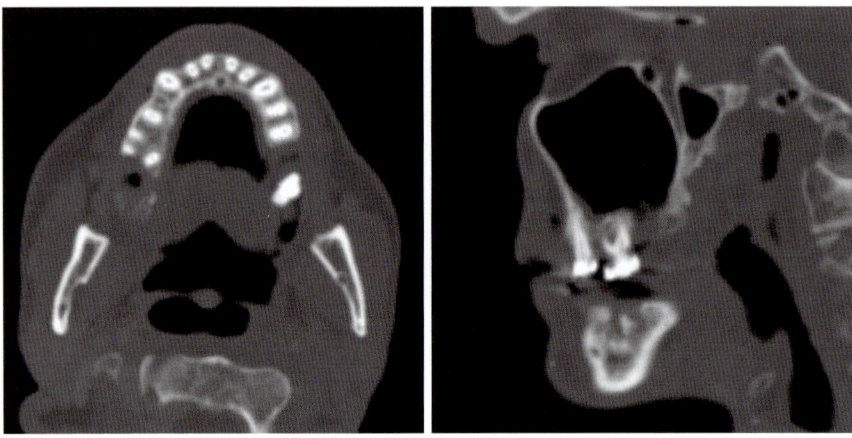

Fig. 11.7 Axial and sagittal computed tomography scan slices. Oroantral fistula, bony defect measuring approximately 10 mm across at site of previously extracted tooth #2

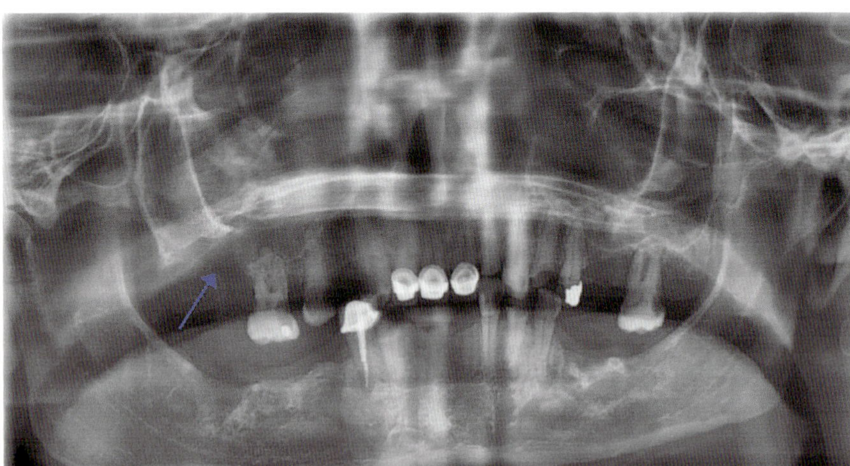

Fig. 11.8 Panoramic tomogram of the same patient, again showing bony communication between right maxillary sinus and oral cavity

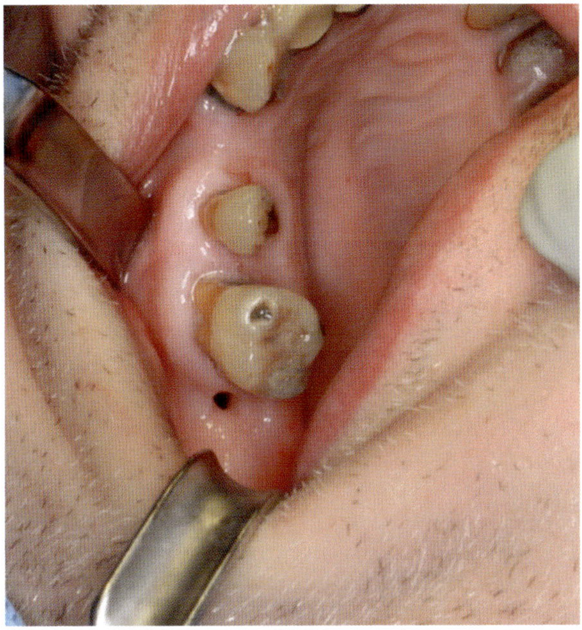

Fig. 11.9 Preoperative photograph revealing oroantral fistula located at the site of previously extracted tooth #2

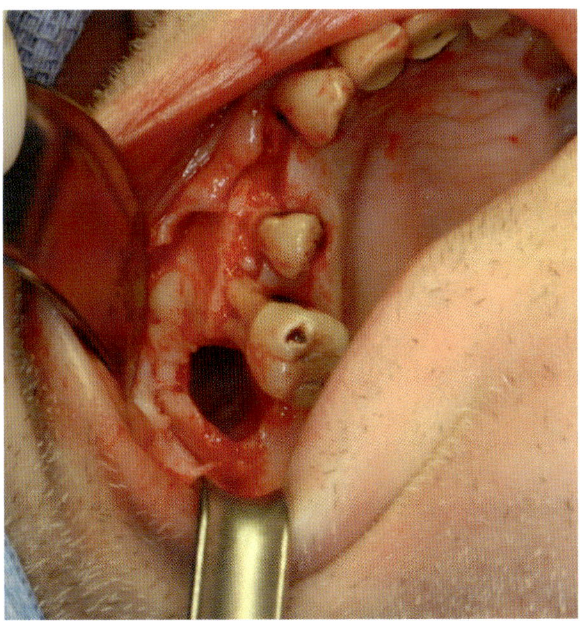

Fig. 11.10 Full-thickness mucoperiosteal flap raised and diseased mucosa excised from the fistula tract revealing the full size of the bony oroantral communication

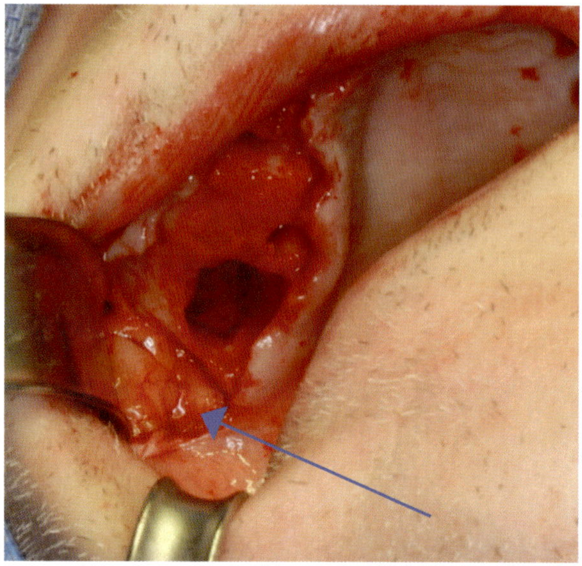

Fig. 11.11 Following the extraction of the adjacent carious teeth, the buccal fat pad capsule was exposed and excised revealing the characteristic pale yellow fat visible in the figure. Note that this patient had extraction of all his remaining teeth due to caries, and the extraction of adjacent teeth is not a necessary part of his fistula closure

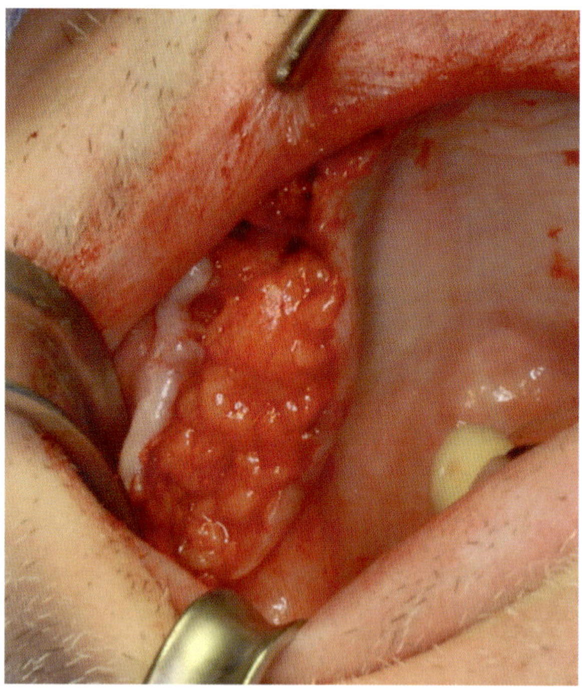

Fig. 11.12 The fat pad was bluntly dissected and gently pulled into the oral cavity to overly the oroantral defect and adjacent molar extraction site. The fat was secured with 4-0 Polysorb sutures to the palatal mucosa

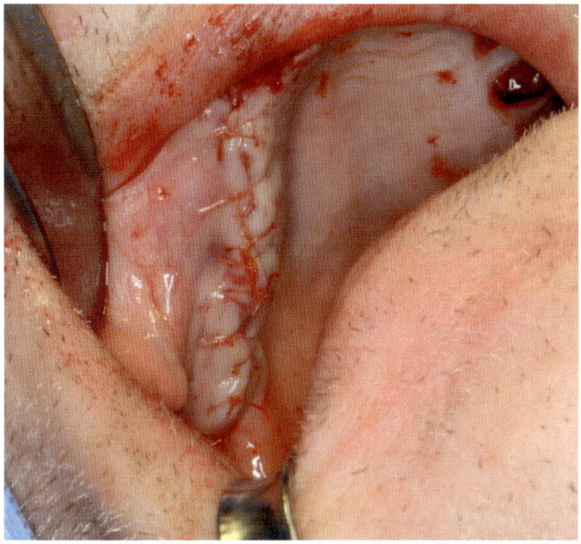

Fig. 11.13 After performing a horizontal scoring incision along the underside (periosteum) of mucoperiosteal flap, a tension-free primary closure was achieved using 4-0 Polysorb suture in interrupted fashion

Case and images courtesy of William L Chung DDS, MD, University of Pittsburgh School of Dental Medicine, University of Pittsburgh Medical Center

Less Common Surgical Approaches

Dorsal Pedicle Tongue Flap

The use of the dorsal tongue flap has been reported for certain applications. Oronasal and oroantral defects associated with clefting have been successfully managed with these flaps. Patients who have received head and neck radiation may benefit from this technique, as the tongue is richly vascularized. Because half of the tongue can be rotated and used without compromising function (speech, mastication swallowing), it offers a large amount of tissue coverage. Many different flap types have been described and used successfully including anteriorly + posteriorly based dorsal flaps, lateral tongue flaps [57].

These procedures are done in at least two stages, because the donor flap is left attached to the tongue to promote vascularization and reinnervation from the recipient site. After the flap is initially attached to the recipient site, patients are on a full liquid diet and sometimes put into maxillomandibular fixation to prevent motion and tearing of the flap. After 9–14 days, the flap is severed from the tongue [57].

Temporalis Flap

Pedicled temporalis flaps have been used for intraoral reconstruction, though this approach requires a coronal incision and thus is more invasive than other techniques. This technique is much less commonly used for OA fistula repair, mainly because the buccal fat technique is adequate for treatment of most large defects. Pourdanesh and colleagues described using coronoid process pedicled on temporalis muscle to repair a 15 × 20 mm defect in a patient [58].

Auricular Cartilage Graft

The use of auricular and nasal cartilage has been described—this involves harvesting a cartilage graft that will cover the bony defect and suturing it in place under the oral mucosa after excising the fistula contents. This technique is used in combination with other flap procedures such as the buccal (Rehrmann) flap or palatal flap. The use of cartilage is intended to create a barrier between oral and sinus mucosa where new bone can form. Cartilagenous and/or bony separation between the oral and sinus mucosa allows for future sinus augmentation procedures if posterior implant therapy is going to be considered [59, 60].

Bone Grafting

Some surgeons have employed bone grafting techniques in an effort to augment the fistula site to make implant placement possible at a later time. Symphysis monocortical block grafts along with particulate xenograft (Bio-oss) has been used to augment the sinus and separate the oral from sinus mucosa. These techniques are very similar to the use of auricular cartilage between sinus and oral mucosa as discussed above [8, 23]. Guided tissue regeneration techniques using type I collagen membrane and demineralized freeze-dried allograft have also been described in the setting of oroantral defects with excellent bone formation that made implant placement possible in the sites [61].

Other Techniques + Materials

Other surgical techniques for management of fistulae have been described but are less commonly used. Biocompatible materials such as gold foil, tantalum, and even aluminum have been used between oral mucosa and sinus mucosa during repair [62]. Hydroxyapatite and polymethylmethacrylate have also been used. Other allografts like fibrin glue and dura can be considered [23]. Finally, some surgeons describe successful closure of OACs with transplanting extracted third molars into the site [63].

Nonsurgical Management of the Oroantral Fistula

It is important to consider the contraindications of surgery, and management options for when surgery is not an option. Patients too ill to safely undergo general anesthesia, patients who refuse surgical intervention, and patients for whom surgery has failed, all may benefit from alternative management strategies.

Acrylic splints can be fabricated to serve as an obturator, preventing passage of air and fluids between the oral cavity and antrum. For patients whom surgery has failed, or patients unable to have surgery, this is an option for symptoms management and to potentially reduce the severity of sinusitis [37]. Patients with larger defects as a result of maxillary resections or complications associated with cleft palate also may benefit from therapy with an obturator. These larger oronasal and oroantral defects may not be amenable to reversal with surgery, and maxillofacial prosthodontic techniques need to be used [64].

Interestingly, a 2016 study was able to demonstrate a nonsurgical method of managing OA fistula and associated rhinosinusitis. In a group of 26 patients, 16 of them showed closure of an OA fistula >3 mm with only local decongestant therapy and 10 days of antibiotics. These results help to illustrate the importance of medical management (decongestants and antibiotics) as adjuncts to surgical techniques. In the study, local decongestants (4% lignocaine and 0.1% xylometazoline) were applied on cotton tipped applicators directly to the middle meatus for 15 min twice weekly, and antibiotics were administered 5 days IV then 5 days PO [38].

Conclusion

Oroantral communications (OACs) are relatively common occurrences in the practice of oral and maxillofacial surgery. They result most commonly from extraction of posterior maxillary teeth, procedures that are done very frequently in the practice of OMFS. A variety of flap techniques have been described to manage pathologic bony communications larger than 5 mm between the mouth and maxillary sinus, the most common of which are the buccal advancement flap, palatal flaps, and pedicled buccal fat graft. These techniques can also be used successfully for repair of oroantral fistulae (OAF). Several newer techniques for repair have been described, including bone-grafting techniques that are designed to allow for future implant placement at the site of the oroantral defect. These techniques show promise for improving the management of OACs and OAFs for the future.

References

1. Bell GW, Joshi BB, Macleod RI. Maxillary sinus disease: diagnosis and treatment. Br Dent J. 2011;201(3):113–8.
2. Ariji Y, Kuroki T, Moriguchi S, Ariji E, Kanda S. Age changes in the volume of the human maxillary sinus: a study using computed tomography. Dentomaxillofac Radiol. 1994;23(3):163–8.
3. Lorkiewicz-muszyńska D, Kociemba W, Rewekant A, et al. Development of the maxillary sinus from birth to age 18. Postnatal growth pattern. Int J Pediatr Otorhinolaryngol. 2015;79(9):1393–400.
4. Mustian WF. The floor of maxillary sinus and its dental, oral and nasal relations. J Am Dent Assoc. 1933;20:2175–87.
5. Tian XM, Qian L, Xin XZ, Wei B, Gong Y. An analysis of the proximity of maxillary posterior teeth to the maxillary sinus using cone-beam computed tomography. J Endod. 2016;42(3):371–7.

6. Abuabara A, Cortez AL, Passeri LA, de Moraes M, Moreira RW. Evaluation of different treatments for oroantral/oronasal communications: experience of 112 cases. Int J Oral Maxillofac Surg. 2006;35:155–8.
7. Punwutikorn J, Waikakul A, Pairuchvej V. Clinically significant oroantral communications—a study of incidence and site. Int J Oral Maxillofac Surg. 1994;23(1):19–21.
8. Cortes D, Rafael MC. Simultaneous oral antral fistula closure and sinus floor augmentation to facilitate dental implant placement or orthodontics. J Oral Maxillofac Surg. 2010;68:1148–51.
9. del Rey-Santamaría M, Valmaseda Castellón E, Berini Aytés L, Gay Escoda C. Incidence of oral sinus communications in 389 upper third molar extraction. Med Oral Pathol Oral Cir Bucal. 2006;11:334–8.
10. Franco-Carro B, Barona-Dorado C, Martinez-Gonzalez MJ, Rubio-Alonso LJ, Martinez-Gonzalez JM. Meta-analytic study on the frequency and treatment of oral antral communications. Med Oral Patol Oral Cir Bucal. 2011;16:682–7.
11. Visscher SH, Van roon MR, Sluiter WJ, Van minnen B, Bos RR. Retrospective study on the treatment outcome of surgical closure of oroantral communications. J Oral Maxillofac Surg. 2011;69(12):2956–61.
12. Lim AA, Wong CW, Allen JC. Maxillary third molar: patterns of impaction and their relation to oroantral perforation. J Oral Maxillofac Surg. 2012;70(5):1035–9.
13. Hasegawa T, Tachibana A, Takeda D, et al. Risk factors associated with oroantral perforation during surgical removal of maxillary third molar teeth. Oral Maxillofac Surg. 2016;20(4):369–75.
14. De carvalho RW, De araújo filho RC, Do egito vasconcelos BC. Assessment of factors associated with surgical difficulty during removal of impacted maxillary third molars. J Oral Maxillofac Surg. 2013;71(5):839–45.
15. Meechan JG. Oro-nasal fistula occurring after a simple dental extraction. Br J Oral Surg. 1983;21(3):229–32.
16. Güven O. A clinical study on oroantral fistulae. J Craniomaxillofac Surg. 1998;26:267–71.
17. Millesie, Gabriele. Complications: Maxilla. Oral and Maxillofacial Surgery, 3rd Ed. Chapter 47. 787-817
18. Oladejo O, Fu B, Sharp H, Hendy C. Oroantral fistula from bisphosphonate induced osteonecrosis of the jaw. J Surg Case Rep. 2010;2010(5):2.
19. Khandelwal P, Hajira N. Management of oro-antral communication and fistula: various surgical options. World J Plast Surg. 2017;6(1):3–8.
20. Nedbalski TR, Laskin DM. Use of panoramic radiography to predict possible maxillary sinus membrane perforation during dental extraction. Quintessence Int. 2008;39(8):661–4.
21. Lopes LJ, Gamba TO, Bertinato JV, Freitas DQ. Comparison of panoramic radiography and CBCT to identify maxillary posterior roots invading the maxillary sinus. Dentomaxillofac Radiol. 2016;45(6):20160043.
22. Dym H, Wolf JC. Oroantral communication. Oral Maxillofac Surg Clin N Am. 2012;24:239–47.
23. Visscher SH, Van minnen B, Bos RR. Closure of oroantral communications: a review of the literature. J Oral Maxillofac Surg. 2010;68(6):1384–91.
24. Sokler K, Vuksan V, Lauc T. Treatment of oroantral fistula. Acta Stomatol Croat. 2002;36:135–40.
25. Rothamel D, Wahl G, d'Hoedt B, Nentwig G, Schwarz F, Becker J. Incidence and predictive factors for perforation of the maxillary antrum in operations to remove upper wisdom teeth: prospective multicentre study. Br J Oral Maxillofac Surg. 2007;45:287–391.
26. Skoglund LA, Pedersen SS, Holst E. Surgical management of 85 perforations to the maxillary sinus. Int J Oral Surg. 1983;12:1–5.
27. Amaratunga NA. Oro-antral fistulae- a study of clinical, radiological and treatment aspects. Br J Oral Maxillofac Surg. 1986;24:433–7.
28. Haanaes HR, Pedersen KN. Treatment of oroantral communication. Int J Oral Surg. 1974;3(3):124–32.
29. Hanazawa Y, Itoh K, Mabashi T, Sato K. Closure of oroantral communications using a pedicled buccal fat pad graft. J Oral Maxillofac Surg. 1995;53:771–5.

30. Awang MN. Closure of oroantral fistula. Int J Oral Maxillofac Surg. 1988;17:110–5.
31. von Wowern N. Correlation between the development of an oroantral fistula and the size of the corresponding bony defect. J Oral Surg. 1973;31:98.
32. Del Junco R, Rappaport I, Allison GR. Persistent oral antral fistulas. Arch Otolaryngol. 1998;114:1315–6.
33. von Wowern N. Frequency of oro-antral fistulae after perforation to the maxillary sinus. Scand J Dent Res. 1970;78:394.
34. Campbell J, Cheung A, Nagy L. Complications of dentoalveolar surgery oral and maxillofacial surgery, vol. 22. 3rd ed. p. 298–310.
35. Borgonovo AE, Berardinelli FV, Favale M, Maiorana C. Surgical options in oro-antral fistula treatment. Open Dent J. 2012;6:94–8.
36. Chambers MD, Chung WL. Oroantral Fistulas. Operative Otolaryngology: Head and Neck Surgery. 3rd ed. Chapter 105: Elsevier; 2017. p. 700–4.
37. Sanas S, Adaki R, Shigli K, Raikar S, Jain P. Prosthodontic management of oroantral fistula: a case report. Int J Sci Stud. 2017;5(2):256–8.
38. Mishra AK, Sinha VR, Nilakantan A, Singh DK. Rhinosinusitis associated with post-dental extraction chronic oroantral fistula: outcomes of non-surgical management comprising antibiotics and local decongestion therapy. J Laryngol Otol. 2016;130(6):545–53.
39. Nemec SF, Peloschek P, Koelblinger C, Mehrain S, Krestan CR, Czerny C. Sinonasal imaging after Caldwell-Luc surgery: MDCT findings of an abandoned procedure in times of functional endoscopic sinus surgery. Eur J Radiol. 2009;70:31–4.
40. Andric M, Saranovic V, Drazic R, Brkovic B, Todorovic L. Functional endoscopic sinus surgery as an adjunctive treatment for closure of oroantral fistulae: a retrospective analysis. Oral Surg Oral Med Oral Pathol Oral Radiol Endod. 2010;109:510–6.
41. Hajiioannou J, Koudounarakis E, Alexopoulos K, Kotsani A, Kyrmizakis DE. Maxillary sinusitis of dental origin due to oroantral fistula, treated by endoscopic sinus surgery and primary fistula closure. J Laryngol Otol. 2010;124:986–9.
42. Joe Jacob K, George S, Preethi S, Arunraj VS. A comparative study between endoscopic middle meatal antrostomy and Caldwell-Luc surgery in the treatment of chronic maxillary sinusitis. Indian J Otolaryngol Head Neck Surg. 2011;63:214–9.
43. Rehrmann A. A method of closure of oro-antral perforation. Dtsch Zahnarztl Z. 1936;39:1136–9.
44. von Wowern N. Closure of oroantral fistula with buccal flap. Rehrmann versus Moczair. Int J Oral Surg. 1982;11(2):156–65.
45. Eneroth CM, Martensson G. Closure of antro-alveolar fistulae. Acta Otolaryngol. 1961;53:4474857.
46. Killey HC, Kay W. Observations based on the surgical closure of 362 oroantral fistulas. Int Surg. 1972;57(7):545–9.
47. Sakakibara A, Furudoi S, Sakakibara S, et al. Tunnel technique for the closure of an oroantral fistula with a pedicled palatal mucoperiosteal flap. J Maxillofac Oral Surg. 2015;14(3):868–74.
48. Salins PC, Kishore SK. Anteriorly based palatal flap for closure of large oroantral fistula. Oral Surg Oral Med Oral Pathol Oral Radiol Endod. 1996;82:253–6.
49. Genden EM, Lee BB, Urken ML. The palatal island flap for reconstruction of palatal and retromolar trigone defects revisited. Arch Otolaryngol Head Neck Surg. 2001;127(7):837–41.
50. Pl E. Utilization of the buccal fat pad for closure of oro-antral and oro-nasal communications. J Max-Fac Surg. 1977;5:41.
51. Fujimura N, Nagura H, Enomoto S. Grafting of the buccal fat pad into palatal defects. J Craniomaxillofac Surg. 1990;18:219.
52. Batra H, Jindal G, Kaur S. Evaluation of different treatment modalities for closure of oro-antral communications and formulation of a rational approach. J Maxillofac Oral Surg. 2010;9(1):13–8.
53. Nezafati S, Vafaii A, Ghojazadeh M. Comparison of pedicled buccal fat pad flap with buccal flap for closure of oro-antral communication. Int J Oral Maxillofac Surg. 2012;41:624–8.
54. Scott P, Fabbroni G, Mitchell DA. The buccal fat pad in the closure of oro-antral communications: an illustrated guide. Dent Update. 2004;31(6):363–4, 366.

55. Kim SG, Kim MK, Han W. The use of the buccal fat pad flap for oral reconstruction. Maxillof Plast Reconstr Surg. 2017;39:5.
56. Colella G, Tartaro G, Guidice A. The buccal fat in oral reconstruction. Br Assoc Plast Surg. 2004;57:326–9.
57. Kim YK, Yeo HH, Kim SG. Use of the tongue flap for intraoral reconstruction: a report of 16 cases. J Oral Maxillofac Surg. 1998;56:716–9.
58. Pourdanesh F, Mohamadi M, Samieirad S, Banimostafaee H, Sadeghi HM. Closure of large oroantral communication using coronoid process pedicled on temporalis muscle flap: a new alternative approach. J Craniofac Surg. 2013;24(4):1399–402.
59. Isler SC, Demircan S, Cansiz E. Closure of oroantral fistula using auricular cartilage: a new method to repair an oroantral fistula. Br J Oral Maxillofac Surg. 2011;49:e86–7.
60. Ozkan A, Durmaz CE. Alternative surgical management of oroantral fistula using auricular cartilage. J Clin Exp Dent. 2015;7(2):e339–41.
61. Sandhya G, Reddy PB, Kumar KA, Sridhar reddy B, Prasad N, Kiran G. Surgical management of oro-antral communications using resorbable GTR membrane and fdmb sandwich technique: a clinical study. J Maxillofac Oral Surg. 2013;12(3):254–9.
62. Steiner M, Gould AR, Madion DC, et al. Metal plates and foils for closure of oroantral fistulae. J Oral Maxillofac Surg. 2008;66:1551.
63. Kitagawa Y, Sano K, Nakamura M, Ogasawara T. Use of third molar transplantation for closure of the oroantral communication after tooth extraction: a report of 2 cases. Oral Surg Oral Med Oral Pathol Oral Radiol Endod. 2003;95(4):409–15.
64. Singh M, Bhushan A, Kumar N, Chand S. Obturator prosthesis for hemimaxillectomy patients. Natl J Maxillofac Surg. 2013;4(1):117–20.

Exposure of Impacted Teeth

12

Killian MacCarthy and Tarryn MacCarthy

Introduction

Most patients with impacted teeth are referred to the surgical practice by an orthodontist. The surgeon has the opportunity to educate the patient on their clinical options and to develop a team-based approach with the general dentist, the orthodontist, the surgeon, and the autonomy of the patient.

After third molars, maxillary canines are the second most commonly impacted tooth [1]. Following the maxillary canine in prevalence of impaction is the mandibular second premolar followed by the mandibular canine. Treatment plans for either extraction of the impacted tooth or exposure and bonding of the impacted tooth should be discussed with the orthodontist prior to surgery to assess the likelihood of success for dental alignment. This decision is made with the aid of a complete workup and accurate diagnosis.

Radiographic Analysis

The workup for surgical management of unerupted teeth requires imaging to guide the consultation. In the past, the buccal shift rule for plain film radiographs (Clarke's rule) was the mainstay for surgical and orthodontic planning of impacted teeth. The SLOB Rule: Same Lingual, Opposite Buccal is a mnemonic device stating that if the X-ray tube shifts and the tooth follows in the same direction as the tube moves in the second image then the impacted tooth is on the lingual. If

K. MacCarthy (✉)
OMS Associates, South Portland, ME, USA
e-mail: killian@maineoralsurgery.com

T. MacCarthy
Mbrace Orthodontic, Falmouth, ME, USA

E. M. Ferneini, M. T. Goupil (eds.), *Office-Based Maxillofacial Surgical Procedures*, https://doi.org/10.1007/978-3-030-22371-7_12

the tooth moves in the opposite direction to the direction of the tube shift then the tooth is on the buccal relative to the adjacent teeth. Lingual and buccal in this example refers to the three-dimensional reference of the impacted tooth relative to the adjacent tooth roots. This rule on 2-dimensional radiographs is unreliable in certain situations in which the tooth is positioned almost directly over the middle of the alveolar ridge or when the crown of the tooth is in one plane and the root apex is in another.

Today current 3D computed tomography allows the dentist to determine the exact position and location of the impacted tooth and with specific accuracy as to the position of the crown and the root apex of the impacted tooth. The discrepancy between the crown and root location can have significant effect on the best direction of orthodontic force and the best location for surgical access. 3D computed tomography allows direct measurement that can be translated to the surgical field with ease (see Fig. 12.1). Limited field view radiographs can isolate the alveolus to 3–4 tooth segments. A full skull cone beam CT can be 3–6 times the radiation dose of a panoramic radiograph [2]. Reduced field views also reduces the possible liability for missed pathology in the skull or spine as those structures can be avoided in the imaged field. With 3D computed tomography the oral surgeon and the orthodontist can more accurately assess for damage to the adjacent teeth and if orthodontic forces might cause further resorption. Lastly, the 3D images can evaluate the palatal bone quality and thickness if temporary anchor screws are going to be used.

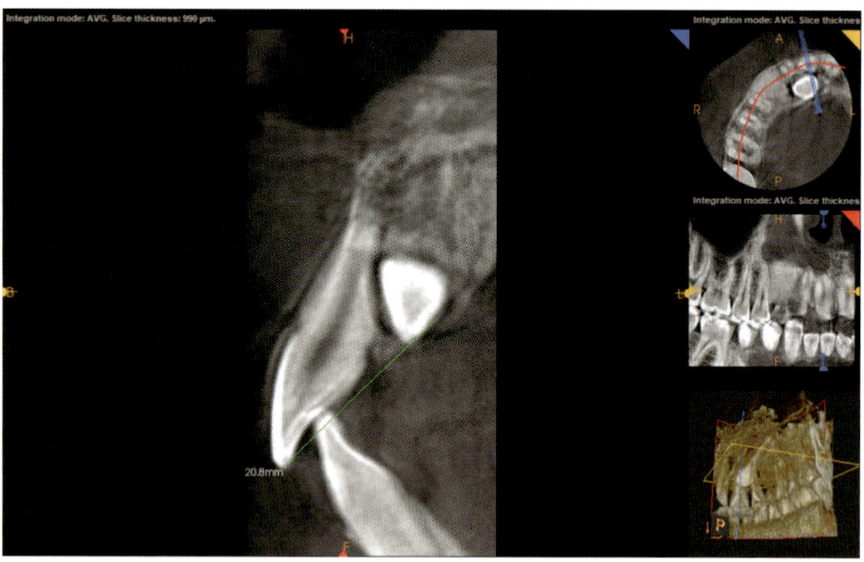

Fig. 12.1 Direct measurement of the canine. Computed Cone Bean Tomography allows direct measurement of the position of teeth that then can be translated to the mouth using a surgical caliper. Measuring from the incisal edge is helpful if the impacted tooth is not easily located. In this particular image the canine is 20 mm from the incisor

Clinical Examination

The clinical exam can suggest the location of an impacted tooth. 85% of impacted maxillary canines are located on the palate [1, 3]. Clinically one might find a bulge in the mucosa to suggest the location of the crown or possibly the root. This hard bulge can be detected on the palate or on the buccal surface of the alveolus, although it is not always perceptible. Mobility of teeth on the mesial or distal of the impacted tooth might indicate root resorption. Root resorption has typically been diagnosed on 2D radiographs. 3D computer tomography is able to discern root resorption in three dimensions much sooner than is shown on the 2D radiographs which will show resorption only at a more advanced stage. Early diagnosis of root resorption of teeth adjacent to impacted teeth is critical in the long-term treatment planning of the orthodontic management of the case. This knowledge could change the treatment plan from a surgical exposure case to an extraction case [4].

Potential Complications

Informed consent is critical. The major and common risks should be reviewed with the patient prior to treatment. The following is a list of the most common (not exhaustive) complications with surgical exposure of impacted teeth:

- Debonding of the bracket can occur for many reasons. If good isolation was not achieved during the surgical exposure or if the bracket was not properly tested for adequate bond strength either situation could result in bracket bond failure. Often bracket bond failure could require a second surgical procedure to reattach the bracket to the tooth.
- The tooth can become nonvital from the exposure procedure requiring root canal therapy. Aggressive exposure of the tooth beyond the CEJ or retractor pressure at or above the CEJ can lead to external resorption of the tooth. High heat or clinical trauma with a high-speed bur to the impacted tooth could also lead to dental devitalization. Surgical limitations for adequate bonding of a bracket to the impacted tooth may require placing a wire ligature around the tooth. This can also lead to external root resorption as the wire is likely to sit at or below the CEJ.
- External root resorption can result from damage to the root during surgery (as described above), as a result of previous trauma to the root of the impacted tooth or to the adjacent teeth (which have stimulated cementoclastic activity), damage to the roots when teeth collide within the bone, and from heavy orthodontic forces.
- Prior to the use of presurgical 3D imaging, there was a higher risk of inadvertently exposing the roots of adjacent teeth during the procedure. It is prudent to still talk about damage to adjacent teeth during the exposure process as this is still a risk.
- Ankylosis of the impacted tooth is also a risk factor. Ankylosis can be a preexisting condition that is better diagnosed with 3D imaging. It is still possible,

however, that ankylosis is not initially diagnosed and only recognized clinically after surgical exposure and once orthodontic forces are applied. Ankylosis can be clinically diagnosed when intrusion or adverse movements of the adjacent teeth occur. It is wise to mention that the impacted tooth might need to be removed if it cannot be moved orthodontically.

- Gingival defects around the impacted tooth subsequent to final orthodontic positioning can later require gingival or connective tissue grafting.

Surgical Treatment

Good surgical technique culminates from presurgical and orthodontic treatment planning. The location of the impacted tooth will dictate the surgical approach. The direction of planned orthodontic forces will also dictate the surgical approach. The younger patient might have interceptive Phase 1 orthodontics (removal of primary teeth, palatal expander, Trans Palatal Arch, etc.) to avoid the need for more involved surgical intervention later in life or to avoid impending root resorption of adjacent teeth [4]. Temporary skeletal anchors can allow the orthodontist to intervene sooner with anchorage that TADS offer compared to the mixed dentition. The chain can be attached to the temporary anchorage device or a fixed orthodontic appliance prior to comprehensive orthodontic treatment. In a patient with mixed dentition an open window technique can be used prior to placement of the orthodontic appliances. The majority of patients in the author's office choose to have this procedure done with moderate sedation or general anesthesia. Though it can be comfortably done under local anesthesia, it is recommended in the case of palatal impacted canines the patient should consider a sedation option. As full patient cooperation will support a better surgical outcome.

Methods that can be used for exposing impacted teeth include (1) gingivectomy, (2) apically repositioned flap, (3) closed eruption technique, or (4) open window technique.

1. The gingivectomy procedure removes the tissue that is covering the impacted tooth. This tissue removal can be accomplished with a scalpel, electrocautery, or a laser. At least 3 mm of attached tissue must remain in order to ensure mucogingival health of the tooth. Adequate anesthesia requires infiltration on the buccal and palatal or anesthetic block. Once anesthetized, retraction or gentle pulling of the lips or cheeks allows proper evaluation for the location of the mucogingival junction. Proper identification of the mucogingival junction will allow accurate measurement of the biologically needed 3 mm of attached tissue [5].
2. An apically repositioned flap creates a finger flap that is elevated and placed in an apical direction to better expose the impacted tooth when it is on the buccal aspect of the alveolus. One risk of using this technique is a nonideal esthetic result of the gingiva. This is a significant concern if considering this technique for an impacted central incisor. If the impacted tooth is positioned very high apically compared to the adjacent teeth this technique can lead to mismatch of attached tissue which is especially obvious in the anterior maxilla. This risk is

increased when the bulk of the crown is above the mucogingival junction. Uncovering the tooth at this location can require a large amount of bone removal that can lead to unstable bony and gingival support of the tooth. There can also be a concern of partial re-intrusion or relapse of the impacted tooth in the retention phase of orthodontics [6].

The surgical technique for an apically repositioned buccal flap involves parallel vertical incisions over the impacted tooth and a midcrestal incision down to the bone. Next, a full-thickness mucoperiosteal flap is elevated. The flap is stabilized apically with 2–4 sutures to the adjacent tissue. If converging incisions (toward the CEJ) are made it can be difficult to suture the narrower flap tip to the wider apical tissue. The surgical exposure ideally leaves two-thirds or more of the clinical crown exposed.

3. For many palatally impacted teeth a closed eruption technique can be used. For access to a palatally impacted canine a neck of tooth incision can be used with release from the 2–3 teeth mesially and distally to the location of the impacted tooth. A full-thickness flap can be elevated. A presurgical 3D radiograph can be used to accurately locate the impacted tooth. Calipers are used to transpose the position of the tooth beneath the bone on the images to the surgical field. A thin shell of bone mostly overlies the impacted tooth and can be easily removed with an elevator or an interproximator elevator (Karl Schumacher New York). If using a handpiece and bur to remove the bone, then judicious bone removal should be employed to ensure only bone is removed and to avoid damage of the impacted tooth and adjacent tooth roots. Once the tooth is located and the covering bone removed, the follicular tissue, which is very vascular, can make bonding of a bracket difficult due to copious oozing. It is wise to remove as much follicular tissue as possible without violating or curetting the CEJ to ensure a drier surgical field to work with, ideally bonding in the first attempt.

   A self-retaining cheek retractor can be used to help hold the lips apart, freeing up a retractor hand. Moisture control is paramount to good bond strength. Sterile cotton rolls keep the field dry by cutting them into thirds or quarters so they can fit easily into the wound. The number of control rolls or cotton roll pieces used is marked on the surgical field with a surgical marker. Confirmation that the presurgical and postsurgical cotton roll count is the same is imperative. A remaining cotton roll in the wound can lead to postoperative infection. If there is concern about accurate counts then a small 1 × 1 cm or 1 × 4 radiopaque neuropatty can be used to help keep the field dry. This will allow for intraoperative or postoperative confirmation of retained sponges with a postoperative radiograph. If cotton rolls or neuropatties are to be used they are placed at the apex of the flap wedging it open and absorbing the apical oozing blood (see Fig. 12.2). Holding the neuropatty or cotton roll in a snap instrument using a sweeping blunt dissection motion can help remove oozing follicular tissue. If not using packing material, then consider suturing the tissue edge of the flap to the mouth prop and having your assistant keep the field dry. Be aware that positioning of the suction tip is important so as not to drag the saliva and blood across the tooth surface which will prevent adequate bonding.

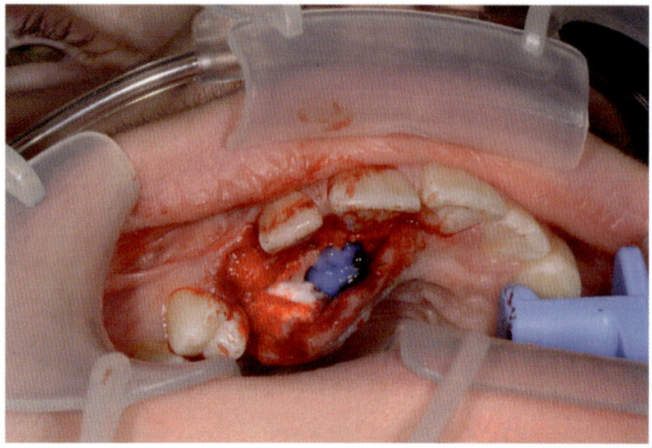

Fig. 12.2 Cotton roll wedge: The cotton roll is being used on the lateral side of the flap as a wedge to hold open the site. Secondarily is helping with hemostasis in the field. The blue etchant is being used to prepare the tooth for bonding of a bracket

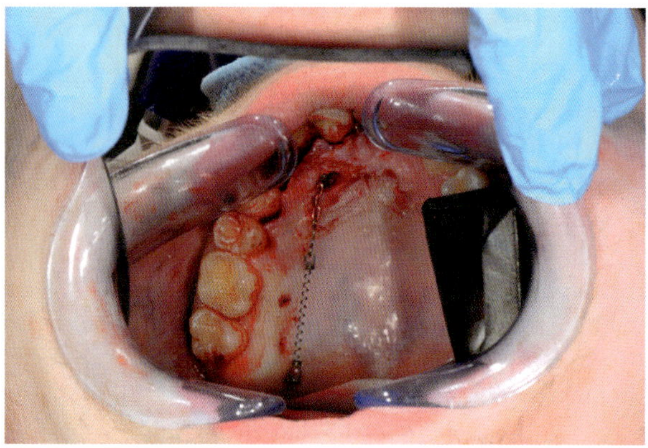

Fig. 12.3 Tissue punch window: If the orthodontist wants an open window then once the tooth is located via an envelope flap a large tissue punch can be used to make a window over the tooth. In this particular image a temporary anchor device is being used to bring this tooth into the mouth

4. If the orthodontist requests an open window exposure, then the same type of tooth incision can be used as in the closed approach. A tissue punch can be used to make a gingival window right over the impacted tooth through the elevated flap (see Fig. 12.3). The elevated flap with a tissue punch through the flap is preferred. This is as opposed to using a tissue punch alone, directly over the impacted tooth, with subsequent laser or electrocautery of the adjacent tissue. There tends to be more tissue removal with the direct punch access and bleeding can be challenging to control. The elevated flap technique leaves a less painful, smaller wound for the patient's recovery. If a directly punched tissue window is used it is recommended to place a dressing over the exposed tooth to be left in place to prevent gingival regrowth [6]. Bracket placement with composite will also lessen gingival regrowth over the impacted tooth. If the periodontal dressing comes loose the gingiva can cover over the bracket within a week. Tissue regrowth might necessitate laser or electrocautery removal to help the final eruption of the tooth.

For successful bonding of a bracket the shape of the tooth and the location of the planned bonding have to be considered. Frequently the palatal surface of an impacted maxillary canine is bonded. Accurate relay of the precise location of bracket bonding on the impacted tooth is valuable for the orthodontist in planning his/her directional forces of eruption. There are several bracket and cleat configurations with chain attached that can be used. If the patient has thick palatal tissue using a tall cleat or bracket can slow tooth eruption. If the bracket is to be placed on the buccal surface of the tooth for a buccally impacted tooth then a low profile bracket should be used, especially if they have a thin gingival biotype (see Fig. 12.4). If a bracket debonds during a closed eruption then it can lead to fenestration of the bracket through the gingiva. If this happens mid-treatment it can lead to gingival defects that will likely necessitate grafting [7].

Bonding of the bracket takes an organized team when keeping the field dry. A mid-surgical time-out before etching the tooth will make sure all instruments and materials are ready to go on the field. Any instrument delay might require another attempt at bonding the bracket if the field gets contaminated with blood. Fuji GC glass ionomer premixed ampules are mixed in a triturator. There are many additional cements on the market that will accomplish the bonding. There are different preparations that can be hand mixed instead of triturated. Premixed cements provide a consistent bond success rate. Time-outs should confirm the correct bracket, tooth, etchant ready, rinse ready, light curing gun turned on and ready to go. Any delay can lead to blood oozing over the field leading to weaker bond strength leading to premature failure. Follow the manufacturer's recommendation for etchant, etching times, and rinse amount. Injecting local anesthesia or trading out the cotton roll with one that is soaked in local anesthesia can control apical bleeding. A firm pull on the bracket will ensure a strong bond to the enamel. A photograph prior to closure or note to the orthodontist will be helpful if there is an unusual bracket placement. Miscommunication about the location of the bracket placement on the tooth might hamper the mechanics of the forced chain eruption.

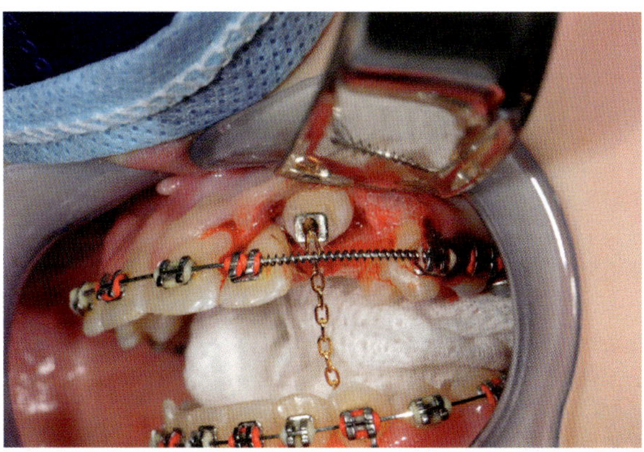

Fig. 12.4 Low profile buccal bracket: This canine is impacted buccally so a buccal flap is used and too high for an open approach. A flat low profile bracket is being deployed to prevent fenestration through the attached tissue

The chain attached to the bracket or cleat can be tunneled under the mucosal flap to the crest of the ridge. For a palatally impacted canine pass the chain through a small nick made in the palatal mucosa where the tooth is located. This allows the orthodontist to see where the tooth is located and how to direct the orthodontic forces.

The next step will be to attach the chain to the arch wire, TAD, or fixed orthodontic appliance. The orthodontist will instruct how to tie the chain and how much force is to be applied to the chain. The chain can be attached with wire, suture, spring, or elastic thread to the arch wire or orthodontic appliance. This preference is dependent on the orthodontist and should be discussed during the treatment planning stage. If there is misunderstanding as to the orthodontist's preference, passive ligation of the chain to the nearest fixed appliance will suffice. The orthodontist will apply the necessary forces to the impacted tooth and in the direction necessitated by the position of the tooth relative to the dental arch.

Closure of the wound can be achieved with vicryl or chromic suture. Chromic sutures risk early resorption and leave inflamed mobile flap edges that take longer to heal. The excess chain links are removed so as to not dangle and bother the patient. One should be careful cutting the chain links as they can fly away from the site and get dislodged under the flap or in the airway if not properly protected.

If the orthodontist wants to use TADS for anchorage, they can be placed either preoperatively or intraoperatively. Both placement times are aided with 3D images that show bone quality, quantity, and location of adjacent roots. If TADS are placed preoperatively, they can be placed at the consultation appointment under local anesthesia.

Consider palatally impacted canines that need to be distalized away from the incisors prior to bringing them into the arch. Two paramedian TADS parallel to the first molar (if adequate bone height allows) can be used for skeletal anchorage in conjunction with a soldered Trans Palatal Arch (TPA) borne on the first molars and the two TADs. Once the TADs have been placed the orthodontist will scan the TADs with an intraoral scanner and send the STL file to the Orthodontic Lab. The lab fabricates an appliance that attaches to the first molars with bands and caps that seat over the TADS with o-caps (see Fig. 12.5). Once the TPA has been cemented in place the patient returns for the surgical uncovering of the impacted tooth or teeth. After surgical exposure of a palatally impacted tooth the tissue is edematous and raw. The sore tissue complicates an accurate scan of the palate and the newly placed TADs due to the bulk of the scanner wand. It is because of this that the surgery is done in two steps: first, placement of the TADs and second, surgical exposure and bond of the impacted tooth/teeth (see Fig. 12.5). TAD placement can happen at the time the impacted tooth is uncovered if no additional orthodontic appliance needs fabrication to fit over the TADs. Once the impacted tooth is uncovered and bonded with a bracket and chain, it can be attached directly to the lone TAD. Palatal skeletal anchorage allows palatally impacted canines to be guided away from the roots of

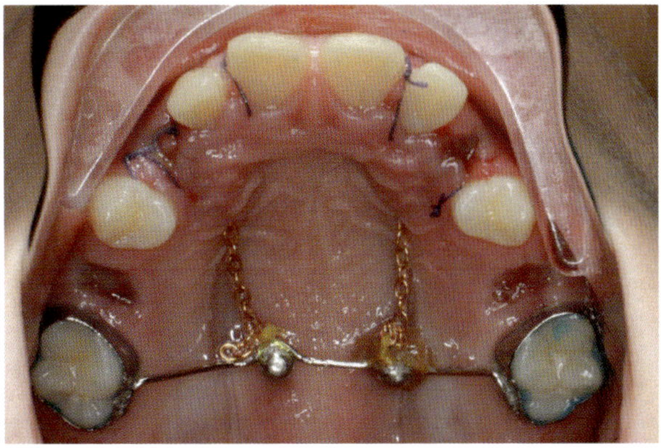

Fig. 12.5 TPA bar with tads: The lab fabricated the TPA bar to attach to the TADS over the comfort caps that sit over the round head of the TAD. The bar does not impede in the surgical exposure

the anterior teeth without the need for buccal fixed orthodontic appliances (braces). This is advantageous for patients who are still in the mixed dentition and are not yet ready for comprehensive orthodontic treatment and for patients who have already experienced root resorption of the anterior teeth. Patients with root resorption will benefit from less time in traditional orthodontic appliances and it is beneficial to remove the assaulting impacted tooth prior to starting comprehensive orthodontics.. Placing two TADs for a TPA allows for a backup should one of the TADs come loose. If you place one TAD and are considering retraction forces directly to the TAD with a nickel-titanium coil spring the TAD location should allow sufficient anterior-posterior distance for the activation of the spring. A nickel titanium spring is attached as close to the bracket as possible along the chain to allow a consistent force on the tooth. The excess gold chain link is removed. The TAD head is protected with a comfort cap that allows the patient's tongue to better tolerate the appliance.

Postsurgical follow-up is scheduled one week to ten days later. This allows for a wound check and removal of the vicryl sutures that might linger for 3–4 weeks more. Coordination with the orthodontist will ensure follow-up with the patient 2–3 weeks after the procedure. The orthodontist will activate or continue the activation of the eruption of the tooth. 6–12 months post-surgery the tooth will erupt into the mouth depending on the age and density of the bone and the position of the canine.

If the surgeon can see the orthodontic issues of treatment, they will have a better understanding of bracket position and the direction of orthodontic forces. Early treatment planning and discussion concerning tissue management can be critical. If the orthodontist understands the issues of incision design, bone quality, and TAD placement he/she will appreciate why, despite previous discussion, the bracket or TAD placement often needs to be decided at the time of surgery. 3D radiographs have taken a lot of the guess work out of the treatments and allow informed discussions between specialists.

References

1. Rayne J. The unerupted maxillary canine. Dent Pract Dent Rec. 1969;19:194–204.
2. Signorellie L, Patacas R, Peltomäki T, Schätzle M. Radiation dose of cone-beam computed tomograph compared to conventional radiographs in orthodontics. J Orofac Orthop. 2016;77(1):9–15.
3. Stellzig A, Badra EK, Komposch G. The etiology of canine tooth impaction-a space analysis. Fortsjer Kieferothop. 1994;55(3):97–f.
4. Bjerklin K, Guitrokh CH. Maxillary incisor root resorption induced by ectopic canines. Angle Orthod. 2011;81(5):800–6.
5. Kockich V, Mathews DP. Impacted maxillary central incisors. In: Kockich V, Mathews DP, editors. Orthodontic and surgical management of impacted teeth. Chapter 1. Hanover Park, IL: Quintessence Publishing Company; 2014. p. 1–25.
6. Mathews DP, Kokich VG. Palatally impacted canines: the case for preorthodontic uncovering and autonomous eruption. Am J Orthod Dentofacial Orthop. 2013;143(4):450–8.
7. Becker A, Casap N, Chaushu S. Conventional wisdom and the surgical exposure of impacted teeth. Orthod Craniofac Res. 2009;12(2):82–93.

Molar Uprighting

13

Daniel Beauvais, Jonny Feldman, and Elie M. Ferneini

Introduction

Surgical uprighting is a technique commonly used to correct the position of an impacted tooth to bring it into stable occlusion. While the mandibular third molar is the most commonly impacted tooth in the mouth, oral and maxillofacial surgeons routinely evaluate impacted teeth elsewhere in the oral cavity for both extraction and alignment purposes. Impacted second molars are of particular interest, as these teeth often can be brought into alignment by utilizing a number of different treatment modalities, thereby preventing the unnecessary extraction of an otherwise healthy tooth. This chapter explores the etiology of impacted molars, indications and contraindications for uprighting, different uprighting methods including advantages and disadvantages, and potential complications of each technique utilized.

Etiology

While the true incidence of impacted mandibular second molars has not been well studied, estimates of approximately three out of every 1000 patients have been cited [1, 2], and the situation usually occurs unilaterally. There are several proposed etiologies for the impacted second molar, including both systemic and local factors. Systemic factors include endocrine conditions such as hypothyroidism and

D. Beauvais (✉)
Department of Oral and Maxillofacial Surgery, School of Dental Medicine, University of Connecticut, Farmington, CT, USA

J. Feldman
Division of Orthodontics, UConn School of Dental Medicine, Farmington, CT, USA

E. M. Ferneini
Beau Visage Med Spa, Greater Waterbury OMS, Cheshire, CT, USA

E. M. Ferneini, M. T. Goupil (eds.), *Office-Based Maxillofacial Surgical Procedures*, https://doi.org/10.1007/978-3-030-22371-7_13

hypopituitarism, febrile diseases, Down syndrome, and irradiation, which may influence permanent teeth impaction. However, these conditions often involve multiple teeth [3, 4]. Local factors include inadequate space for eruption due to arch-length deficiency, excessive distance between the first and second molars resulting in lack of guidance by the distal root of the first molar, prolonged primary tooth retention, lack of mesial movement of the permanent first molar, supernumerary teeth, and tumors, which can obstruct eruption [4–9]. It is essential to determine the cause of impaction in each case that is evaluated in order to properly sequence the treatment, especially if other specialists are involved with the patient's oral care.

Evaluation

Evaluation of impacted molars is done through clinical examination and use of radiographs. When multiple teeth are found to be impacted, the clinician should suspect and evaluate for a systemic cause. The ideal age of uprighting of mandibular second molars varies, but is typically between ages 11 and 14, or before root formation is complete [7]. Radiographic evaluation is essential for determining tooth position and level of impaction, as well as root formation. Common modalities include panoramic and periapical films, though the use of in-office cone beam computed tomography (CT) scans has become commonplace for determining tooth shape, crown-root relationship, and tooth inclination [10]. Conventional radiographs can be used to determine the three-dimensional position of an impacted tooth by utilizing the principle commonly referred to as the SLOB rule, or same-lingual, opposite-buccal. A common method is to use two separate periapical films, and shift the tube horizontally between exposures. The unerupted tooth will appear to move in the same direction as the tube if it is lingually positioned, and will appear to move in the opposite direction as the tube if it is buccally positioned. This is not always required when evaluating an impacted tooth, but becomes useful when the position of the tooth and surgical access are in question. Additionally, a thorough medical history will aid in determining if any systemic causes should be suspected.

Indications for Uprighting

For the majority of non-third molar impactions, the most ideal treatment outcome is aligning the tooth in a functional position. Alignment utilizes both surgical and orthodontic treatment strategies, and it is essential to coordinate between specialists during the surgical planning process. Extraction of the impacted tooth is necessary if there is evidence of root pathology or association with pathologic lesions, based on clinical and radiographic exam. Additionally, if the tooth is tipped lingually or buccally, the tooth should not be surgically uprighted since intact buccal and lingual plates are necessary for stability.

Advantages of molar uprighting include improved function, periodontal health, and decreased caries risk for the impacted molar and adjacent teeth. In addition, the presence of a functional molar prevents the supraeruption of the opposing dentition. Periodontitis is a major concern with partially erupted teeth, as pseudopocket formation makes teeth exceedingly difficult to cleanse. By uprighting an impacted molar, the pseudopocket is minimized and the crown becomes more easily cleansable, creating an environment for a healthy gingival attachment and better plaque control [11].

Treatment Options

Techniques for uprighting impacted second molars include surgical uprighting and orthodontic repositioning. Some of the major advantages of surgical uprighting are immediate repositioning, low cost, and a relatively high rate of success with proper surgical technique.

Surgical exposure and bonding of an orthodontic appliance allows for active guidance of the impacted tooth into a functional position. The disadvantages of orthodontic repositioning are, the patient must have orthodontic treatment underway in order to deliver an appropriate force system to upright the impacted tooth, sufficient space must be present in the dental arch for the eventual position of the impacted tooth, and the extended treatment time for repositioning. Advantages to orthodontic repositioning include a lower incidence of ankylosis, pulp necrosis, and root resorption when compared to surgical uprighting. The literature for both surgical uprighting and orthodontic repositioning is limited to mostly case reports, though results have demonstrated reliable success with long-term stability for both treatment categories.

Surgical Uprighting

Surgical uprighting can be safely performed with local anesthesia, with supplementation by intravenous sedation when appropriate. Following adequate anesthesia, a full-thickness mucoperiosteal flap is elevated to expose the site of the impacted molar. There are different opinions regarding extraction of the third molar when uprighting an impacted second molar. Some authors state that it is important to extract the third molar at the time of uprighting a second molar, as the presence of the third molar may limit the movement of the second molar [12–14] (Figs. 13.1a, b and 13.2a, b). However, it has also been advocated to keep

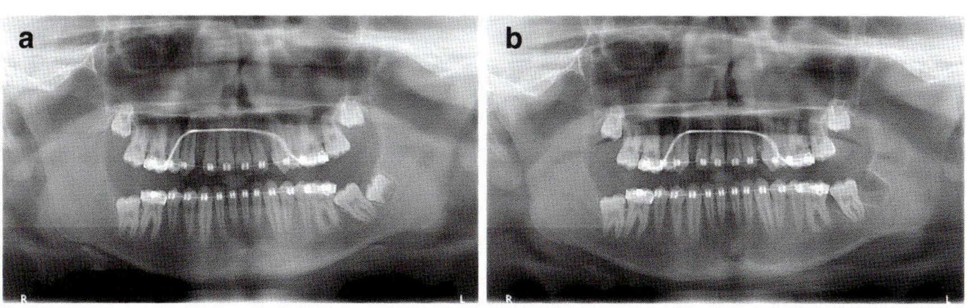

Fig. 13.1 (**a**) Preoperative panoramic imaging of impacted teeth #17 and 18. Note the mesioangular angulation of tooth #18. (**b**) Postoperative panoramic imaging after removal of tooth #18 and surgical uprighting of tooth #17

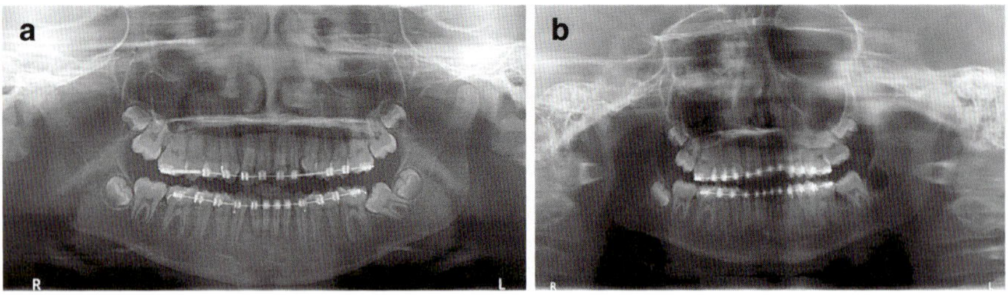

Fig. 13.2 (**a**) Preoperative panoramic imaging of impacted teeth #17 and 18. Note the mesioangular angulation of tooth #18. (**b**) Postoperative panoramic imaging after removal of tooth #18 and surgical uprighting of tooth #17

the third molar, if possible [1]. It is theorized that the third molar may provide some immediate stability to the uprighted second molar, and furthermore, if the second molar eventually needs to be extracted, the third molar can be used to replace it via transplantation or orthodontic repositioning. Either strategy may be employed, though discussion should take place with the patient during the surgical planning process. Alveolar bone is then removed around the crown of the second molar with a bur, allowing for exposure of the height of contour of the crown. A dental elevator is then used to apply distal and occlusal forces in order to position the mesial marginal ridge of the second molar at the same level as the distal marginal ridge of the adjacent first molar. The uprighted molar should not be tipped more than 90° [11]. If the third molar was not previously extracted and limits the elevation of the second molar, the third molar should then be extracted at this time. Once the second molar has been successfully elevated into the desired position, the occlusion is checked to ensure that no occlusal forces are present on the uprighted molar [11]. The surgical site is then irrigated with normal saline and gingiva is closed with 3-0 chromic gut sutures. In order to achieve added stability, in the case of gross mobility on the elevated second molar, orthodontic brackets may be utilized. Attachments can be bonded onto the second molar and the adjacent first molar, if the patient does not already have orthodontic appliances. A 28-gauge ligature wire tied in a figure-eight fashion can be used to splint the first and second molar together. Alternatively, the teeth can be splinted using a wire that is secured to the first and second molars using acid etched composite resin. A postoperative panoramic radiograph should be obtained to provide a baseline for follow-up evaluation. Postoperative instructions for the patient are similar to those of other extractions. Swelling, bleeding, and pain are normal in the immediate postoperative period, and postoperative analgesics may be prescribed. Importantly, it is paramount that the patient avoids bite forces to the uprighted tooth during the initial healing period, or approximately two weeks [1]. The patient should be seen for follow-up in one week to re-evaluate the stability of the uprighted molar, and again in 6 months for repeat panoramic radiograph [6].

Orthodontic Repositioning

In general, orthodontic molar repositioning consists of an attachment that is bonded to the surgically uncovered buccal or distobuccal surface and the subsequent application of an uprighting force along with an appropriate anchorage unit to counteract the uprighting forces. The application of the uprighting force may involve elastics or elastomeric chains, NiTi-coil springs, superelastic NiTi wires, a variety of uprighting springs, or wires. The anchorage for the repositioning forces may involve mini-implants, surgical plates, partial or comprehensive orthodontic appliances. The orthodontic repositioning of a molar is complicated by its distal position in the arch and the difficulty in applying the correct force system for repositioning. The use of mini-implants (MIs) has increased in recent years. The main advantages are their ability to reposition teeth with minimal orthodontic appliances and their ability to limit applying unwanted forces to anchor teeth [15]. MIs may require less intra-oral hardware, which may lead to better patient satisfaction [16].

A systematic review done by Magkavali-Trikka et al. discussed the use of MIs with direct and indirect anchorage. Direct anchorage occurs when the application of the uprighting force is on the Mi or surgical plates. When the MIs or surgical plates are used to counteract the forces on the anchorage unit it is called indirect anchorage. The use of MIs with direct anchorage was studied in 15 papers included in this systematic review, and were used in situations that called for correction of molars in the sagittal plane. The MIs were placed in either the retromolar area, vertically in the alveolar ridge of a mesial edentulous site, or mesial to the mandibular molar and between the roots of the adjacent teeth to achieve direct anchorage. Forces were created using either coil springs or by buttons and elastomeric chains. For mesially tilted second molars, buttons were placed on the buccal, lingual, and mesial surfaces, and elastic chains were attached to a MI in the retromolar area, thus creating a distalizing uprighting force. Other treatment options utilizing direct anchorage include using uprighting springs, a cantilever or archwires on the MI or plate delivering the appropriate force on the molar.

A different scenario occurs when there is lingual eruption of the mandibular second molars. This can be caused by an arch-length discrepancy in the posterior segments [17]. While surgical uprighting should not be performed in this situation, orthodontic alignment has been shown to be successful. Two options for correcting this scenario are: interarch cross elastics and MI anchorage. Interarch cross elastics can be used to correct a lingually tipped mandibular second molar and a buccally tipped maxillary second molar simultaneously if both molars need repositioning. However, if the upper second molar is in an ideal position, the lingual and extrusive forces applied to the maxillary second molar are not ideal. In addition, extrusive forces applied to both molars can create occlusal trauma or complicate the buccal lingual correction of the molars. An alternative option is to use MIs placed in the alveolar bone palatal to the maxillary second molar and buccal to the mandibular second molar to generate palatal and intrusive forces on the maxillary molar and buccal and intrusive forces on the mandibular molar. The procedure utilizes MIs in the maxillary and mandibular alveolar bone, with elastics attached in order to create lateral forces. This treatment method described by Park and colleagues [17] has the benefit of minimal hardware placement and is potentially better tolerated by patients than the interarch cross elastics approach.

Indirect anchorage has also been studied, albeit less extensively. In one case, [18], a MI placed between the second premolar and the first molar was connected to the anchorage unit by a rigid stainless steel wire, helping to counteract the forces felt on the anchor unit. An appropriate repositioning force system is placed on the anchorage unit reinforced by the MI and applied to the molar for uprighting.

Complications

Complications following surgical uprighting of second molars have been well documented and include infection, osteitis, pulp calcification, root resorption, and ankylosis. In a study done by Pogrel and colleagues, an 18-month follow-up period revealed mostly positive results. In a study where 22 second molars were uprighted, one was lost due to infection in the early postoperative period. In this patient, a periodontal infection around the uprighted tooth developed into an osteitis that resulted in bone loss and subsequent gross mobility of the tooth. The molar was extracted, as it appeared non-vital with a radiographic bony defect. The other patients in this case series demonstrated no mobility with stable occlusion, as well as adequate bone formation such that no pocketing depths were greater than 3 mm. Root formation following uprighting has been shown to be variable, with just over half of patients showing continued root formation. However, the root apices appear to be closed in all cases. Likewise, vitality tests using an electronic pulp tester has inconsistent results. Pulp calcification was seen in approximately one-third of cases, though none of these patients were symptomatic. Furthermore, none of the teeth studied required root canal treatment by the 18-month follow-up [19].

The appearance of postoperative radiographs is also a potential concern, due to the potential for root resorption, ankylosis, or pulp calcification. Padwa et al. describes a rate of abnormal postoperative radiographs as 47.3% in a study that examined surgical uprighting results over a 2-year period [1]. However, no pain, swelling, or other symptoms during the follow-up period were seen, nor were any new periodontal defects created. Thus, the radiographic findings of pulpal changes have not been shown to be indicative of clinical failure.

Complications associated with orthodontic repositioning include reduction in amount of keratinized gingiva, gingival recession, gingivitis, ankylosis, devitalization, root resorption, injury to the periodontium, and marginal bone loss [20–23]. While no studies have directly compared surgical uprighting with orthodontic repositioning of impacted molars, careful exposure of the impacted tooth and the appropriate application of external forces will minimize the risk of complications in either treatment option.

Conclusion

Surgical uprighting of molars has been demonstrated to be a safe and reliable means of repositioning teeth into a functional position. Traditional methods of uprighting include immediate surgical repositioning, conventional orthodontic repositioning, or orthodontic repositioning combined with the use of mini-implants or surgical plates. While both options have demonstrated efficacy, the decision-making process should include an informed discussion of the treatment protocols between the patient, surgeon, and orthodontist.

References

1. Padwa BL, et al. Surgical uprighting is a successful procedure for management of impacted mandibular second molars. J Oral Maxillofac Surg. 2017;75:1581–90.
2. Grover PS, Lorton L. The incidence of unerupted permanent teeth and related clinical cases. Oral Surg Oral Med Oral Pathol. 1985;59:420.
3. Bishara SE. Impacted maxillary canines: a review. Am J Orthod Dentofacial Orthop. 1992;101:159–71.
4. Levy I, Regan D. Impaction of maxillary permanent second molars by the third molars. J Paediatr Dent. 1989;5:31–4.
5. Shapira Y, et al. Uprighting mesially impacted mandibular permanent second molars. Angle Orthod. 1998;68:173.
6. Boynton T, Lieblich SE. Surgical uprighting of second molars. Atlas Oral Maxillofac Surg Clin North Am. 2013;21:235.
7. Raghoebar GM, et al. Eruption disturbances of permanent molars: a review. J Oral Pathol Med. 1991;20:159–66.
8. Jacoby H. The etiology of maxillary canine impaction. Am J Orthod. 1983;84:125–32.
9. Varpio M, Wellfelt B. Disturbed eruption of the lower second molar: clinical appearance, prevalence, and etiology. ASDC J Dent Child. 1988;55:114–8.
10. Bodner L, et al. Image accuracy of plain film radiography and computerized tomography in assessing morphological abnormality of impacted teeth. Am J Orthod Dentofacial Orthop. 2001;120:623–8.
11. Ness GM. Impacted teeth. In: Miloro M, editor. Peterson's principles of oral and maxillofacial surgery. 3rd ed. USA: People's Medical Pub. House-USA; 2011.
12. Vig KW. Some methods of uprighting lower second molars—II. Br J Orthod. 1976;3:39–44.
13. Johnson JV, Quirk GP. Surgical repositioning of impacted mandibular second molar teeth. case report Am J Orthod Dentofacial Orthop. 1987;91:242–51.
14. McAboy CP, et al. Surgical uprighting and repositioning of severely impacted mandibular second molars. J Am Dent Assoc. 2003;134(11):1459–62.
15. Trikka M, et al. Mandibular molar uprighting using orthodontic miniscrew implants: a systematic review. Prog Orthod. 2018;19:1.
16. Sohn D, et al. Minor tooth movements using microimplant anchorage: case reports. Implant Dent. 2008;17:32–9.
17. Park HS, et al. Uprighting second molars with micro-implant anchorage. J Clin Orthod. 2004;38:100–3.
18. Yun SW, et al. Molar control using indirect miniscrew anchorage. J Clin Orthod. 2005;39:661–4.
19. Pogrel MA. The surgical uprighting of mandibular second molars. Am J Orthod Dentofacial Orthop. 1995;108:180–3.
20. Proffit WR. Contemporary orthodontics. St. Louis: Mosby; 1993.

21. Boyd RL. Clinical assessment of injuries in orthodontic movement of impacted teeth, II: surgical recommendations. Am J Orthod. 1984;86:407–18.
22. Vanarsdall RL, Corn H. Soft-tissue management of labially positioned unerupted teeth. Am J Orthod. 1977;72:53–64.
23. Di Biase DD. Mucous membrane and delayed eruption. Dent Pract Dent Rec. 1971;21:241–50.

Management of Impacted Teeth

14

Frank de Latour and Vernon Burke

Introduction

Removal of impacted teeth is one of the most common procedures performed by OMS on a daily basis. Referrals commonly come from a variety of sources as part of a comprehensive orthodontic or restorative treatment plan from dental colleagues. Impacted teeth can be defined as those teeth which fail to erupt into the dental arch by the middle of the third decade of life. Common reasons for failure of tooth eruption include lack of adequate arch space for eruption, the presence of adjacent teeth blocking the path of eruption, dense overlying bone, or excessive overlying soft tissue. Impacted teeth must be differentiated from unerupted teeth which are those that are in the process of eruption and will most likely erupt by the middle of the third decade into a functional position. Unerupted teeth are commonly seen in younger patients and if a referral is made for removal of a tooth in an adolescent it may be prudent to wait a period of time before removal as these may erupt over time.

The most commonly impacted teeth are third molars, both maxillary and mandibular. Due to the fact that these teeth are last to erupt there is frequently insufficient arch space because of the presence of the rest of the teeth leading to third molar impaction. Impaction of third molars is followed by maxillary canines and mandibular premolars. Failure of eruption of the canine and premolars is commonly

The views expressed in this article (book, speech, etc.) are those of the authors and do not reflect the official policy or position of the US Army Medical Department, Department of the Army, DoD, or the U.S. Government

F. de Latour
William Beaumont Army Medical Center, Ft Bliss, TX, USA

V. Burke (✉)
High Desert Oral and Facial Surgery, El Paso, TX, USA
e-mail: burke@hdofs.com

E. M. Ferneini, M. T. Goupil (eds.), *Office-Based Maxillofacial Surgical Procedures*, https://doi.org/10.1007/978-3-030-22371-7_14

related to insufficient arch length, as these teeth are among the last to erupt in the permanent dentition. Maxillary premolars, incisors, and first and second molars may also become impacted, but these are the most infrequent teeth to fail to erupt.

Once a tooth has been evaluated and it determined that it will not erupt it should be considered for removal unless contraindicated. Leaving an impacted tooth in place until it causes significant issues may lead to increased patient morbidity. The least morbidity for removal of impacted teeth occurs when the patient is between the ages of 15 and 25. Early removal of a known impacted tooth is frequently recommended as this is known to decrease postoperative complications [1, 2].

These teeth are removed for a variety of indications which have been outlined in the Parameters of Care by AAOMS which include [3]:

- Pain
- Facilitate the management of limit progression of periodontal disease
- Ectopic position
- Facilitate prosthetic rehabilitation
- Facilitate orthodontic tooth movement and promote dental stability
- Tooth interfering with orthognathic and/or reconstructive surgery
- Fractured tooth
- Nonrestorable caries
- Internal or external resorption of tooth or adjacent teeth
- Tooth involved in tumor resection
- Prophylactic removal in patients with certain medical conditions, surgical condition, or treatments
- Patient's informed refusal of non surgical treatment options
- Nontreatable pulpal lesion
- Acute or chronic infection
- Abnormalities of tooth shape or size
- Findings of periodontal disease
- Findings of periapical disease
- Elective therapeutic removal
- Tooth in line of jaw fracture complicating fracture management
- Pathology associated with tooth follicle
- Insufficient space to accommodate erupting tooth or teeth

Contraindications for Removal of Impacted Teeth

Although all the above are accepted indications for removal of impacted teeth, there are several contraindications to their removal. There are situations in which the risks outweigh the benefits and removal should be deferred.

One such contraindication is related to the extremes of age. Removal of impacted teeth should be delayed in children and adolescents until a definitive diagnosis of impaction can be made. Also, as patients advance in age the risk of increased postoperative morbidity increases. If an impacted tooth has remained within the alveolar process without any evidence of periodontal disease, caries, or pathology for an extended period, then removal should not be performed to prevent unnecessary patient morbidity.

In patients with a compromised medical status, removal of impacted teeth should be undertaken only if there is a definitive reason for their removal. Elective removal of asymptomatic teeth is unnecessary in individuals with significant cardiovascular and respiratory disease. However, if symptoms or definitive reasons exist for removal then consultation with the patient's medical team should be considered to ensure patient safety during the perioperative period.

Classification Systems for Impacted Third Molars

Several classification systems have been used to help the surgeon determine the difficulty in removal of impacted third molars and they are presented below. The Pell and Gregory classification system addressed the relationship of the mandibular third molar to both the occlusal plane of the mandible as well as the relationship of the crown to the anterior border of the ramus [4]. During assessment of case difficulty those teeth with deeper impactions, Pell and Gregory Class C, and those completely within the ramus, Pell and Gregory Class III, should be considered more difficult as increased bone will need to be removed prior to tooth delivery. This may assist the surgeon during the preoperative discussion with the patient regarding the expected postoperative course. The Winter's Classification system addresses the angulation of the third molar in relation to the second molar. Those teeth with mesioangular impactions are considered easier to remove than those with distoangular due to the surgical approach needed for delivery. Application of both of these systems on a routine basis can assist in guiding the surgeon in not only surgical planning, but also preoperative discussions with the patient at to the expected postoperative course. Finally, application of the Rood's Classification of the relationship of the mandibular third molar roots to the inferior alveolar nerve should be routinely employed [5]. In the study seven radiographic signs were mentioned as possibly indicative of a close relationship of the tooth roots to the IAN. It was determined that based on their study only diversion of the IAN, darkening of the root, and interruption of the white line of the IAN were statistically significant predictors of postoperative IAN injury or disruption. The surgeon should pay close attention for these three markers and ensure that patients with them are properly counseled regarding the risks of tooth removal.

Pell and Gregory Classification of Third Molars

Class A–C: Based on relationship of tooth crown to the occlusal plane

A: Occlusal plane of third molar is even with occlusal plane of second molar (Fig. 14.1)
B: Occlusal plane of third molar is between the occlusal plane of second molar and CEJ of second molar (Fig. 14.2)
C: Occlusal plane of third molar if below the CEJ of second molar (Fig. 14.3)

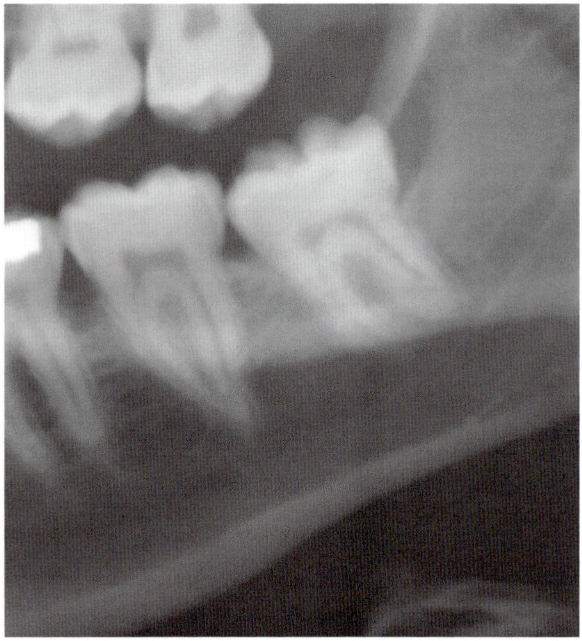

Fig. 14.1 Pell and Gregory classification A

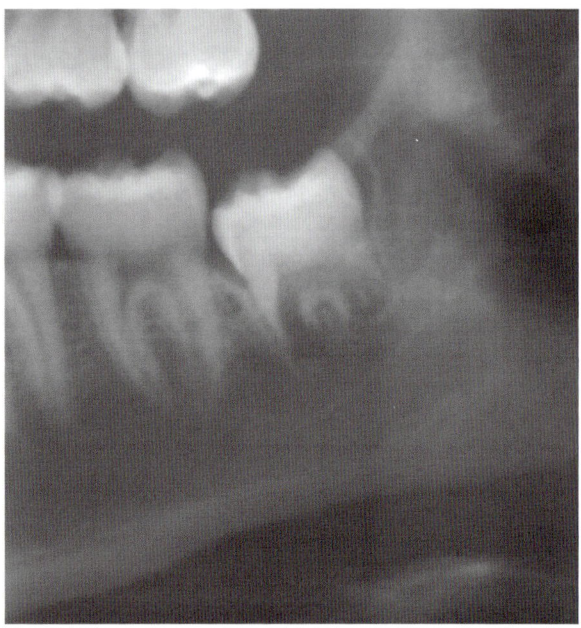

Fig. 14.2 Pell and Gregory classification B

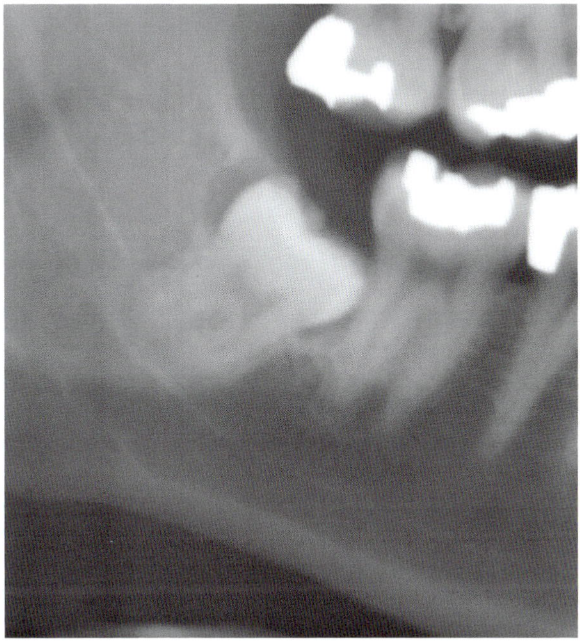

Fig. 14.3 Pell and Gregory classification C

Class I–III: Based on relationship of tooth crown to the anterior border of mandibular ramus

I: Crown is completely anterior to the anterior border of the ramus (Fig. 14.4)
II: Approximately one half of the occlusal surface if anterior to the anterior border of the ramus (Fig. 14.5)
III: Tooth if completely located within the mandibular ramus (Fig. 14.6)

Winter classification of third molars

- Mesioangular (Fig. 14.7)
- Vertical (Fig. 14.8)
- Distoangular (Fig. 14.9)
- Horizontal (Fig. 14.10)

Rood's classification of third molar relation to IAN

- Darkening of the root
- Deflection of the root
- Bifid root
- Narrowing of the root
- Interruption of the white line
- Deflection of the inferior alveolar canal
- Narrowing of the canal

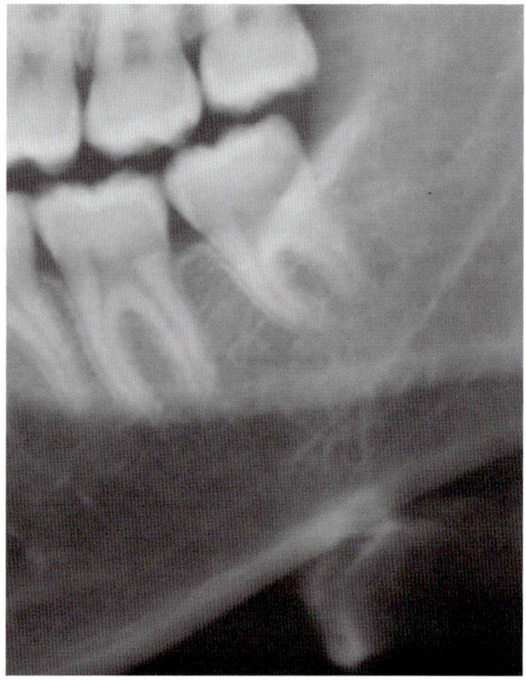

Fig. 14.4 Pell and Gregory classification 1

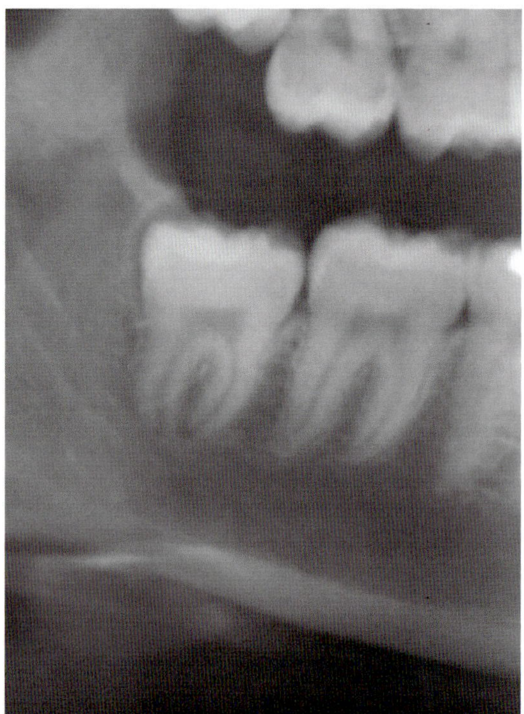

Fig. 14.5 Pell and Gregory classification 2

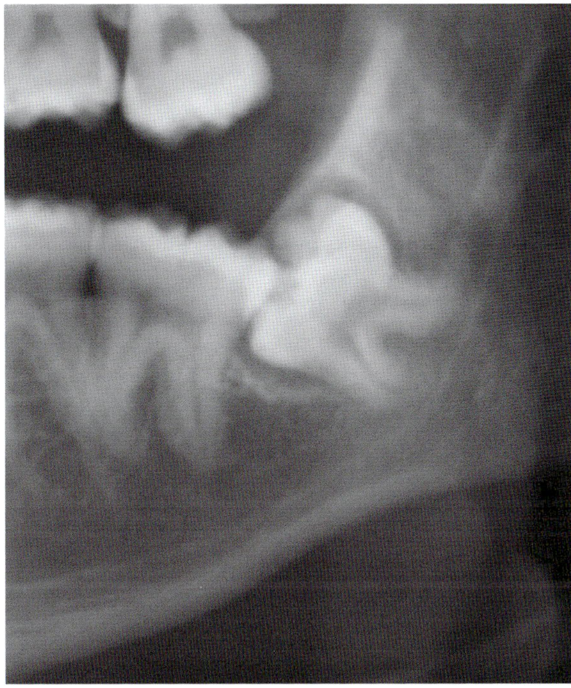

Fig. 14.6 Pell and Gregory classification 3

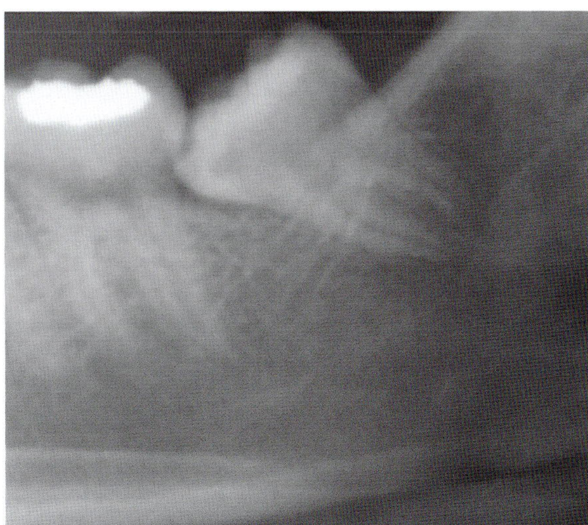

Fig. 14.7 Mesioangular inclination

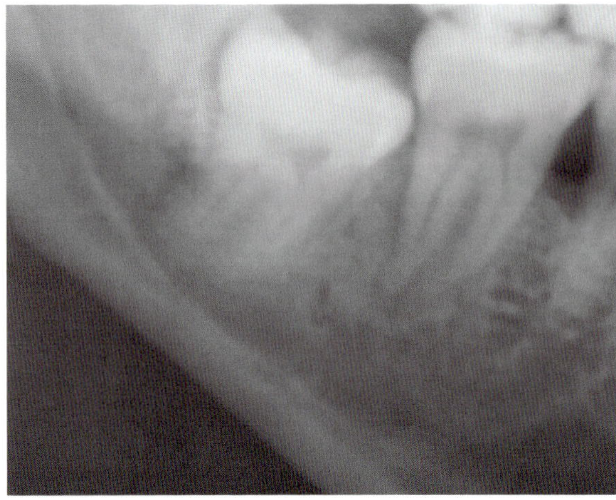

Fig. 14.8 Vertical inclination

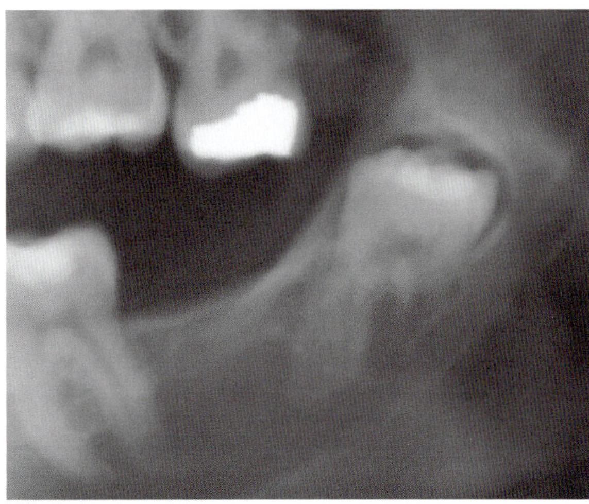

Fig. 14.9 Distoangular inclination

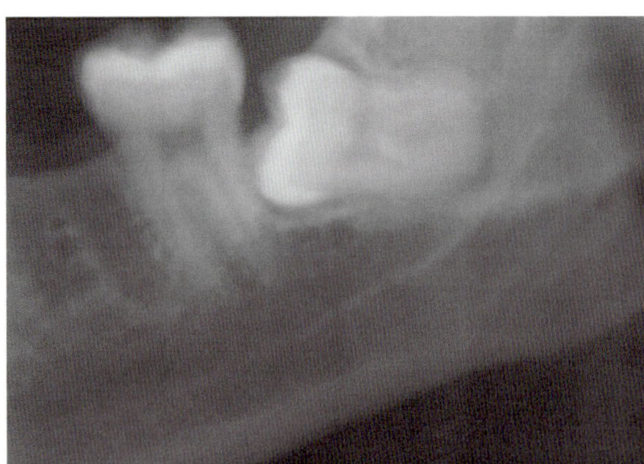

Fig. 14.10 Horizontal inclination

Technique for Removal of Third Molars

Removal of impacted teeth should follow a systematic approach during the removal process. The first step is proper armamentarium to facilitate safe and efficient removal. The following represents a list of the authors' commonly used instrumentation for removal of impacted teeth. This list may vary from provider to provider, but this represents the authors' essentials.

Armamentarium

- Aspirating syringe
- Bite block or mouth prop
- Sweetheart tongue retractor
- Minnesota cheek retractor
- Copeland and Frasier suction
- #9 Periosteal elevator
  - Elevators: narrow, wide, Cogswell A, Cogswell B, and others as preferred
- Forceps: #150, #151, and Cowhorn
  - Rongeur
  - Molt Curette
- Bone file
- Needle driver
- 3-0 chromic gut suture
- Irrigation
- Surgical handpiece
- #702/703 bur or #8 round bur

Identify the Setting for Removal of Teeth and the Depth of Anesthesia Needed

Preoperative patient medical assessment, oral cavity evaluation, and radiographic evaluation will guide this process. Patients must be evaluated individually to determine the most appropriate setting for removal of teeth when indicated. In some instances, local anesthesia may be all that is needed for removal while others may require a full general anesthetic in the operating room due to the position of the teeth or patient concerns. Although a complete discussion of perioperative patient management is outside the scope of this chapter several key points must be addressed (see Chapter 1). All patients must undergo a focused history and physical during preoperative evaluation. Significant medical conditions should be discussed in detail during the interview process. The surgeon must pay close attention to cardiovascular, pulmonary, and psychologic issues as they may impact the overall anesthetic and surgical plan. Appropriate consultations to additional medical providers should be used when deemed appropriate to ensure patient safety. A full list of patients' medications, allergies, family history, and social history should be evaluated as well. It is recommended to ask the patient to bring a list of all medications with complete dosing schedules during evaluation. The surgery is then discussed in detail to include the risks, benefits, and complications. Both verbal and written information is provided to the patient to ensure full comprehension.

After discussions with the patient, the surgeon must determine the best and safest anesthetic plan for the patient. The patient's medical conditions, anxiety regarding the surgery, and the extent of the surgery must all be considered. Evaluation and planning on a case-by-case basis is critical as no two patients or cases are the same. Regardless of the setting, patient safety and attempts to limit the overall morbidity must be paramount in the decision-making process.

Technique for Extraction of Mandibular Third Molars

Incision Design

Proper patient positioning and preparation are essential first steps in efficient removal of impacted teeth. The authors prefer to have the patient in a semi reclined seated position. After getting the patient and chair into the proper position, a medium to large bite block is placed on the contralateral side from the surgical area. After bite block placement then a throat screen consisting of a 4×4 gauze and a sweetheart retractor are placed. A Minnesota retractor is preferred for retraction of the cheek and exposure of the area. Retraction in a lateral and inferior direction will allow for both visualization of the site and ease of incision through the "tented out tissues." Many different designs have been proposed in the literature for removal of impacted third molars and each based on the surgeon preference. The common theme among all is adequate access and visualization of the surgical site which in turn will facilitate efficient removal of the tooth. The authors prefer an incision with both distobuccal and mesiobuccal releasing incisions. Some surgeons prefer an envelope flap with a distobuccal release. The incision preferred by the authors with distobuccal and mesiobuccal releases provides wide access, limits tension on the soft tissues, and allows for protection of the tissues during the bone removal process. The flap is made with a #15 Blade and is full thickness down to the alveolar bone. A critical point in making the distal portion of the incision is to ensure that there is a buccal angulation of the incision. Failure to do this may place the lingual nerve at risk for damage and lead to unnecessary postoperative complications.

Flap Reflection

A #9 periosteal elevator is then used to reflect the flap to allow for visualization of the impacted tooth or the area where the tooth is present. A Minnesota retractor is then placed into the flap with lateral retraction, and the foot of the retractor against the alveolus (see Fig. 14.11). This allows for protection of the tissues as well as visualization of the surgical site. Attempt to avoid unnecessary and excessive flap reflection as this may increase postoperative pain and complications. Reflection of only a few millimeters past the external oblique ridge is all that is required for most impactions. It must be reinforced that excellent visualization of the surgical field is

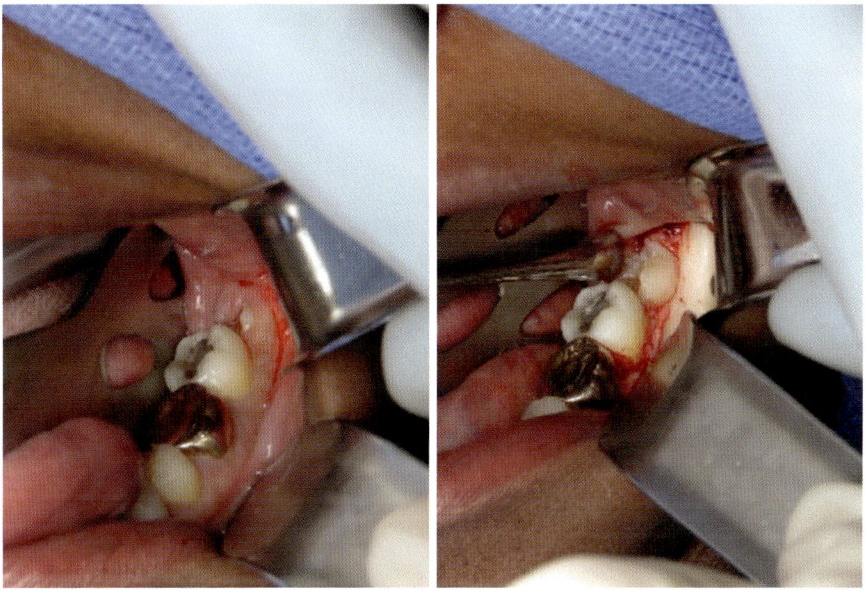

Fig. 14.11 Incision and flap retraction

required. Insufficient flap reflection is a common cause for difficulty in removal of teeth as inability to see the surgical sites results in inefficient crown uncovering and sectioning.

Crown Uncovering

A surgical handpiece with a #702/703 bur is then used to uncover the crown of the tooth. Some surgeons may prefer a larger bur or a round bur for bone removal and tooth sectioning. The surgeon should take into account the specifications of their armamentarium as this can help guide their surgical approach. The average #702 bur has an average diameter of the head approximately 1.5 mm and the working length of the shaft of 5 mm. Copious irrigation with sterile saline should be used throughout the boner removal process to prevent overheating the bone and allow for removal of debris.

Generally, the uncovering process begins on the buccal surface of the tooth and proceeds to the distal as indicated based on crown morphology and tooth angulation. Bone should be removed to uncover the entire clinical crown of the tooth to the cemento-enamel junction (see Fig. 14.12), as this will facilitate efficient tooth removal. Avoid bone removal on the lingual aspect of the tooth as this puts the lingual nerve at risk for unnecessary damage. It is paramount to remove the appropriate amount of bone to allow for easy delivery of the tooth and sectioning of the tooth if deemed necessary.

Pitfalls in the exposure of teeth are easily identified than correcting in some instances. In training surgeons identified certain issues that repeat. Even experienced surgeons fall victim to these issues occasionally. The most common of these issues is the lack of exposure of the clinical crown. This leads to disorientation and difficulty when elevating the tooth as the attempt at extraction is "working down a hole."

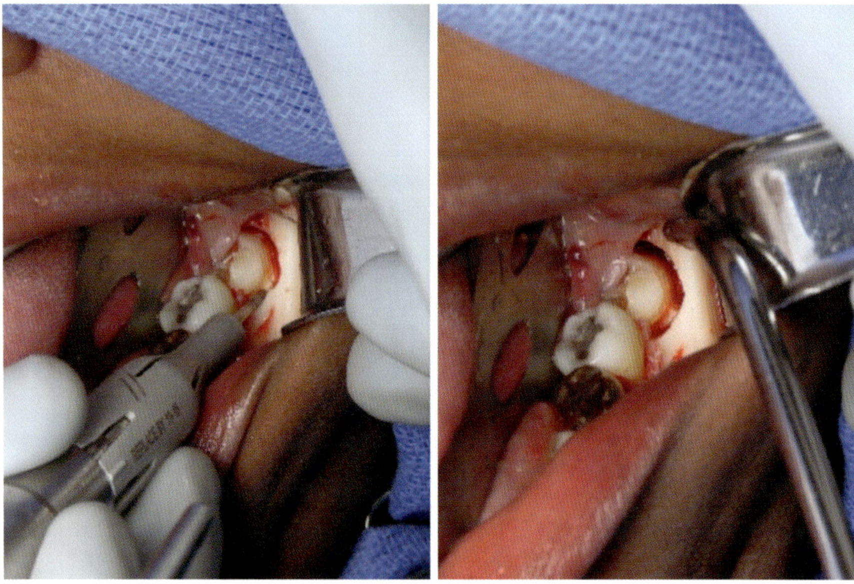

Fig. 14.12 Troughing

As stated earlier, one should expose the impacted tooth to the CEJ on the buccal and distal sections. The knowledge of dental anatomy guides the approach to bone removal. Creating a buccal trough to the depth and width of the #702/703 bur around the mesial, buccal, and distal surfaces of the crown is generally sufficient to allow for appropriate exposure. Appropriate space should be made for both visualization of the landmarks as well as insertion and use of elevators for delivery.

On mesially angled third molars, a common mistake is stopping short of exposure of the mesial aspect of the crown. Stopping short of the line angle does not allow for the elevation of the tooth once sectioned. It also impedes path of withdrawal of the tooth. Crown exposure requirements are similar on horizontally impacted teeth, the practitioner must remove sufficient bone to allow for identification of the CEJ as well as the buccal groove. Exposure of these landmarks is critical to ensure appropriate sectioning of the tooth, which is addressed in the next section. Uncovering of distoangular teeth is perhaps the most critical as improper exposure can lead to incorrect sectioning and difficulty in removal. The surgeon must remember that the path of delivery for the tooth is into the ramus. Careful attention must be paid to bone removal on the distal portion of the tooth. This can be difficult in many situations due to the angulation which the bur and handpiece must be inserted. The surgeon and assistant must be cognizant of the surgical equipment at all times as there may be instances, especially with distal and horizontal teeth. The angulation required from the bur and handpiece may put the lip at risk for a surgical burn or laceration when crowns are being uncovered during these and all impactions.

Crown and Root Sectioning

Elevation of the tooth should be attempted after uncovering of the crown. In some instances, such as mesial or vertically impacted teeth, simple elevation may be all that is needed for delivery of the tooth. The authors prefer the use of a simple straight elevator for this initial elevation. The buccal trough created during uncovering with the #702 should be sufficient for seating of the elevator and allow for controlled forces to be applied to the tooth.

If the tooth movement is minimal with elevation, then the practitioner should consider sectioning the crown and/or the roots to facilitate delivery. As previously discussed, the crown should have been previously uncovered to appropriately identify the relevant clinical anatomy such as the buccal groove and the mesiobuccal cusp. Failure to identify these landmarks may lead to sectioning the tooth in an unfortunate way, which will lead to increased difficulty in removal. The surgeon should make every effort to section the tooth parallel to the long axis of the tooth through the buccal groove. The authors prefer to fully bury the #702 bur within the tooth following the appropriate angulation. The bucco-lingual width of the tooth is approximately 10 mm and the depth to the furcation is approximately the same. With full use of the bur the surgeon can ensure that a cut of at least 5 mm is made, but the authors will routinely increase the depth of the sectioning approximately 2–3 mm past the flutes of the bur to ensure that a proper split of the tooth may be achieved. The sectioning of the crown should not be done fully through the tooth lingually to prevent inadvertent damage to the lingual nerve. Many practitioners' goal is to section three-quarters of the way through the crown. This provides protection to the lingual nerve which may lie directly against the lingual alveolus of the third molar.

Once the surgeon has achieved appropriate sectioning of the crown using the surgical bur, they then transition to use of elevators for completion of the sectioning. A Cogswell A elevator is commonly used to complete the fracture of the crown. It is placed to the depth of the section and force applied to the tooth. This allows for splitting of the tooth and fragment removal. Depending on the angulation of the tooth and the depth of the sectioning, the roots may be removed at the same time as the crown, while in other cases the roots may need to be removed individually.

The following paragraphs address the individual surgical techniques for each of the four most common impactions of mandibular molars.

Sectioning and removal of mesioangular teeth is the easiest to accomplish due to their angulation. After removal of bone to expose the crown on the buccal and distal surfaces, the surgical handpiece is used to section off the distal half of the crown (see Fig. 14.13). After removal of this fragment a small straight elevator can be used to remove the tooth or a purchase point and Cogswell B may be used to elevate and remove the tooth.

Horizontal impactions are considered the next easiest impaction to remove. After exposure of the majority of the crown and the superior part of the distal root, the handpiece is used to section the crown from the roots at the CEJ. The crown is then removed at this time if possible. In some instances, the crown may need to be further sectioned to facilitate delivery from the site. After crown removal there should be

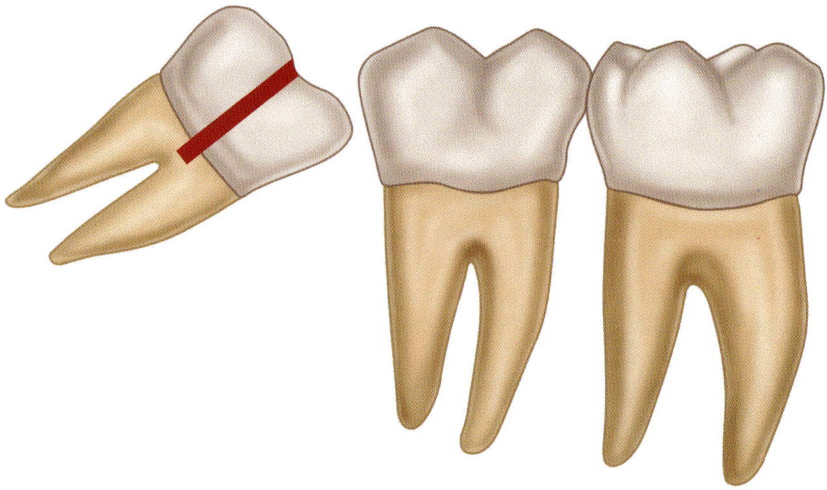

Fig. 14.13 For a mesioangular impacted tooth, the tooth is sectioned into two pieces, preferably at the root furcation

sufficient space for delivery of the roots (see Fig. 14.14). The author prefers to place a purchase point in the superior aspect of the distal root and then use a Cogswell B for delivery. In the cases where the roots are divergent, further sectioning of the roots may be needed to facilitate delivery.

Teeth that are vertically positioned are approached in a similar fashion to those mesioangularly impacted (see Fig. 14.15). However, additional bone must be removed on the mesial aspect of the tooth to facilitate the use of a small straight elevator. This is sometimes challenging due to the proximity of the second molar. Close attention should be pain in these circumstances to prevent inadvertent trauma or damage to the second molar.

Distoangular teeth are considered the most difficult impaction to remove. This is primarily due to path of delivery for the tooth. Sufficient bone in the vicinity of the distal portion of the tooth should be removed to allow for delivery (see Fig. 14.16). The crown is then commonly sectioned along the buccal groove and then a horizontal cut is made to allow for complete delivery of the crown. Cogswell A elevators are commonly used for the process of crown removal. After delivery of the crown the roots are delivered using small straight and Cogswell B elevators. If resistance is met during attempted root delivery, then sectioning of the roots is recommended.

Irrigation and Closure

Once the tooth has been fully removed then the socket should be carefully inspected. Irrigation should be carried out and then evaluation for the presence of the IAN, lingual perforation, or damage to the dentition. After irrigation, hemostasis must be

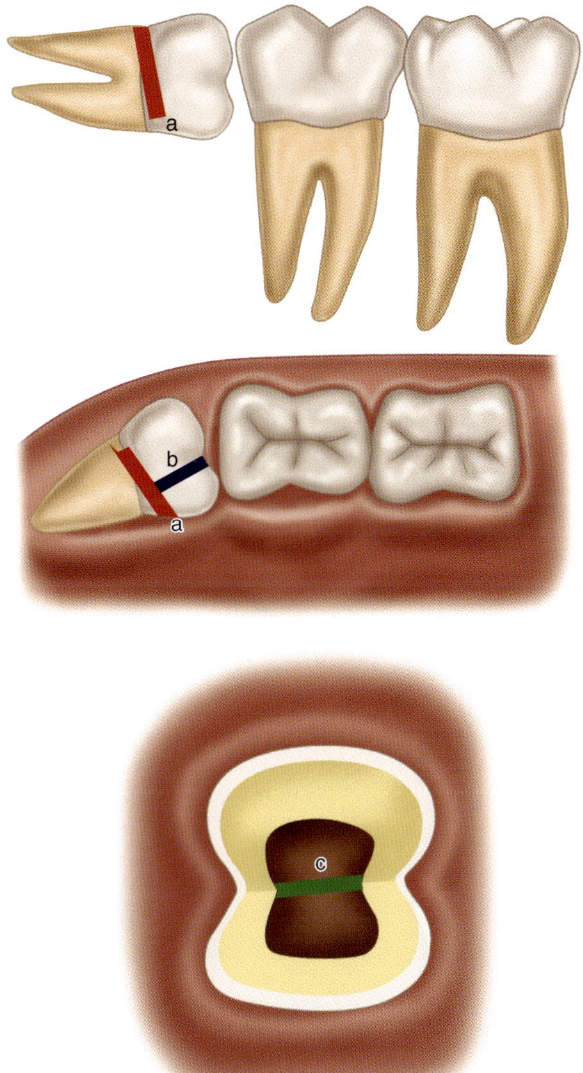

Fig. 14.14 For a horizontal impacted tooth the crown is sectioned from the roots. The angle for the section cut is made from posterior-superior to anterior-inferior ("A" cut). The crown may need to be sectioned further ("B" cut). For multiple rooted teeth further sectioning may be required ("C" cut)

achieved. Although infrequent, the surgeon must be prepared to control any significant postoperative bleeding. Commonly, direct pressure in the area of the bleed with a damp gauze is sufficient for control. When applying direct pressure, the surgeon must exercise patience and maintain pressure for a minimum of 5 minute prior to inspection of the site. If pressure is unable to control the bleeding, then use of a gelatin sponge or oxidized cellulose may be applied to the area. Both may be left in the extraction site and closure achieved over the area with the use of resorbable sutures. Oxidized cellulose should not be used in sites where the nerve visualized

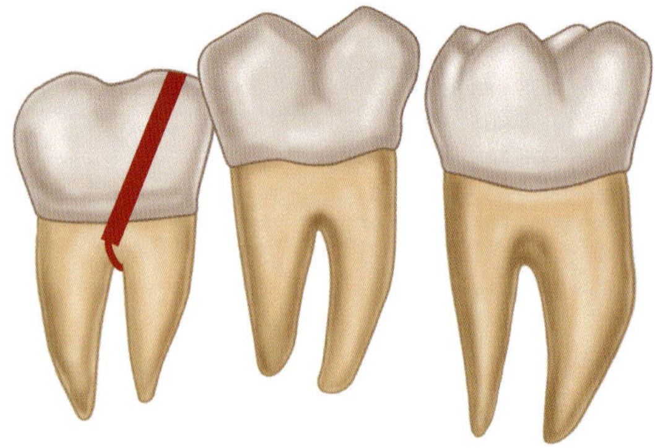

Fig. 14.15 For vertically impacted teeth, the tooth is sectioned into two pieces

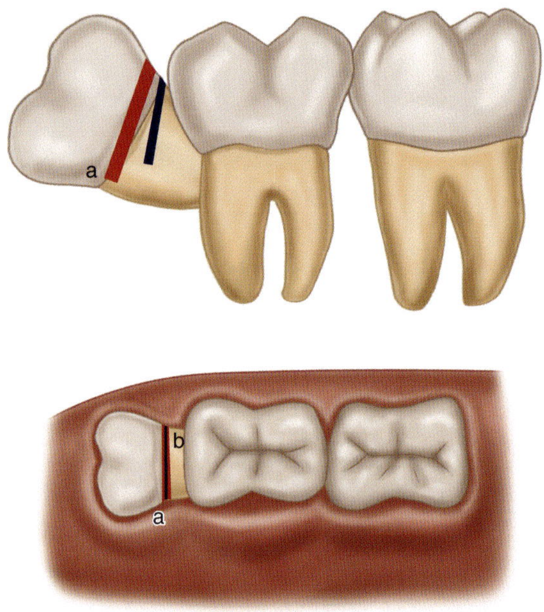

Fig. 14.16 For distally angled impacted teeth, the crown is separated from the root. Occasionally the crown may need to be "T" cut similar to the "B" cut used for horizontal impactions. A purchase point "B" will aid in removal

as its breakdown products have been noted to damage nerves. A further discussion of bleeding associated with impacted teeth is addressed in a further section of this chapter. In general, the sutures may or may not be used based on surgeon preference. Studies have shown there is a decreased incidence of postoperative pain, edema, and trismus associated with a suture-less technique during third molar extractions [6]. However, many surgeons prefer to place sutures to reapproximate the flap edges and allow for primary closure of the area. Lastly, gauze packing or tonsil sponges are placed and the patient is instructed to maintain pressure on the area for 30–45 min after discharge from the office.

Technique for Extraction of Maxillary Third Molars

Incision Design

As with mandibular third molars, visualization of the surgical site is paramount to ensure removal of the maxillary third molars. A small to medium sized bite block is placed on the contralateral side. After placement of the bite block a gauze throat screen and sweetheart retractor are placed. The patients head is then turned toward the opposite side, there by placing the surgical site in a more direct line of sight. After these preparatory steps then a Minnesota Retractor is placed in the posterior maxilla and upward and lateral retraction is performed to allow for maximal visualization of the surgical site. The surgical site is then inspected for the presence or absence of the crown as this may assist in guiding the incision. Fully erupted teeth require no incisions as they may be moved with simple elevation. Those teeth with partial or full impaction require an incision to facilitate removal. The authors prefer an incision midline and posterior on to the tuberosity with a distobuccal release or sulcular. The incision is taken from the tuberosity and extends to the distal of the second molar. Once the second molar is encountered then a sulcular incision is made and this is continued until the distobuccal line angle of the first molar. Alternatively, at the distobuccal line angle of the second molar a releasing incision is made into the maxillary vestibule. For most cases, approximately 1 cm releasing incision will allow adequate visualization of the surgical site and prevent tearing of the tissues. All incisions are made full-thickness down to the alveolar bone with a #15 blade.

Flap Reflection

After the creation of the incision, a #9 periosteal elevator is used to reflection of the flap. This is performed in a subperiosteal plane directly against the bone. To ease visualization, reflection proceeds anterior to posterior and inferior to superior. After reflection of the flap a Minnesota retractor is repositioned to allow for flap reflection and visualization of the surgical site. It is critical at this point to place the Minnesota in the proper position. It must be placed posterior and superior to the crown of the tooth. This positioning prevents inadvertent displacement of the tooth into the infratemporal fossa as the retractor acts as a stop during elevation of the tooth. Once the flap is raised then the area is inspected, and the surgeon then transitions to uncovering or elevation of the tooth.

Crown Uncovering

The crown must be evaluated and the decision for bone removal made at this point. Elevators must be able to be positioned below the CEJ to allow for removal. If the positioning of the elevator is not possible due to the presence of bone, then bone must be removed. Bone is removed using chisels, rongeur, or surgical burs to allow seating of the appropriate elevator. Bone is removed on the buccal as well as coronal using the aforementioned instruments. As with mandibular third molars, the clinical crown should be easily identified as this will make elevation of the tooth significantly easier.

Tooth Delivery

Appropriate elevators should be seated and with the use of controlled force, the tooth removed. The authors prefer the use of a small straight elevator for initial elevation. This is seated and pressure applied in a distal and occlusal fashion. In many cases this is sufficient to allow for delivery of the tooth. In some cases, this will initially allow the tooth to move, but delivery may not be achieved. In these instances, Miller or Potts elevators are positioned and similar forces applied to facilitate removal. It should be stated, rarely do maxillary third molars need to be sectioned and all attempts should be undertaken to avoid this if possible.

Irrigation and Closure

Once the tooth is removed the alveolus should be carefully inspected. Irrigation is carried out and then evaluation for the presence of the sinus perforations or damage to the dentition. After irrigation, hemostasis is achieved and digital pressure applied to the alveolus for compression of the socket. The authors do not routinely close these sites as most heal without issues.

Management of Impacted Maxillary Canines

The canine tooth is considered the cornerstone of the dental arch and is critical in determining overall function. The average eruption time frame is between 11 and 14 years old. Maxillary canines are the most commonly impacted teeth behind third molars. Studies have shown that canine impaction is seen within 1–2% of the population. They may be impacted either labially or palatally within the alveolus. Palatal impaction has been noted to occur approximately 85% of the time and labial impactions accounting for the other 15% [7, 8]. Labial positioning of the canine is most likely related to a deficiency in overall arch length which leads to labial positioning of the tooth during development. Palatal impactions are associated with early eruption of the lateral incisor which interrupts the normal path of eruption of the canine.

Impacted maxillary canines are a common source of referrals to OMS offices. The teeth can be managed by either extraction or via exposure and ligation with subsequent orthodontic therapy to bring the tooth into the correct position within the alveolus. When possible, it is advisable to attempt to avoid extraction of the canine as this leads to significant changes within the arch and the occlusion. Multiple treatment strategies have been attempted to facilitate this process in the past, but today modern dental materials have allowed for predictable treatment of impacted canines via the use of bonded brackets and orthodontic forces.

A CBCT should be considered on all patients with impacted canines. It allows for precise localization of the tooth and alerts the surgeon to any potential interferences or difficulties which may be missed on a standard panoramic radiograph. If unable to obtain a CBCT then at a minimum a panoramic radiograph along with PA radiographs employing SLOB rule should be taken.

Clinically, patients with impacted canines may present with retained primary canines, absence of labial bulge from the permanent canine, a palatal bulge, and a possible distal positioning of the lateral incisor. Confirmation of the labio-palatal position, relation of the crown to the mucogingival junction, and amount of keratinized gingiva are all essential in the preoperative workup. Discussion with the referring provider is crucial in the treatment planning process and the plan agreed upon by all parties prior to surgery. As the process of exposure and ligation is discussed elsewhere is this book the following will address primarily removal of these teeth.

Technique for Extraction of Palatally Impacted Canines

Incision

The patient should be positioned reclined in the surgical chair to allow for surgeon visualization of the palate. A medium to large bite block should be placed in the contralateral side. As with all extractions, a throat screen is placed to prevent aspiration. A #15 Blade is then used to make a sulcular incision on the side of the impaction. The length and amount of reflection of the flap will be dictated by the position and amount of exposure needed to facilitate the procedure.

Reflection

A #9 periosteal elevator is used to elevate the flap in a subperiosteal plane. The authors prefer to start the dissection in the anterior and proceed to the posterior. During the elevation process the surgeon looks for the presence of the crown or any bulges in the palatal bone. Dissection is carried out in all directions to ensure no tearing of the palatal mucosa and to protect soft tissues during the use of the surgical handpiece. If the neurovascular bundle from the incisive canal is encountered this can be transected, if necessary, without issues and hemostasis achieved prior to continuing with the procedure. After adequate elevation of the palatal tissues a Seldon is placed medial to the crown of the tooth to allow for visualization of the crown and protection of the soft tissues.

Crown Exposure

Once the tissues have been reflected the area is further assessed for the exact position of the crown. Regardless of whether extraction or exposure and ligation is planned, the crown must be fully uncovered. Failure to remove bone past the height of contour of the tooth will lead to inability to elevate and deliver the tooth. With exposure and ligation, it is crucial not to remove bone past the CEJ as this may lead root resorption.

A surgical bur of surgeon's preference is used for full uncovering of the crown. The authors prefer to use a #702 bur for crown exposure and to create a trough which will allow for elevator placement. Controlled force with a small straight elevator should be applied to the tooth at this time to see if delivery is possible. If it is not possible, then the crown of the tooth should be sectioned at the CEJ. Sectioning at the CEJ should be made nearly through the tooth and then a Cogswell A Elevator used to complete the section. The crown can then be removed with minimal issues. If not, the crown can be further sectioned in a longitudinal fashion. Removal of the crown creates space for delivery of the root. Simple elevation with a small straight elevator may be attempted to see if this allows for delivery. If this is unsuccessful then a purchase point should be placed into the superior portion of the root and a Cogswell B used for delivery. It should be noted that procedure is commonly necessary in patients with moderate to severe crowding. The crowding places the roots of adjacent teeth in close proximity to the surgical site. It is essential that good visualization and proper technique are adhered to avoid damage to the adjacent dentition.

Closure

After inspection of the extracted tooth fragments to ensure that all have been removed, copious irrigation should be carried out in the surgical site. Any areas of sharp bone or small fragments should be removed to ensure no postoperative issues. Hemostasis should then be achieved in the area. It is essential to make sure that a hematoma does not form under the palatal flap as this may lead to unnecessary postoperative complications such as infections. After achieving hemostasis, full reapproximation of the flap is critical. All papilla should be reapproximated and the flap secured with resorbable sutures. Postoperatively the authors routinely prescribe a chlorhexidine mouth rinse and antibiotics for 7 days. Patients are then seen for a scheduled follow-up approximately 7–10 days after surgery to ensure routine healing without complications.

Technique for Extraction of Buccally Impacted Canines

The decision for an OMS to remove a buccally impacted canine comes only after thorough consultation with the referring doctor. As mentioned before the canine is the cornerstone of the arch. The maxillary canine's role in both function and esthetics cannot be overstated and should only be removed after development of a thorough treatment plan. As buccal impaction of maxillary canines is commonly associated with significant crowding, the surgeon must be supremely aware of the adjacent teeth in order to ensure their protection during the extraction process. If adjacent teeth are damaged in the extraction process this could lead to the unfortunate consequence of loss of additional teeth in the anterior maxilla.

Incision

If the crown of the tooth is not immediately visible during the preoperative assessment, then a CBCT is essential for localization of the tooth. Not only will it give the precise location of the tooth, but this will aid in the surgical planning and provide the surgeon with information to ensure atraumatic removal of the tooth.

Incisions are based on the position of the crown. The authors prefer an envelope flap with either mesial or distal releasing incisions for access. In most cases, it is possible to use only a distal release which is more esthetic and, in our opinion, less painful. This provides good visualization and allows for easy repositioning of the tissues. In higher impactions a papilla sparing technique may be employed to prevent periodontal issues postoperatively. Incision placement must be made based on crown position and to ensure that healing without unnecessary complications occurs.

Flap Reflection

Reflection of the tissues is initiated with a #9 periosteal elevator in a subperiosteal plane. Dissection continues in anterior, posterior, and superior directions to ensure complete visualization of the crown. The surgeon must ensure no tearing of the buccal mucosa as this may lead to bleeding and postoperative issues with scarring of the gingiva or loss of papilla. The tissue in the anterior maxilla is tightly bound and thin making it easy to button hole. Often a Woodson, #7 periosteal or other fine instrument is better suited. The reflection must be adequate to allow for bone removal and full crown uncovering.

Crown Exposure

A Minnesota retractor is placed at the base of the flap to allow for visualization of the crown or the approximate location of the crown. Some surgeons prefer a smaller retractor in this area. Once retraction is adequate, the surgeon must then undertake the process of bone removal and full crown exposure. Occasionally, a rongeur can be used. If this is inadequate a surgical handpiece is used to remove bone to below the height of contour of the tooth. The authors prefer the use of a #702 bur for this process, but round burs may be used based on surgeon preference. After complete exposure of the crown, elevation is attempted. If unsuccessful then the tooth is sectioned with a surgical bur and a Cogswell A. The crown is then removed to allow space for root delivery. A purchase point is commonly placed into the remaining tooth structure and a Cogswell B is used to remove the tooth. In some instances, further sectioning is needed to remove the tooth in as atraumatic fashion as possible. Pitfalls in this area include the proximity of the roots of the adjacent teeth. It is possible to create considerable obility of adjacent teeth during in vigorous elevation. In the medially impacted teeth, the crown may be close or across the midline. This bone is very dense and may require significant bone removal

Closure

The tooth fragments should be inspected to ensure full removal. In addition, the adjacent teeth and structures should be evaluated to ensure no damage during the removal process. Once completed, irrigation to the site is carried out to remove debris. After irrigation, hemostasis should be achieved. Reapproximation of the tissues with resorbable sutures should be carried out in a standard fashion. Primary closure should be obtained, if possible, to facilitate efficient healing.

Management of Other Impacted Teeth

Although the majority of impacted teeth encountered will be third molars and maxillary canines, there will be instances where they are called upon to remove other impacted teeth. The management of other impacted teeth follows the same principles which have been discussed throughout the chapter.

First, a through clinical evaluation should be performed to allow for possible visualization of parts of the tooth or any signs which may help determine its precise location. Following the clinical evaluation is a comprehensive radiographic evaluation. The authors routinely perform a CBCT on all these cases to allow for precise localization of the tooth and its relation to other teeth and vital structures. After evaluation with the surgeon, discussion with the referring dentist should be had to formulate and finalize the treatment plan. Commonly, surgeons will see these referrals from our orthodontic colleagues as part of a comprehensive orthodontic plan. It is essential that all parties are fully understanding of the plan.

Surgical options for impacted teeth are commonly extraction or exposure and ligation. Patients must understand the plan as well as the risks, benefits, and alternatives. The following will discuss the extraction of other impacted teeth as exposure and ligation is discussed elsewhere. Each impacted tooth must be treated as a single entity and although common surgical principles should be followed in each case the surgeon must remain flexible as these teeth may present different challenges. As mentioned before, localization of the tooth is the first step in the process. Clinical and radiographic evaluation will help guide the remainder of the surgical plan.

Maxillary bicuspid impacted teeth are most frequently located on the palatal aspect of the arch. Removal of such teeth presents a particular issue with visualization. Preoperative assessment includes the ability of the patient to tolerate a procedure such as this in a clinic situation. Once a proper venue is decided, a good plan is the key for a smooth procedure. Proper positioning of the patient demands the upper maxillary arch be at least perpendicular to the floor. Good ergonomics will decrease surgeon fatigue as well as decrease surgery time. Once the patient is properly positioned, local anesthesia is provided in order to achieve patient comfort as well as a degree of hemostasis during procedure. By using a sulcular incision a subperiosteal flap is raise. Good technique will avoid brisk bleeding which can be difficult to manage in the sedated patient and alarming in the awake patient. Precise use of electrocautery will prevent palatal necrosis. The palatal soft tissue is firm and does not stretch well so broad exposure is often necessary. A Seldon retractor often works well to retract the palatal soft tissue and is held by the operator on the left side of the patient and the assistant on the right. In our experience, these teeth are often tucked under the erupted teeth in the arch. If one is unable to elevate the tooth at this point, a round bur is used to unroof the tooth of any bone and a trough is made around the crown. The majority of the time this is all that is required. Rarely, does one need to section these teeth, which is fortunate as it is a challenging location to position a drill. If sectioning is undertaken, damage to adjacent roots is a real concern. Once the tooth is removed, visualization of the residual alveolus to inspect for perforation into the antrum or nasal cavity is assessed. If perforation is found, sinus precautions should be instituted after watertight closure of the flap. The authors prefer closure with interdental suturing of 3.0 Chromic.

Maxillary bicuspid teeth which are buccal, or positioned in the arch and impacted can usually be approached by a buccal route. Buccal approach should be performed as described in this chapter previously or by surgeon's preference. Consideration should be given to bone grafting these defects if large interdental defects are left after extraction, especially for patients in active orthodontics.

Mandibular bicuspid teeth are another common impaction which is referred to the OMS. These teeth may be impacted on the buccal or lingual and both present challenges in removal due to the anatomy present in the region. As mentioned before, the first step in treatment is determining the setting of care for the patient, taking into account patient comfort, patient morbidity, and which setting will facilitate efficient and safe removal. Those with deep impaction which may require significant retraction and bone removal may be better suited for an operating room where the surgeon can have maximal access. While those which are partially impacted may be performed in a clinic setting. Regardless of the setting, the surgical approach remains the same.

Patient preparation for removal of lingually impacted bicuspids is paramount to ensure delivery. The patient is commonly positioned with mandibular occlusal plan parallel to the floor to allow for good visualization and ease of use of the handpiece by the surgeon. After chair adjustment, a medium or large bite block is placed on the contralateral side of the occlusion. A throat screen and a sweetheart retractor are then positioned to allow for tongue retraction and to prevent aspiration. Once completed then mandibular blocks are performed as well as local infiltration of the lingual tissues in the vicinity of the impaction. This local infiltration will assist with hydrodissection of the tissues and enable easier flap elevation. Once completed a sulcular incision is created using a #15 blade. The overall length will need to be broad and is dictated by the depth of the impaction. It is essential to limit tension on the flap and for this reason incisions are usually made from second molar to approximately the canine with extension anterior as needed. Dissection is then carried out in a subperiosteal plane using a #9 molt elevator or finer instrument. The dissection must remain subperiosteal to prevent damage to the lingual nerve which is in close proximity to the alveolus in this region. The crown of the tooth should be localized if possible. In those cases where the tooth is fully impacted, CBCT imaging is essential for localization of the tooth and the initial site of bone removal. A Seldon retractor is then placed adjacent to the impacted tooth and positioned against the alveolus. This retractor performs two essential tasks in removal of these teeth. The first being retraction of the tissues allowing for adequate visualization of the surgical site. The second task is protection of these tissues. The surgeon and assistant must be constantly vigilant during the use of the handpiece to ensure that the seldon is fully protecting the tissues as failure to do this may cause tearing of the tissues and significant damage to the lingual nerve. Bone removal is performed with either a round bur or a #702, depending on surgeon preference. The crown is fully exposed, and a trough created around the tooth. Elevation may them be attempted with small straight elevators. As these teeth are commonly impacted with a mesial or vertical inclination, simple elevation maybe all that is needed for removal. However, there are some cases of deep impaction where the delivery of the tooth is blocked out by overlying bone and removal of this bone may lead to an increased change of damage to the roots of the adjacent teeth or significant adjacent root exposure. The authors recommend at this point to section the crown off the tooth, thereby creating space for delivery of the root. This is accomplished in the fashion previously discussed. Roots may then be delivered via simple elevation or with the use of a purchase point in the root. After removal, the site is fully inspected and irrigation carried out. Bone grafting to the area is based on the clinical judgment of the surgeon. If concern exists for postoperative interdental or bone defects, then grafting should be performed in these sites. Closure is carried out with the use or resorbable sutures placed interdentally at each papilla that was reflected during reflection of the flap. This will allow for excellent reapproximation of the flap and efficient healing.

Removal of buccally impacted mandibular bicuspids begins a similar fashion to removal of lingual canines. Patients need to be counseled preoperatively at the risk for postoperative hypoesthesia in the lip and chin on the side of the extraction due to possible manipulation of the mental nerve during the extraction process. Due to the presence of the mental nerve the authors recommend a wide sulcular incision to prevent flap tension and allow for adequate visualization and protection of the mental nerve. Dissection is carried out in an inferior fashion to expose the impacted tooth and the mental nerve. After visualization of the mental nerve it is imperative that it is protected throughout the remainder of the procedure. Once appropriate dissection is completed to allow for bone removal a Minnesota retractor is placed to allow for retraction of the flap buccally. A Seldon or similar retractor is used for protection of the mental nerve. A surgical handpiece under copious irrigation is used for bone removal around the entire crown of the tooth with special care to prevent damage to the adjacent dentition or the mental nerve. After sufficient bone removal, elevators and forceps are used for removal of the tooth. If unable to deliver, then careful sectioning of the crown and removal of the roots is recommended. Irrigation and inspection are carried out followed by full reapproximation of the flap.

Mandibular canines are commonly impacted buccally and should be approached from the buccal aspect of the alveolus. Depending on the depth of the impaction and the position of the crown these teeth may be accessed from sulcular or vestibular incisions. The vestibular incision should be placed within the unattached gingiva inferior at least a few millimeters from the mucogingival junction to allow for closure. After creation of the incisions dissection if used to locate the tooth and a surgical handpiece is used for crown exposure and sectioning if needed. Removal with a combination of elevators and forceps will allow for tooth delivery. Closure of the sulcular incision is performed via reapproximation of each papilla. Vestibular incisions are closed in a layered fashion with Vicryl sutures used for resuspension of the mentalis muscle and closure of the gingiva with resorbable sutures.

Maxillary and mandibular incisors are rarely impacted. In instances where they are noted to be impacted every attempt should be used to use exposure and ligation via a comprehensive orthodontic treatment plan to maintain the tooth. In cases where this is not possible, or significant pathology exists then the surgical plan follows that previously outlined. Teeth should be localized within the alveolus and a surgical plan formulated. Impactions near the alveolar ridge may be accessed via a sulcular incision, whereas deeper impaction may require a vestibular incision. Dissection is similar to all other impactions in a subperiosteal plane. Bone removal is commonly necessary and protection of the tissues via the use of a Minnesota elevator allows for retraction as well as tissue protection. Elevators and forceps are generally sufficient for delivery of the tooth.

Complications with Removal of Impacted Teeth

The process of removal of bone to facilitate the extraction commonly causes patients more postoperative discomfort than that seen with other routine extractions. Patients should be counseled that their activity may be limited first 3–5 days postoperatively due to the sequelae of the surgical process. The swelling and inflammation associated with removal of impacted teeth usually subsides within the first week and patients commonly have a rapid improvement and may return to normal activities after this time period. The vast majority of patients recover in an uneventful fashion; however, it is documented that approximately 10% of patients have some form of complication postoperatively after third molar removal [9]. These complications have a wide range from very mild such as alveolar osteitis to more severe such as jaw fracture. It is noted that complication rates are increased in a variety of circumstances to include surgeon experience, age of patient, depth of impaction, and position of tooth [10, 11]. Patients presenting with factors which may increase complications rates should be counseled preoperatively that the postoperative period may differ from that of other friends or family members.

Bleeding

Prevention of postoperative bleeding starts with a thorough history and physical. Patients with possible bleeding disorders, family history of bleeding disorders, on systemic anticoagulation or antiplatelet therapy should be identified preoperatively and the appropriate labs, medication adjustments, and premedications provided prior to initiation of surgery. Significant postoperative bleeding is a rare occurrence during removal of impacted teeth. Good surgical technique and careful manipulation of the soft tissues will assist in prevention of unnecessary bleeding in the surgical site. However, if bleeding does occur the first step in the process of control should be direct pressure with gauze to the site. If direct pressure is unsuccessful at control of the bleeding, then a variety of hemostatic agents are available to assist the surgeon in control. The use of a gelatin sponge and oversuturing the site is commonly sufficient for bleeding control at the site. In addition, oxidized cellulose may be packed into the surgical site, but due to reports of neurotoxicity during breakdown it should be used with caution near the IAN. Microfibrillar collagen may also be packed into the site in cases of uncontrollable hemorrhage. Bone bleeding is controlled by pressure on the bone with the back side of a curette or bone wax.

Nerve Damage

Surgical removal of impacted teeth puts at risk several branches of the trigeminal nerve, specifically the lingual and inferior alveolar nerves. Manipulation of the tooth roots may lead to neurosensory disturbances in the IAN, whereas reflection of tissue flaps may lead to issues with the lingual nerve. It is reported that only about 3% of cases result in a nerve injury and the vast majority are transient in nature [12–14]. Even though these disturbances are transient they may be extremely disconcerting to the patient and subsequently these patients must be followed until full resolution. Patients reporting neurosensory disturbances postoperatively are seen at regular intervals to track the progress of the injury. As previously stated, many of these are minor paresthesia or hypoesthesia's and spontaneously resolve within the first few weeks. Complete management and timing is outside the scope of this chapter, but all cases of NSD should be carefully monitored and thorough documentation undertaken.

Displaced Roots

During the extraction process teeth and roots may become displaced into unwanted areas. Prevention of this is paramount as removal is quite challenging. Visualization of the entire surgical field is a key first step as well as use of controlled forces for removal. Maxillary teeth or root tips may become displaced into the maxillary sinus or the infratemporal fossa. If displacement into the infratemporal fossa occurs the surgeon should use finger pressure to pull the tooth forward followed by careful suctioning. If this is unsuccessful then it may be prudent to wait approximately 4–6 weeks for fibrosis to occur prior to further attempted removal. If asymptomatic and no other indication exists, the surgeon and patient may elect to leave the tooth in place. Displacement into the maxillary sinus may require the use of a Caldwell-Luc Antrostomy for visualization and removal of the root tip is displacement occurs.

Displaced fragments during removal of mandibular third molars commonly enter the submandibular space. Gentle finger pressure in an anterior direction may allow for retrieval of the root, but if this is unsuccessful then as, previously mentioned, a waiting period of 4–6 weeks may be needed to allow for fibrosis. Imaging will be needed to localize the fragment and surgical plans can be formulated after confirmation of the exact location.

Sinus Perforations

Perforation of the maxillary sinus is a possibility with removal of impacted maxillary teeth as they lie in close proximity to the sinus walls and membrane. Failure to recognize this communication or perforation may lead to the formation of a fistula at this site. The incidence of this occurs most frequently with removal of maxillary first molars as their palatal root is in close proximity to the sinus membrane. The incidence of oral-antral communication with removal of third molars is reported to be approximately 0.25% [15, 16]. The low reported rate is possibly due to lack of recognition at time of surgery.

As previously mentioned after removal of teeth the alveolus must be carefully inspected. Communications of 2 mm or less will commonly resolve and heal without any further treatment or interventions. The authors recommend replacement of the flap and closure of all sites, regardless of visualization of the sinus membrane to ensure healing and patient comfort. If a larger exposure is identified, then a variety of techniques exist for repair of the area. Communications of 3–5 mm may be addressed with closure of the site and strict sinus precautions. In areas with communications of 6+ mm the use of buccal flaps, gold foil, palatal flaps, and tongue flaps are possible options. The authors prefer the use of a buccal flap. The ease of access and ability for quick and predictable repair and healing of the area with minimal additional discomfort to the patient. If persistent fistula is noted, the authors prefer secondary treatment with a buccal fat pad flap in the presence of a three layered closure. The buccal fat pad is accessed by the use of blunt dissection in the superior aspect of a flap commonly used for third molars. This blunt dissection is directed toward the cheek through the periosteum. Once identified the fat pad is gently teased from the area until it can be positioned over the site with no tension. It is secured to the palatal mucosa with Vicryl sutures and the mucosal flap positioned over top of the area and secured in place. Primary closure of the site is preferred, but not required as the fat pad will epithelialize within a few weeks postoperatively.

Patients with sinus communications or fistulas are placed in strict sinus precautions which include no nose blowing, no straws, no smoking, and sneezing with an open mouth for 4 weeks. Furthermore, saline sinus rinses and decongestants such as Sudafed are prescribed to improve patient comfort. Additionally, Augmentin or Clindamycin are prescribed for patients to prevent any postoperative infections. Patients are closely followed postoperatively to ensure routine healing of the areas and compliance with the sinus precautions. Complete healing must be ensured to prevent formation of a fistula and further surgical interventions (see Sect. 2, Chap. 4)

Alveolar Osteitis

Alveolar osteitis (AO) or “dry socket” is the most common postoperative complication related to removal of third molars. Literature reports the presence of AO as somewhere between 3% and 25% [15]. It is thought to be related to the premature fibrinolysis of a blood clot, most commonly in the mandibular third molar extraction sites. Prior to replacement with granulation tissue the blood clot is lost leading to increased pain and odor within the sites. The overall pathogenesis is not well understood and the literature concerning prevention and treatment strategies is inconsistent. Use of 0.12% Chlorhexidine rinse immediately prior to surgery followed by use in the immediate postoperative period has been shown to decrease the presence of alveolar osteitis [17]. Furthermore, decreasing surgical trauma, use of a handpiece, and copious irrigation are all established recommendations for minimizing the incidence of AO.

Treatment is aimed at reducing the patient's symptoms and improving their postoperative course. Many different medicaments, dressings, and agents exist, but there is little evidence as to the superiority of one over the others. In the authors practice the site is irrigated with chlorhexidine to reduce the overall bacterial load and clear any food or debris from the area. Finally, a dressing consisting of a collagen sponge and eugenol is placed into the socket. Eugenol acts to interrupt neural transmission and assists in pain control but should be used with caution in sites with exposure of the IAN due to the potential for neurotoxicity. Patients are then seen for follow-ups every 48–72 h for dressing changes and evaluation of healing. Additional NSAIDS may be prescribed but the use of additional narcotics is not always necessary with the use of medicaments. The patient will continue to follow up until full resolution of symptoms.

Infection

Surgery within the oral cavity is considered a clean-contaminated procedure. Literature reports infection rates of clean-contaminated procedures at 3.94% [18]. The incidence of infection postoperatively from removal of impacted third molars ranges from 0.8% to 4.2% [15]. Infections maybe classified as early or late based on the postoperative time during which they are seen. Risk factors increasing the infection rate include increased age of the patient, depth of impaction, presence of inflammation—gingivitis or pericoronitis, experience of the surgeon, and location of surgery [15]. Routine use of antibiotics is not recommended as there appears to be little evidence to suggest a significant decrease in infections with their use.

Early postoperative infections are considered a mixed infection with the presence of both aerobic and anaerobic species which is consistent with the normal oral flora. Infections typically spread along fascial planes to the adjacent spaces. Infections from maxillary third molar sites typically are seen in the maxillary vestibule, buccal space, and the temporal areas. Those resulting from mandibular surgical sites have the ability to spread to the mandibular vestibule, buccal space, masseteric space, pterygomandibular space, and submandibular space. Spread to the submandibular, pterygomandibular, and lateral pharyngeal spaces has the potential to be life threatening via airway compromise and spread to deeper spaces.

All patients reporting persistent or increasing swelling after the initial healing period of 4–7 days should be evaluated in office by the surgeon for the potential presence of postoperative infection. After determination of the severity of the infection, patients should be placed on the appropriate antibiotic regimen. Debridement and irrigation of the area is critical if an infection is suspected. After appropriate surgical intervention, penicillins are an excellent choice as the first line antibiotics in non-allergic patients. Due to the presence of increased beta-lactamase resistance, the authors commonly prescribe Augmentin due to its increased profile and twice a day dosing. Clindamycin remains an excellent choice as its spectrum includes both aerobic and anaerobic organisms. However, the dosing schedule is more cumbersome, so compliance is decreased. In some rare instances, severe infections may present postoperatively and hospital admission may be needed. These circumstances should be rapidly identified, and all appropriate steps taken to identify the source of the infection, immediate surgical intervention, and appropriate administration of IV antibiotics.

A significant percentage of infections are considered late infections. They are related to retained debris under the surgical flap not removed during the surgical process. They commonly present three to four weeks postoperatively and are considered subperiosteal abscesses. Patients will commonly report full resolution of symptoms, but then a small area of swelling appears at the three to four week time frame. In these instances, the authors recommend surgical site irrigation and a course of antibiotics. If failure to resolve symptoms after this treatment, we recommend debridement of the area.

For infection rates to remain low it is critical that surgeons exercise good surgical technique with copious irrigation throughout the tooth removal process. All patients with complaints of continued postoperative swelling should be quickly and thoroughly evaluated. Postoperative antibiotics should be used in the appropriate circumstances with the provider taking into account the most likely source of the infection and the most common microorganisms. Surgical debridement and irrigation are cornerstones of source control in postoperative infections. Furthermore, patients should be regularly seen throughout the process to ensure full resolution of healing and prevention of complications such as osteomyelitis.

References

1. Bui C, Seldin EB, Dodson T. Types, frequencies, and risk factors for complications after third molar extraction. J Oral Maxillofac Surg. 2003;61:1379–89.
2. Phillips C, White R, Shugars D, et al. Risk factors associated with prolonged recovery and delayed healing after third molar surgery. J Oral Maxillofac Surg. 2003;61:1436–48.
3. Stuart EL, Harry D, David F. AAOMS parameters of care dentoalveolar surgery. J Oral Maxillofac Surg. 2017;75(Suppl 1):e50–73.
4. Pell G, Gregory G. Report on a ten-year study of a tooth division technique for the removal of impacted teeth. Am J Orthod. 1942;28:660.

5. Rood J, Shehab A. The radiologic prediction of inferior alveolar nerve injury during third molar surgery. Br J Oral Maxillofac Surg. 1990;28:20–5.
6. Osunde O, Adebola R, Saheeb B. A comparative study of the effect of suture-less and multiple suture techniques on inflammatory complications following third molar surgery. Int J Oral Maxillofac Surg. 2012;41:1275–9.
7. Rayne R. The unerupted maxilary canine. Dent Pract Denr Rec. 1969;19:194–205.
8. Stellzig A, Basadra E, Komposch G. The etiology of canine tooth impactions—a space analysis. Fortsher Kieferorthop. 1994;55(3):97–103.
9. Goldberg M, Nemarich A, Marco W. Complications after mandibular third molar surgery: a statistical analysis of 500 consecutive procedures in private practice. J Am Dent Assoc. 1985;111:277–9.
10. Hinds E, Frey K. Hazards of retained third molars in older persons: report of 15 cases. J Am Dent Assoc. 1980;101:2460250.
11. Sisk A, Hammer W, Shelton D, Joy E. Complications following third molar surgery: the role of the experience of the surgeon. J Oral Maxillofac Surg. 1986;44:855–9.
12. Wofford D, Miller R. Prospective study of dysesthesia following odontectomy of impacted third molars. J Oral Maxillofac Surg. 1987;45:15–9.
13. Manson D. Lingual nerve damage following lower third molar surgery. Int J Oral Maxillofac Surg. 1988;17:290–4.
14. Robinson P. Observations on the recovery of sensation following inferior alveolar nerve injuries. Br J Oral Maxillofac Surg. 1998;26:177–89.
15. Bouloux G, Steed M, Perciaccante V. Complications of third molar surgery. Oral Maxillofac Surg Clin N Am. 2007;19:117–28.
16. Punwutikorn J, Waikakul A, Pairuchvej V. Clinically significant oroantral communications: a study of incidence and site. Int J Oral Maxillofac Surg. 1994;23:19.
17. Larsen P. The effect of chlorhexidine rinse on the incidence of alveolar osteitis following surgical removal of impacted mandibular molars. J Oral Maxillofac Surg. 1991;49:932–7.
18. Ortega G, et al. An evaluation of surgical site infections by wound classification system using the ACS-NSQIP. J Surg Res. 2012;174(1):33–8.

Coronectomy

15

Regina Landesberg

Introduction

The removal of mandibular third molars is associated with temporary paresthesia/anesthesia in 0.26–8.4% of cases while the incidence of permanent nerve damage is reported to be as high as 3.6%. Multiple factors are associated with an increased risk of IAN damage, including patient age, operator experience, difficulty of surgical procedure, and the anatomic relationship of the tooth to the inferior alveolar canal (IAC) [1–3]. Coronectomy was first described by Knutsson [4] as a procedure to decrease the potential for IAN injury in high-risk patients. The surgical technique involves an atraumatic removal of the third molar crown, leaving the root fragment(s) undisturbed with little to no trauma to the IAN (Fig. 15.1). The limited number of RCT, CCT, and case reports suggest that coronectomy results

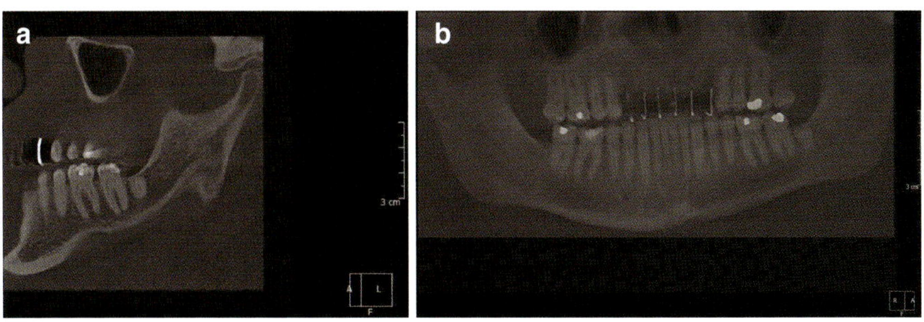

Fig. 15.1 Cone beam CT of 23-year-old male who had a successful coronectomy performed 6 years prior. Note that the roots of #17 are covered by bone. Courtesy of Dr. Aditya Tadinada. (**a**) Lateral view, (**b**) Panoramic view

R. Landesberg (✉)
Oral/Maxillofacial Surgery, Simsbury, CT, USA
e-mail: Elferneini@uchc.edu

E. M. Ferneini, M. T. Goupil (eds.), *Office-Based Maxillofacial Surgical Procedures*, https://doi.org/10.1007/978-3-030-22371-7_15

in a significant decrease in IAN deficits in high-risk patients (0.00–1.3%) when compared to complete surgical extraction of third molars [5, 6]. In the only two RCT (discussed below) where coronectomy was compared with a control group of patients who had complete surgical extractions, infection rates were not statistically different. Complications unique to coronectomy include a failed procedure requiring complete tooth removal. This is most often due to the inadvertent mobilization of root(s) [7, 8]. Additionally, the migration of retained root fragments with the potential for a second surgical procedure remains a concern; however, in a recent study of 612 coronectomies followed for up to five years, the incidence of root exposure was 2.3% [9].

Indications

The major indication for performing a coronectomy as opposed to complete surgical removal of a tooth is to avoid injury to the IAN resulting in temporary/permanent paresthesia/anesthesia. Appropriate patient selection appears to be paramount to a successful outcome. Perhaps the most important risk factor in predicting the risk of nerve damage is the radiographic proximity of the IAN to the third molar. Panoramic radiographic findings that suggest increased risk for IAN injury include interruption of the lamina dura of the Inferior IAC, displacement of the IAC, narrowing of the IAC, and darkening and/or deflection of the tooth root(s) [10, 11]. While there are no defined quantitative parameters, several authors, most notably Matzen et al. [12], recommended obtaining a cone beam CT (CBCT) when panoramic radiographs show one or several of the above findings. While the authors acknowledge that CBCT adds an additional expense as well radiation exposure, it was felt to provide a more accurate assessment of the relationship of tooth roots to IAN as well as give the surgeon additional guidance should the coronectomy fail necessitating complete root removal [13].

Contraindications

Teeth with active decay that extends into the pulp are not candidates for coronectomy. Periapical pathology is another contraindication for this procedure. Coronectomy is contraindicated in patients who are immunocompromised, including those receiving chemotherapy, radiation, or immunotherapy. Additionally, this procedure is not recommended in poorly controlled diabetics. Horizontally impacted teeth where the crown is located close to the IAN are not good candidates for this procedure as there may be a higher risk of IAN injury than complete removal [14–17]. Other contraindications include patients who are scheduled for orthognathic surgery or orthodontic distalization of second molars. The incidence of root migration requiring a second surgical is reported to be low (2.3%) and can usually be performed under local anesthesia. The majority of root migration in coronectomy patients slows to a minimum at 24 months and most authors recommend a follow-up of at least 6 months [9]. Therefore, this procedure may not be the best choice for those patients that are unwilling to commit to a longer period of postoperative observation than what is required for those who undergo complete surgical removal of third molars.

Procedure

Multiple authors have reported various minor modifications of the original technique for coronectomy [7, 8, 13–17]. The tooth is exposed with a mucoperiosteal flap, similar to that used for complete surgical removal of the third molars. Most surgeons describe the use of a release incision. The overwhelming majority of surgeons favor a buccal approach; however, the technique described by Pogrel (Fig. 15.2) involves raising both buccal and lingual flaps with placement of a lingual retractor to protect the lingual nerve while the crown is sectioned in total with a fissure bur at a 45° angle [16, 17]. If exposure of the tooth is necessary, a minimal amount of buccal bone should be removed with a fissure bur that will allow access to the cemental enamel junction. Renton et al. [8] and Gleeson [18] described partial sectioning of

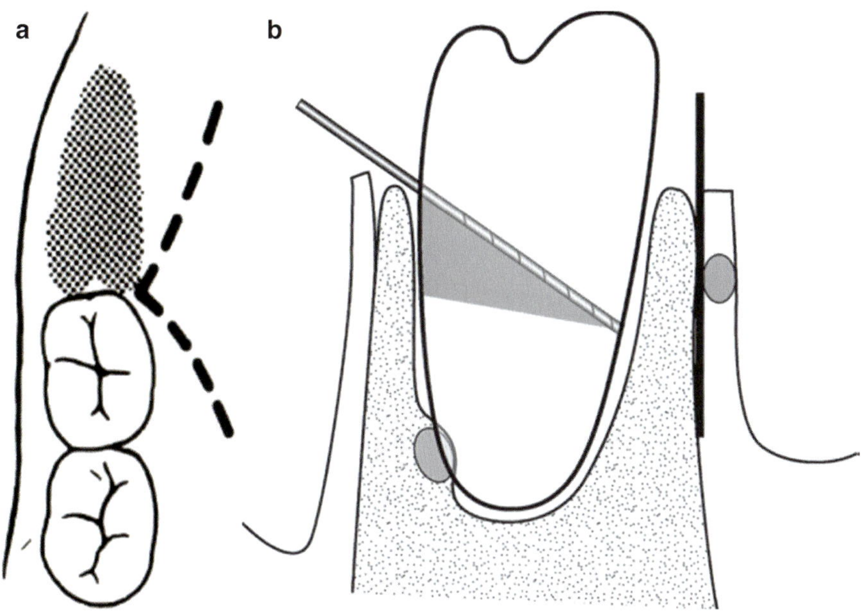

Fig. 15.2 Coronectomy technique as described by Pogrel [17]. (**a**) A conventional buccal incision left side along the external oblique ridge to the distobuccal line angle of the second molar and a releasing incision into the sulcus. (**b**) Diagrammatic representation of coronectomy technique. A lingual retractor is in place to protect the lingual soft tissues, including the lingual nerve, and the fissure bur is used at approximately 45° to section the crown completely. The gray area is then removed secondarily to place the apical portion of the tooth at least 2–3 mm below the crest of bone. Reprinted from Oral Surg Clin NA: 19, Pogrel MA, Partial Odontectomy 85-91 (2007) with permission from Elsevier

the crown with a fissure bur and completing the decoronation with the use of elevators. There is significant concern among several authors that the force generated during elevation may predispose to mobilization of the root fragment(s) and failed coronectomy, resulting in the need for complete surgical extraction. This concern has led Monaco et al. [13] to section the crown in mesiodistal and buccolingual directions. All authors perform reduction of root fragment(s) so they sit 2–4 mm below the crest of the alveolar bone after removal of the crown. No pulp treatment is necessary as the studies have shown that root fragments remain vital [19, 20]. Primary closure of the surgical incision is uniformly recommended regardless of surgical technique.

Complications

Most of the reported complications associated with performing a coronectomy are similar to those seen with surgical removal of third molars, including pain, swelling, bleeding, infection, delayed healing, and dry socket. A systemic review by Long et al. [6] reported inconsistent use of pre- and postoperative antibiotics.

Coronectomy was developed as an alternative to complete surgical removal of mandibular third molars that would eliminate or significantly decrease temporary/permanent paresthesia/anesthesia due to injury of the IAN. While the reported incidence of temporary paresthesia/anesthesia is 0.26–8.4%, permanent nerve damage is reported to be as high as 3.6% for surgical extraction of mandibular third molars [1–3]. With the exception of a 2004 study by O'Riordan [21] who reported sensory loss in 3/52 coronectomy patients, the incidence of nerve injury for coronectomy ranges from 0.00% to 0.09%. A 2012 systemic review of the best available studies (two RCT and two CCT) reported the incidence of IAN deficits between 00.0% and 065% and the incidence of lingual nerve injury (LNI) appears to be extremely low (0.05%) [6]. Pogrel [16, 17] reported one case of transient LNI likely due to their surgical exposure involving both buccal and lingual approaches with the use of a lingual retractor (see Procedure section). The only other report of LNI was a study by Pederson et al. where 5/231 coronectomies had evidence of LNI one week after surgery. All LNI had had resolved by the final postoperative visit [22].

While some degree of root migration is reported in the overwhelming majority of patients following coronectomy, most reports follow patients for a limited period of time, typically 6–24 months with panoramic radiographs. Yeung et al. [23] evaluated root migration patterns 4–8.5 years after coronectomy of 57 mandibular third molars by CBCT and found that the mean amount of migration was 2.82 mm. Consistent with that reported by others, the roots predominantly migrated mesially (76.8%) and the degree of migration had a negative correlation with the age of the patient. Most studies found that the majority of root migration occurred during the first 24 months following coronectomy and the roots tended to migrate away from the IAC. The incidence of root eruption that required subsequent removal is reported to be between 0% and 9%; however, none of these cases resulted in damage to the IAN [22–25].

Failed coronectomy requiring complete surgical extraction has been reported to be as high as 38.3% in a 2004 study by Renton et al. [8]; however, other RCT and CCT had an incidence between 2.3 and 9.4% [5]. The need to convert a coronectomy procedure into a complete surgical removal most often is due to mobilization of the tooth root while sectioning the crown. The procedure is technique sensitive and may explain some of the large deviations in failure rates reported in the literature. Other factors that may increase the likelihood of root mobilization include type and depth of impaction. One study reported that females with conical roots had the highest risk of root mobilization [8].

Review of Literature

Since the original description in 1989 there have been multiple articles in the literature describing coronectomy as an alternative to surgical removal of mandibular third molars where a high risk for IAN exists. While many of the publications have been case reports, several prospective and retrospective studies exist (Table 15.1). These as well as the only two RCT and two CCT available to date have been analyzed in several systemic reviews and meta-analysis [5, 24]. A systemic review by Long et al. cited limitations due to few studies that met criteria for inclusion, no high-quality studies and short periods of follow-up [6].

In the larger of two RCT performed by Leung and Cheung in 2009 [7], 349 mandibular third molars with close proximity to the IAN were randomized (171 coronectomies, 178 complete surgical removals). Patients with radiographic criteria

Table 15.1 Summary of outcomes of coronectomy

Author (year)	Study type	#CSR	Coronectomies		Transient injury			Permanent injury		
			Successful	Failed	CSR	Suc Cor	Failed Cor	CSR	Suc Cor	Failed Cor
Renton (2005)	RCT	102	58	36	19	0	3	NR	0	2(8)
Leung (2009)	RCT	178	155	16	9	1	1	3	0	0(7)
Hatano (2009)	CC	–	98	4	–	1	0	–	0	0(25)
Cilasun (2011)	CC	–	86	2	–	0	0	–	0	0(26)
Pogrel (2004)	PCS	–	47	3	–	0	0	–	0	0(30)
Goto (2012)	PCS	–	49	3	–	0	0	–	0	0(29)
Kohara (2015)	PCS	–	101	10	–	1	0	–	0	0(28)
Monaco (2015)	PCS	–	108	8	–	0	0	–	0	0(13)
Pederson (2018)	PCS	–	231	NR	–	5	NR	–	3	0(22)
Kouwenberg (2016)	PCS	–	134	17	–	0	0	–	0	0(27)
O'Riordan (2004)	RCS	–	49	3	–	3	0	–	1	0(21)

RCT randomized control trial, *CC* case controlled study, *PCS* prospective cohort study, *RCS* retrospective cohort study, *NR* not reported (as detailed in Indications above) were randomized to one of two procedure groups. Procedures were carried out by surgical residents at the University of Hong Kong. IAN deficits, lingual nerve deficits, postoperative pain, infection, and dry socket were evaluated at 1 week and 1, 3, 6, 12, and 24 months. Panoramic radiographs were taken postoperatively for coronectomy patients at 1 week and at 3, 6, 12, and 24 months and the degree of root migration was calculated. Sixteen cases (9.4%) resulted in loosening of roots during the coronectomy procedure and the procedure was switched to a complete surgical removal. These cases were considered "failed coronectomies" and were analyzed as a separate group. IAN deficit accounted for 9/178 (5.10%) in teeth that received complete surgical removal of third molars and 1/155 (0.65%) in teeth that underwent a coronectomy. These results were statistically significant ($p = 0.023$). There was one case (1/16, 6.25%) of IAN deficit in the failed coronectomy group. No lingual paresthesia/anesthesia was noted in any group. The IAN defect in the coronectomy patient recovered after 6 months while 6/9 patients in the surgical removal group recovered after 1 month. The remaining three patients had persistent hypoesthesia. The patient in the failed coronectomy with an IAN deficit was reported to have a full recovery at 6 months.

The percentage of patients who reported pain at one week was significantly lower in the coronectomy group (57.3% 101/178, 41.9% 65/155 $p = 0.005$). There was also a significantly lower mean VAS score in the coronectomy group at one week (3.7 vs. 3.1 $p = 0.026$) but there were no differences in pain at any of the subsequent time periods. Infection rates were not different between groups. While there were no cases of dry socket in the coronectomy group, 5/178 (2.8%) cases were reported in the extraction group. Root migration was followed in this study for 24 months and was seen in 62.2% of patients in 3 months. The total amount of migration at 24 months ranged from 0 to 6 mm. The authors have continued to follow long-term root migration with panoramic and CBCT in this patient population for upwards of 8.5 years (see Complications). This study, the larger of the only two available RCT, demonstrates that coronectomy was successful in significantly decreasing IAN injury in high-risk patients; however, there are several methodological shortcomings of note. Surgical procedures were performed by the resident staff and the number of different surgeons or their level of training was not reported. Furthermore, it does not appear that the evaluation of IAN defects was blinded as to procedure.

In the only other RCT by Renton et al. [8], 128 patients who had radiographic evidence of proximity of third molars to the IAC were randomized into one of the two groups, coronectomy ($n = 94$) or complete surgical extraction ($n = 102$). All procedures were performed by three surgeons with the assistance of senior house officers. During the coronectomy procedure, 36/94 patients had roots that were mobilized, necessitating complete surgical removal. These patients were therefore assigned to a subgroup designated "failed coronectomy" and analyzed as a distinct group. The mean follow-up period was 25 months. IAN injury was reported in 19 patients (18.6%) in the extraction group and 3 patients (8.3%) in the failed coronectomy group. There were no cases of IAN reported in patients that had received a coronectomy. No significant differences in infection or dry socket rates were noted and none of the patients in the study had eruption of retained roots that required removal. Of note was the large number of failed coronectomies (38.3%) in this study, which was significantly higher than that reported by Leung and Cheung as well as others [3, 5–7]. This may be attributed to differences in surgical protocol as the technique described by Renton et al. [8] appears to rely on a greater use of elevation than that described by others.

In a meta-analysis by Cervear-Espert et al. [24] the 2 RCT (above) as well as the 2 CCT that compared coronectomy to complete surgical extraction all showed a significant decrease in IAN deficit (89% decrease, 95% CI). A systemic review by Long et al. [6] of pooled data from the same 4 studies determined that the relative risk of IAN injury was 0.11 (95% CI) which indicates that complete surgical removal is nearly 10 times more likely than coronectomy to suffer paresthesia/anesthesia. Several other prospective and retrospective cohort studies have demonstrated a low incidence of IAN injury following coronectomy when compared to that reported in the literature for complete surgical removal of third molars (Table 15.1). A recent systemic review by Dalle Carbonare et al. [5] surveyed publications between January 1990 and October 2016 and evaluated IAN and lingual nerve injuries in successful and failed coronectomies. Fourteen papers, including 2 RCT (reviewed above), 2 CCT (Hatano et al. [26], Cilausn et al. [27]), 2 retrospective cohort studies, and 8 prospective cohort studies met the criteria for inclusion in their analysis. Of 2087 coronectomies there were 152 failures (7%). The incidence of IAN and lingual nerve injury was 0.5% and 0.05%, respectively, for successful coronectomies while failed coronectomies had a 2.6% incidence of IAN injury. Permanent IAN paresthesia was seen in 0.05% of successful coronectomies and in 1.3% of coronectomies that failed. No permanent lingual nerve paresthesias were seen in successful or failed coronectomies. Root mobility, root migration or root exposure were found to be the most common causes for failure of coronectomies. The authors conclude that since the incidence of permanent IAN paresthesia following coronectomy is lower than that seen with complete surgical removal of third molars (1.3% and 3.6%, respectively), coronectomy is a safe alternative to complete surgical removal of deeply impacted third molars. It is however essential to discuss potential complications, including the 7% incidence of failed coronectomy when obtaining preoperative consent. Furthermore, these investigators strongly recommend development of a standardized protocol for patient follow-up as presently there is no consensus on the length of postoperative observation or radiographic evaluation for coronectomy patients [5].

Conclusions

Coronectomy appears to be a viable alternative to complete surgical removal of mandibular third molars where the risk of IAN temporary/permanent nerve damage is high. Patients must be carefully selected as there are several postoperative complications (root migration and exposure) unique to this procedure. Furthermore, coronectomy appears to require a longer follow-up period than that of surgical removal of third molars. The availability of good RCT is severely limited which likely explains the lack of a more widespread acceptance of this procedure in clinical practice.

References

1. Queral-Godoy E, Valmaseda-Castellón E, Berini-Aytés L, Gay-Escoda C. Incidence and evolution of inferior alveolar nerve lesions following lower third molar extraction. Oral Surg Oral Med Oral Pathol Oral Radiol Endod. 2005;99(3):259–64.
2. Leung YY, Cheung LK. Risk factors of neurosensory deficits in lower third molar surgery: an literature review of prospective studies. Int J Oral Maxillofac Surg. 2011;40(1):1–10.
3. Cheung LK, Leung YY, Chow LK, Wong MC, Chan EK, Fok YH. Incidence of neurosensory deficits and recovery after lower third molar surgery: a prospective clinical study of 4338 cases. Int J Oral Maxillofac Surg. 2010;39(4):320–6.
4. Knutsson K, Lysell L, Rohlin M. Postoperative status after partial removal of the mandibular third molar. Swed Dent J. 1989;13(1-2):15–22.
5. Dalle Carbonare M, Zavattini A, Duncan M, Williams M, Moody A. Injury to the inferior alveolar and lingual nerves in successful and failed coronectomies: systematic review. Br J Oral Maxillofac Surg. 2017;55(9):892–8.
6. Long H, Zhou Y, Liao L, Pyakurel U, Wang Y, Lai W. Coronectomy vs. total removal for third molar extraction: a systematic review. J Dent Res. 2012;91(7):659–65.
7. Leung YY, Cheung LK. Safety of coronectomy versus excision of wisdom teeth: a randomized controlled trial. Oral Surg Oral Med Oral Pathol Oral Radiol Endod. 2009;108(6):21–7.
8. Renton T, Hankins M, Sproate C, McGurk M. A randomised controlled clinical trial to compare the incidence of injury to the inferior alveolar nerve as a result of coronectomy and removal of mandibular third molars. Br J Oral Maxillofac Surg. 2005;43(1):7–12.
9. Leung YY, Cheung KY. Root migration pattern after third molar coronectomy: a long-term analysis. Int J Oral Maxillofac Surg. 2018;47(6):802–8.
10. Rood JP, Shehab BA. The radiological prediction of inferior alveolar nerve injury during third molar surgery. Br J Oral Maxillofac Surg. 1990;28(1):20–5.
11. Sedaghatfar M, August MA, Dodson TB. Panoramic radiographic findings as predictors of inferior alveolar nerve exposure following third molar extraction. J Oral Maxillofac Surg. 2005;63(1):3–7.
12. Matzen LH, Christensen J, Hintze H, Schou S, Wenzel A. Influence of cone beam CT on treatment plan before surgical intervention of mandibular third molars and impact of radiographic factors on deciding on coronectomy vs surgical removal. Dentomaxillofac Radiol. 2013;42(1):98870341.
13. Monaco G, Vignudelli E, Diazzi M, Marchetti C, Corinaldesi G. Coronectomy of mandibular third molars: a clinical protocol to avoid inferior alveolar nerve injury. J Craniomaxillofac Surg. 2015;43(8):1694–9.
14. Patel V, Gleeson CF, Kwok J, Sproat C. Coronectomy practice. Paper 2: complications and long term management. Br J Oral Maxillofac Surg. 2013;51(4):347–52.
15. Gady J, Fletcher MC. Coronectomy: indications, outcomes, and description of techniqueAtlas Oral Maxillofac Surg Clin North Am. 2013;21(2):221–6.
16. Pogrel MA. Coronectomy: partial odontectomy or intentional root retention. Oral Maxillofac Surg Clin North Am. 2015;27(3):373–82.
17. Pogrel MA. Partial odontectomy. Oral Maxillofac Surg Clin North Am. 2007;19(1):85–91.
18. Gleeson CF, Patel V, Kwok J, Sproat C. Coronectomy practice. Paper 1. Technique and troubleshooting. Br J Oral Maxillofac Surg. 2012;50(8):739–44.
19. Patel V, Sproat C, Kwok J, Beneng K, Thavaraj S, McGurk M. Histological evaluation of mandibular third molar roots retrieved after coronectomy. J Oral Maxillofac Surg. 2014;52(5):415–9.
20. Vignudelli E, Monaco G, Mazzoni A, Marchetti C. Root fragment vitality after coronectomy: histological evidence in a case. J Oral Maxillofac Surg. 2015;73(11):2093.
21. O'Riordan BC. Coronectomy (intentional partial odontectomy of lower third molars). Oral Surg Oral Med Oral Pathol Oral Radiol Endod. 2004;98(3):274–80.

22. Pederson MH, Bak J, Matzen LH, Hartlev J, Bindslev J, Schou S, Nørholt SE. Coronectomy of mandibular third molars: a clinical and radiological study of 231 cases with a mean follow-up period of 5.7 years. Int J Oral Maxillofac Surg. 2018;47(12):1596–603.
23. Yeung AWK, Wong NSM, Bornstein MM, Leung YY. Three-dimensional radiographic evaluation of root migration patterns 4-8.5 years after lower third molar coronectomy: a cone beam computed tomography study. Int J Oral Maxillofac Surg. 2018;47(9):1145–52.
24. Cervera-Espert J, Pérez-Martínez S, Cervera-Ballester J, Peñarrocha-Oltra D, Peñarrocha-Diago M. Coronectomy of impacted mandibular third molars: a meta-analysis and systematic review of the literature. Med Oral Patol Oral Cir Bucal. 2016;21(4):e505–13.
25. Hatano Y, Kurita K, Kuroiwa Y, Yuasa H, Ariji E. Clinical evaluations of coronectomy (intentional partial odontectomy) for mandibular third molars using dental computed tomography: a case-control study. J Oral Maxillofac Surg. 2009;67(9):1806–14.
26. Cilasun U, Yildirim T, Guzeldemir E, Pektas ZO. Coronectomy in patients with high risk of inferior alveolar nerve injury diagnosed by computed tomography. J Oral Maxillofac Surg. 2011;69(6):1557–61.
27. Kouwenberg AJ, Stroy LP, Rijt ED, Mensink G, Gooris PJ. Coronectomy of the mandibular third molar: respect for the inferior alveolar nerve. J Craniomaxillofac Surg. 2016;44(5):616–21.

Part III

Maxillofacial Cosmetic Procedures

Scar Revision in the Office Setting

16

Neel S. Joshi, Zulara N. Wahla, and Charles L. Castiglione

Modern surgical techniques rely upon the regenerative capacity of tissue to restore baseline function and appearance. A surgical wound undergoes a well-documented physiologic process that can be divided into four dynamic and overlapping phases that include vascular response, inflammatory response, proliferation, and maturation. The primary vascular response consists of vasoconstriction, platelet aggregation, and initiation of clot formation. During the inflammatory response, macrophages and white blood cells move to the area of injury with a focus on removing damaged cells, pathogens, and bacteria. The markers of inflammation—rubor, calor, tumor, and dolor—are seen during this phase. In the proliferative phase, myofibroblasts rebuild the wound with new collagen and extracellular matrix, causing wound contracture. This is the period during which re-epithelialization is known to occur. The final remodeling phase consists of a transition from type III to type I collagen and full maturation of the scar [1]. A derangement of this intrinsic healing process may lead to aberrant scarring.

Cicatrix, or scar tissue, is the fibrous tissue that replaces normal tissues that are destroyed following injury or disease or that are divided after an incision [2]. Scar tissue is important for many reasons ranging from function to aesthetic outcomes. The maximum tensile strength of a scar is 80% that of unwounded skin. This has ramifications for basic functionality as well as repair after subsequent insults. Additionally, the location of scar tissue can have extensive impact for patients. For example, scar tissue that crosses joints can cause joint contracture and severely limit range of motion. Location also bears a significant impact on facial aesthetics. People are adept at recognizing even subtle facial irregularities and asymmetry,

N. S. Joshi · Z. N. Wahla
Department of Surgery, University of Connecticut School of Medicine, Farmington, CT, USA
e-mail: nejoshi@uchc.edu; wahla@uchc.edu

C. L. Castiglione (✉)
Hartford Hospital, Connecticut Children's Medical Center, Hartford, CT, USA

E. M. Ferneini, M. T. Goupil (eds.), *Office-Based Maxillofacial Surgical Procedures*, https://doi.org/10.1007/978-3-030-22371-7_16

and as such facial scarring can have profound psychological and behavioral consequences. There are five unique areas that affect patients' attitudes: physical comfort and functioning, acceptability to self and others, social functioning, confidence in the nature and management of the condition, and emotional well-being [3]. It is therefore paramount that the approach to a patient with unsatisfactory facial scarring addresses these five areas, and often treatment of the scar itself is but one component of a holistic process.

Classification of Scars

Scars can be classified in several different ways including clinical morphology (color/depth), etiology, and histopathology. Color classification consists of red scars (persistent inflammation or dilated capillaries), brown scars (melanin or hemosiderin deposition) or white scars (absence of melanin or dermal fibrosis) [4]. The depth of the scar can be broken down into either elevated or depressed. Elevated scars are the result of excessive collagen deposition and fibrosis at the site of injury. Elevated scars can further be characterized into hypertrophic and keloid scars. Hypertrophic scars demonstrate vertical growth only and do not extend beyond the confines of the original defect. Alternatively, keloid scars demonstrate both vertical and lateral growth and extend beyond the original defect. The subtypes of the depressed scars are icepick, boxcar, and rolled. Icepick scars are small (<2 mm in width and <1 mm in depth) and have an acute angle at the base and usually occur in multiples. A common example of an icepick scar is due to prior inflammatory acne. Boxcar scars occur at right angles and appear crater-like and are larger than icepick scars. Rolled scars are much larger in diameter with shallow, rolled, nonangled borders that are often the result of involuted or retracted cysts or nodules [4].

Factors Contributing to Scar Formation

Both local and systemic factors contribute to scar formation, and an understanding of these is necessary in order to appropriately strategize a revision. Local factors include the amount of moisture in a wound, infection, maceration, presence of devitalized tissue, pressure and resultant tissue ischemia, radiation, trauma, and edema. Systemic factors that may play a role in wound healing include patient age, weight, skin type and pigmentation, chronic diseases, immunosuppression, nutritional status, and vascular insufficiency [5]. The role of patient genetics has also been studied for its involvement in wound healing and subsequent scar formation. Keloids in particular have been an area of focus. To date, there have been multiple pathways reported to be involved, including apoptosis, mitogen activated protein kinase (MAPK), transforming growth factor beta (TGF-β), interleukin 6 (IL-6), and plasminogen activator inhibitor 1 (PAI-1) [6]. The coumarins decursin and decursinol angelate have also recently been implicated in upregulating transcription genes in keratinocytes and are intimately involved in extracellular matrix remodeling [7]. As research evolves, new clinical and treatment modalities will arise.

Table 16.1 American Society of Anesthesiologist (ASA) physical status classification system

Class	Characteristics
ASA 1	A normal, healthy patient Example: fit, BMI <30, nonsmoker
ASA 2	A patient with mild systemic disease Example: no functional limitation, well-controlled disease (e.g., treated hypertension, obesity with BMI <35, frequent social drinker or smoker)
ASA 3	A patient with a severe systemic disease that is not life-threatening Example: patient with some functional limitation as a result of disease (e.g., poorly controlled hypertension or diabetes, morbid obesity, chronic renal failure, bronchospastic disease, stable angina, implanted pacemaker)
ASA 4	A patient with a severe systemic disease that is a constant threat to life Example: patient with unstable angina, poorly controlled COPD, symptomatic CHF, MI or stroke within the past 3 months
ASA 5	A moribund patient who is not expected to survive beyond the next 24 h without the operation
ASA 6	A brain-dead patient who organs are being removed for transplant

Patient Safety

Scar revision is an important growing sector of maxillofacial surgery. In 2016, Americans collectively spent over $3 billion on cosmetic plastic surgery and minimally invasive procedures for scar revision, including but not limited to soft tissue fillers, dermabrasion, and laser treatments for facial scarring [8]. There are numerous treatment approaches for facial scars ranging from at-home treatments to extensive surgical procedures. In this chapter, we will focus on therapies that are appropriate for the office setting.

While there are no explicit criteria to determine a procedure's appropriateness for the office, a surgeon should consider the technical aspects of the proposed treatment, the type of anesthesia required, and the patient's overall health before deciding how to proceed. Patient safety takes precedence, and all patients undergoing general anesthesia should have a preoperative risk stratification performed by their primary care. In patients with known pulmonary or cardiac dysfunction, it is always safer to perform procedures in a hospital operating room. The American Society of Anesthesiologists (ASA) classification system (Table 16.1) provides a more concrete way to stratify patients. Generally speaking, patients above an ASA class 2 would be inappropriate for general anesthesia in the office.

Planning Scar Revision

Scarring is an unavoidable part of wound healing, and not all scars will be amenable to nor benefit from revision. As such, appropriate patient selection is critical both for managing expectations as well as providing a good outcome. For example, the ideal scar is typically a fine line, flat, and matches the pigmentation of surrounding skin. In a best-case scenario, it may also fall within a skin fold or at a boundary between facial subunits, such as the alar-facial groove. Scars that meet or come very close to these criteria are unlikely to benefit substantially from revision, and may in fact become more cosmetically problematic. At the other end of the spectrum, scars that are the result of injuries with significant tissue loss and are now characterized by thin, atrophic dermis may be exceptionally limited in terms of options, and revision may be best left for cases of functional impairment or disfigurement.

There are, however, a number of patients in whom scar revision may provide worthwhile cosmetic or functional benefits. Such indications for revision are as follows:

1. Restriction of movement/function
2. Contracture/distortion of features
3. Keloids and/or hypertrophic scarring
4. Aberrant color or texture

It is worth noting that while a patient's expectation of scar revision may include removal of all scar tissue, this may in fact not be the best cosmetic approach for many patients. Particularly in patients with facial scarring resulting in disfigurement, the emphasis should remain on return of facial features to their appropriate positions and recovering compromised function.

Given that normal wound healing involves a multi-phase process, it is important to delay surgical scar revision until after it has had an opportunity to run its course. Typically, this can take 6–18 months before the remodeling phase is completed. While not an objective measure, a scar that has turned white is generally more appropriate for revision than one that remains reddened. That having been said, for patients with functional impairment involving the eyelid or oral cavity, waiting months for revision may not be a viable option. In these cases, waiting until the proliferative phase completes (typically at 21 days) can still help improve the likelihood of a positive outcome.

A thorough history that includes how the scar was acquired and any previous treatments is also key in developing an appropriate approach to revision. Whereas a traumatic wound that was allowed to heal by secondary intention may respond well to surgical revision, a scar that has been operated on in the past with a poor outcome is likely to require an alternative approach.

Topical and Over-the-Counter Treatments

A significant portion of patients who present in the office setting for scar revision may have tried or may have questions about available over-the-counter options. Additionally, there are prescription topical treatments that can be attempted on an outpatient basis in patients who would prefer not to undergo a procedure. As many topical treatments impact the remodeling phase of wound healing, they are often used as a first-line treatment and initiated before the scar has fully matured. While the effectiveness of these therapies alone—particularly for advanced scarring—may be limited, they can have some benefit as adjuncts to other approaches as well as preemptive use in the early phases of wound healing.

Aloe Vera

Perhaps the most recognizable ingredient in over-the-counter skin creams and lotions, *Aloe vera* has a long history of use in traditional medicine. While controversy remains over the active substance in *A. vera,* it has long been used for treatment of burns and scar tissue [9]. A prevailing belief is that *A. vera* has a moisturizing effect on tissue [10, 11], which may explain its soothing effects. Nonetheless, studies on *A. vera*'s impact on wound healing and scarring remain decidedly split. *A. vera* does appear to improve the rate of wound healing, but there is no evidence to suggest this translates into a more favorable aesthetic outcome [12, 13]. Furthermore, as studies on *A. vera*'s effectiveness have been on its use in the immediate postoperative setting, it is unclear what, if any, impact it might have on a mature scar.

Vitamin E

A frequently appearing ingredient in over-the-counter creams and ointments, vitamin E is often promoted in marketing as a strong antioxidant that can improve scarring. Early studies of vitamin E preparations in rat models showed a decrease in collagen accumulation—similar to corticosteroids—but this came at the cost of decreased tensile strength [14]. In human studies, the results have been even more concerning, as vitamin E has been either ineffective at modifying scar appearance [15, 16] or has in fact resulted in worse outcomes [17]. Furthermore, contact dermatitis has been a frequently reported complication. This has held true when vitamin E has been used either as monotherapy or alongside other treatments.

One area where vitamin E has shown benefit is when used in conjunction with silicone therapy [18], and as such there may be a role for a combination therapy involving the two. Nonetheless, given the potential for worsening of scar aesthetics, the incidence of dermatitis, and the weakening of healed tissue, vitamin E monotherapy is generally inadvisable.

Pressure Therapy

Pressure therapy has been shown to have beneficial effects in diminishing hypertrophic scarring; however, the face poses a challenge in crafting a pressure dressing that is not unduly bulky or restrictive. In lieu of pressure dressings, massage therapy may actually offer many of the same benefits while additionally breaking up the disorganized scar and offering an opportunity for remodeling [19]. Massage can also improve a patient's overall sense of well-being [20], which can affect his or her attitude toward the scar itself.

Onion Extract Gel

Onion extract gel (Mederma; Merz Pharmaceuticals) has gained popularity among patients and physicians as a treatment for burns and postsurgical scarring. This extract contains the flavonoid quercetin, which has been shown to have antioxidant properties as well as the ability to inhibit fibrosis, decrease histamine release, and promote wound remodeling in in vitro studies [21, 22]. In randomized trials, onion extract gel has demonstrated benefits in appearance and scar softness as compared to untreated controls [23, 24], but comparison against petroleum emollient in a separate study showed no relative improvement [25].

Silicone Gel

Coming in a variety of formulations, including gels, creams, and sheeting, silicone has been in use as a scar and burn treatment since 1981 [26]. Since its initial application in the burn setting, silicone gels have been studied extensively as a treatment for hypertrophic scarring and keloids. There is evidence that silicone gel sheeting can improve scar thickness and color [27], but whereas elsewhere in the body silastic sheeting can be more easily applied, the face again presents a challenge in this regard. The rise of 3D printing may be able to assist, however. Recent research involving individually designed and printed facemasks lined with silicone allow for pressure therapy to be used in conjunction with silicone on the face. This has had the effect of improving scar thickness, scar hardness, and patient satisfaction in a small study [28].

Imiquimod

Imiquimod is a prescription immunomodulator available for topical administration in a variety of formulations, most commonly as a 5% cream. FDA approved for treatment of genital warts, actinic keratoses, and primary superficial basal cell carcinoma, the use of imiquimod for scarring remains off-label. In several case studies of patients undergoing keloid excision of the earlobe, the use of imiquimod cream postoperatively was shown to reduce recurrence and improve cosmetic appearance [29–32]. However, a similar benefit has not been identified for primary scarring. An eight-week course of nightly 5% imiquimod cream has been most commonly described in the literature.

Minimally Invasive Procedures

Intralesional Injections

Corticosteroids

In patients who have failed topical therapies such as silicone and pressure, intralesional injections can be an effective tool, especially for those not yet appropriate for surgical revision. Several agents have been studied for this purpose, the most frequently used of which is triamcinolone acetonide, often administered in conjunction with lidocaine as the injection can be painful. Used as a first-line treatment for keloids and hypertrophic scarring as early as two weeks postoperatively, triamcinolone can be given every 2–4 weeks for several months if necessary [33]. Given as a 10 mg/mL solution, a dose of 0.5 mL (5 mg) per cm^2 is recommended, with a maximum dose of 30 mg/day. Triamcinolone monotherapy has a highly variable response rate, with reports ranging from 50% to 100% and recurrence from 9% to 50% [34]. In conjunction with surgical excision, corticosteroid injections can potentially yield recurrence-free rates of over 90% [35].

Corticosteroids such as triamcinolone act via TGF-β1 inactivation, causing inhibition of fibroblast growth and promotion of collagen degeneration by collagenase [36, 37]. They are also potent anti-inflammatory agents and can cause vasoconstriction of the wound bed leading to diminished oxygen and nutrient delivery [38]. As such, they do present potential risks of skin atrophy and hypopigmentation, which patients should be counseled on prior to treatment. Additionally, subcutaneous rather than dermal injection of corticosteroid can increase the risk of wound dehiscence [33].

Antineoplastic Agents

Another agent worth consideration in patients refractory to triamcinolone therapy is 5-fluorouracil (5-FU). 5-FU is perhaps best known as an antineoplastic agent that acts by blocking thymidine synthesis through inhibition of thymidylate synthase. This, in turn, prevents DNA replication, blocking cellular overgrowth [39]. When administered intralesionally, 5-FU has shown some positive results with pain and hyperpigmentation as the primary side effects. Efficacy seems tied to the age of the scar in question, as patients with scar age >5 years have been noted to be less likely to respond [40], and recurrence has been correlated with increased scar age as well [41].

Like 5-FU, bleomycin is another antineoplastic agent that has found success in patients who have failed triamcinolone therapy. Bleomycin causes cell cycle arrest in the G_2 phase and induces apoptosis. In dark-skinned patients, bleomycin may be a desirable first-line alternative to intralesional corticosteroid as it is more likely to cause hyperpigmentation and may be more easily hidden in these individuals [42].

Cryotherapy

First attempted in 1993, intralesional cryotherapy involves the passage of liquid nitrogen through a cryoprobe inserted into the deeper layers of a scar. When used in scars that have been refractory to other agents, it can have a potentially significant impact on scar volume, with reduction as high as two-thirds reported in the literature [43]. Unfortunately, the effect is inconsistent, as in some case series, fewer than 50% of patients showed a 50% or better reduction while others experienced progression following cryotherapy [44]. The application of cryotherapy is generally limited to smaller scars due to technical considerations: the cryoprobe must be able to pass entirely through the lesion, and the effect is relatively localized. Perhaps its greatest value, however, comes from the impact it has on scar organization, as seen from histological studies that have shown increased parallelization of collagen, similar to normal dermis [43]. This, in turn, may make treated scars more responsive to other intralesional treatments.

Soft Tissue Fillers

Beneficial particularly for depressed scars, hyaluronic acid-based soft tissue fillers can not only add volume—leading to a smoother contour—but also may have an impact on the inflammatory response in the area of scar tissue. In vitro studies of fetal vs. adult skin have noted increased concentrations of hyaluronic acid in fetal skin along with glycoproteins that stimulate its production [45]. This, in turn, appears to inhibit white blood cell chemotaxis and random migration as well as phagocytic activity. As healed fetal wounds demonstrate relatively less inflammatory infiltrate, it has been theorized that this effect of hyaluronic acid may directly contribute to scarless wound healing.

Clinically, fillers can be injected into the deep dermis, breaking up adhesions and restoring appropriate contour in mildly depressed or inverted scars. Best results may be achieved with needle passes to lyse dermal adhesions prior to injection [33]. Although generally well tolerated, care should be taken to avoid overcorrection, as increased pressure can result in skin necrosis.

In addition to hyaluronic acid fillers, injectable calcium hydroxylapatite and poly-L-lactic acid fillers exist on the market as well. As these fillers are degraded and absorbed over time, their effect is temporary, but can last well over six months.

Fat Grafting

Harvesting patients' adipose tissue through liposuction before reinjecting into an area of scarring has shown some success in multiple applications, including acne scarring [46] and radiated surgical wounds [47]. While the results of fat grafting can partly be attributed to its role as a filler in depressed scars [48], this does not fully explain the effects of these injections, as they are believed to promote angiogenesis [47], decrease fibrosis, reduce collagen thickness, and improve scar pliability [49]. More recent trials have investigated in vitro culture of adipose tissue-derived stem cells isolated from a patient's own tissue and which was then re-differentiated into adipocytes for injection [48].

There are a few techniques for fat grafting in the facial region, but the differences among them are small. Fundamentally, each involves harvesting fat, isolating viable adipocytes and preadipocytes, and injecting this aspirate in the area of desired treatment [50]. LipoStructure® is one such technique that involves harvesting under low suction, centrifuging the aspirate to separate a dense cellular concentrate from ruptured cell supernatant, and injection at the site of scarring. Cell-assisted lipotransfer is very similar, though processing involves adding collagenase prior to centrifugation, and the processed cells are added to additional aspirated fat before reinjecting. LipoKit® (Medi-Khan) is an all-in-one device that allows for larger scale harvesting and injection of adipocyte-derived stem cells. Overall, fat grafting has shown some promise in the treatment of scar tissue, though further investigation is still necessary [37].

Dermabrasion

As the name suggests, dermabrasion is a technique that involves exfoliating the epidermis and a partial thickness of the dermis using a rotating abrasive instrument, called a diamond fraise. Often used in smoothing rough contours or non-hypertrophic scars, blending skin grafts with poor pigment matching, or camouflaging unevenly healed surgical wounds, dermabrasion can either be used alone or as an adjunct to surgical revision.

Using a dermabrader attached to a foot pedal, the diamond fraise can spin at up to 20,000–30,000 rpm. With gentle pressure, the epidermis and a partial thickness of the papillary dermis should be abraded. Care should be taken to stay within the mid to deep papillary dermis and avoid the reticular dermis to prevent recurrent or worse scarring. When performing dermabrasion near the eye or lip, aim the fraise so that the direction of rotation is toward the free margin (eyelid or vermillion border) to prevent unintentional abrasion of these sensitive areas. A metal eye shield should also be placed over the eye to protect it.

Effective over a wide area of scarring, dermabrasion works by allowing the exposed dermis to re-epithelialize, smoothing out irregularities in the process. In order to promote appropriate healing and epithelialization, a petroleum-based ointment or petroleum gauze should be kept over the wound to keep it moist.

A notable risk of dermabrasion is reactivation of facial herpes virus. As a result, pre-procedural antiviral prophylaxis with valacyclovir for 2–3 days is recommended. Other complications include changes in pigmentation, and caution should be exercised before treating patients with darker skin tones (Fitzpatrick V–VI) as hypopigmentation can be difficult to treat. Hyperpigmentation in fairer skinned patients can be managed with a topical whitening agent such as hydroquinone.

Laser Therapy

The original studies of laser therapy on fibroblasts were performed using a 1064-nm neodymium:yttrium-aluminum-garnet (Nd:YAG) laser. In vitro testing demonstrated that exposure to this wavelength caused fibroblasts to decrease their production of collagen [51]. Used alongside argon and CO_2 lasers in the treatment of hypertrophic scars and keloids in the 1980s and early 90s, initial results were promising, but recurrence rates were high [52]. In the mid-90s, pulsed dye lasers (PDLs) were studied, and the vascular-specific 585-nm wavelength in particular was noted to have benefit in the treatment of hypertrophic scars and keloids [53]. Studies have shown PDLs inhibit TGF-β expression, fibroblast proliferation, and type III collagen deposition [54]. In mouse models, they can cause selective thermolysis of scar microvasculature [55]. Still other studies have explored PDL effects on mast cell activation and breaking of disulfide bridges in collagen. As the exact in vivo mechanism of PDL activity on scar tissue remains uncertain, any combination of these effects may explain its use for revision.

The application of laser recontouring extends to atrophic scars as well, and both ablative and nonablative lasers with longer wavelengths can aid in this purpose. CO_2 and erbium:yttrium-aluminum-garnet (Er:YAG) lasers are two preferred ablative options. Both work by heating and vaporizing superficial skin, effectively serving a similar function as dermabrasion without as much operator dependence. They also provide an opportunity for skin tightening and neocollagenesis at the treated site [56]. By contrast, nonablative lasers, which include 1320-nm Nd:YAG, 1450-nm diode, and 1064-nm Nd:YAG, utilize longer wavelengths to achieve deeper penetration without disrupting the overlying epidermis. This has the benefit of fewer side effects—such as erythema, edema, or herpes simplex reactivation—but comes at the cost of decreased efficacy. Both ablative and nonablative lasers tend to require multiple treatments to achieve an optimal result, which led to the development of fractional treatment systems that produce microscopic thermal zones surrounded by unaffected tissue. This approach leads to faster re-epithelialization and less dyspigmentation [52], while serial treatments allow for evening out of the treatment areas.

Surgical Scar Revision

Though a great number of nonsurgical options exist for management of scarring, definitive management of hypertrophic scars and keloids typically requires surgical excision (Fig. 16.1). Likewise, surgical intervention may be of great benefit to patients with contracted or disfiguring facial scars. There are a multitude of approaches to surgical scar revision, not all of which are appropriate for the office setting. While the ability to administer general anesthesia in the office expands the possibilities, cases where extensive undermining and dissection is expected may pose too high of a bleeding risk. Similarly, patients in whom medical comorbidities increase the potential for anesthesia complications may be better managed in a formal OR setting.

Despite a number of noninvasive and minimally invasive options for scar revision, many cases will not show a satisfactory response to these therapies. In these patients, excision—or re-excision—and closure would be an appropriate choice (Fig. 16.2). There are a few technical considerations to keep in mind when planning and performing a scar excision [57]. First, the skin should be marked when relaxed, as applying tension can distort features. Second, incisions should be made under extreme four-point tension. Third, as slightly raised scars tend to be easier to manage in the postoperative period than depressed scars, leaving a thin dermal bed rather than violating subcutaneous soft tissue is recommended. Finally, closure should involve a deeper subcutaneous layer as well as an intracuticular layer that together yields a well-approximated closure with slight eversion (Fig. 16.3).

In areas that demonstrate sufficient laxity, a simple excision can be performed to remove a scar and revise it to a fine-line incision. If, however, the result of this

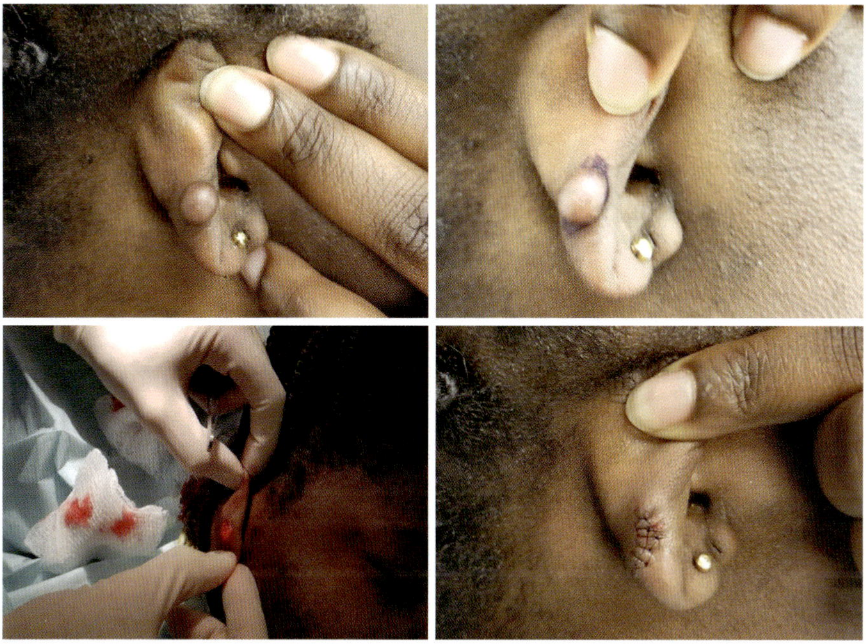

Fig. 16.1 An 18 year old female with a small keloid of the posterior ear after infection of a pierce site. Elliptical excision with layered closure is performed

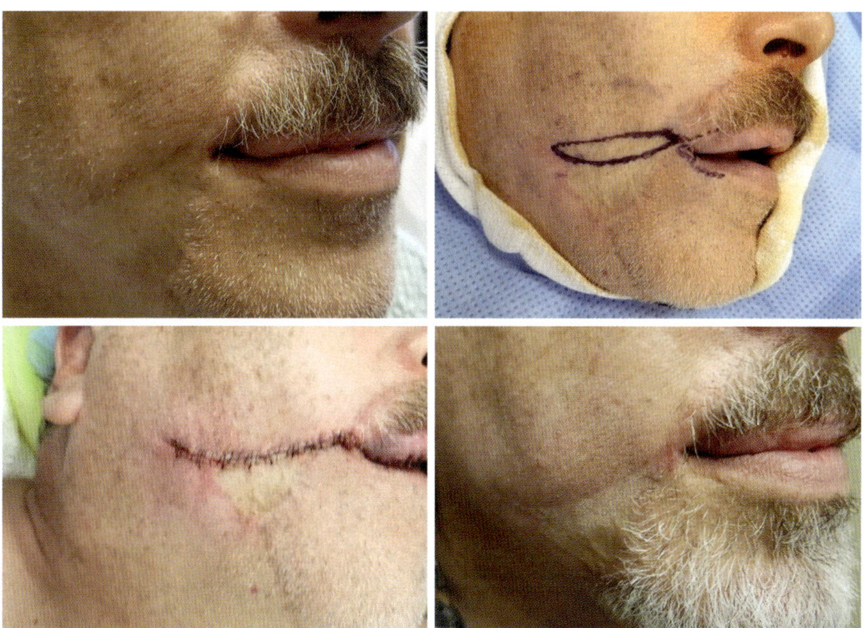

Fig. 16.2 A 62 year old male who had prior split thickness skin grafting for a full thickness radiator burn. His oral commissure is wide and retracted inferiorly causing drooling. Simple excision of a portion of the graft as well as a minor commissure repair improve his appearance and function

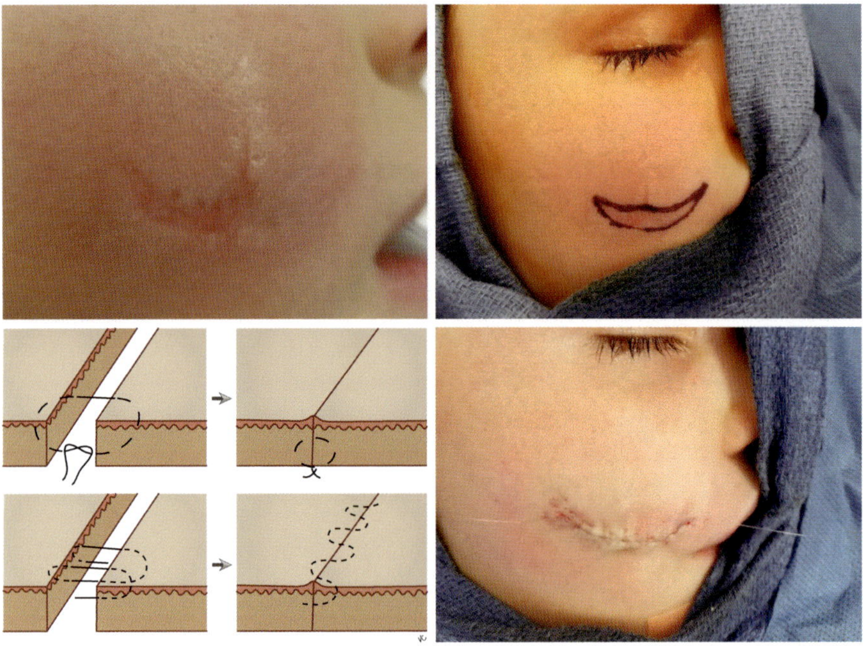

Fig. 16.3 A 10 year old female 1.5 years after a right cheek dog bite, now with a depressed and widened stellate scar. The area of concern including some of the vertical scar extension is excised and closed in layers with slight eversion using intracuticular sutures

would be a long, conspicuous scar that cannot be easily camouflaged by resting skin tension lines or facial anatomy, there are techniques to help visually break up a scar to make it less noticeable.

W-Plasty and Geometric Broken Line Closure

The W-plasty and geometric broken line closure (GBLC) are two methods of scar irregularization that can make scars less apparent, especially when making facial expressions. Both involve complete excision of the preexisting scar, but instead of making an ellipse around the lesion, the edges are made irregular, resulting in a non-linear scar (Fig. 16.4).

The W-plasty is performed by drawing a zig-zag pattern along the desired margin of excision. Depending on the length of the scar that needs to be excised, this could be a single W-shaped pattern, or a running W. Each limb of this pattern should be at minimum 5 mm, though choosing a significantly longer length comes with the downside of removing excessive healthy skin. It is worth recognizing that as the scar contracts, the limbs will naturally shorten as well. The same principles of the W-plasty apply to GBLC, with the only difference being the pattern itself. Instead of simply a zig-zag pattern, GBLC uses a series of triangles, rectangles, and

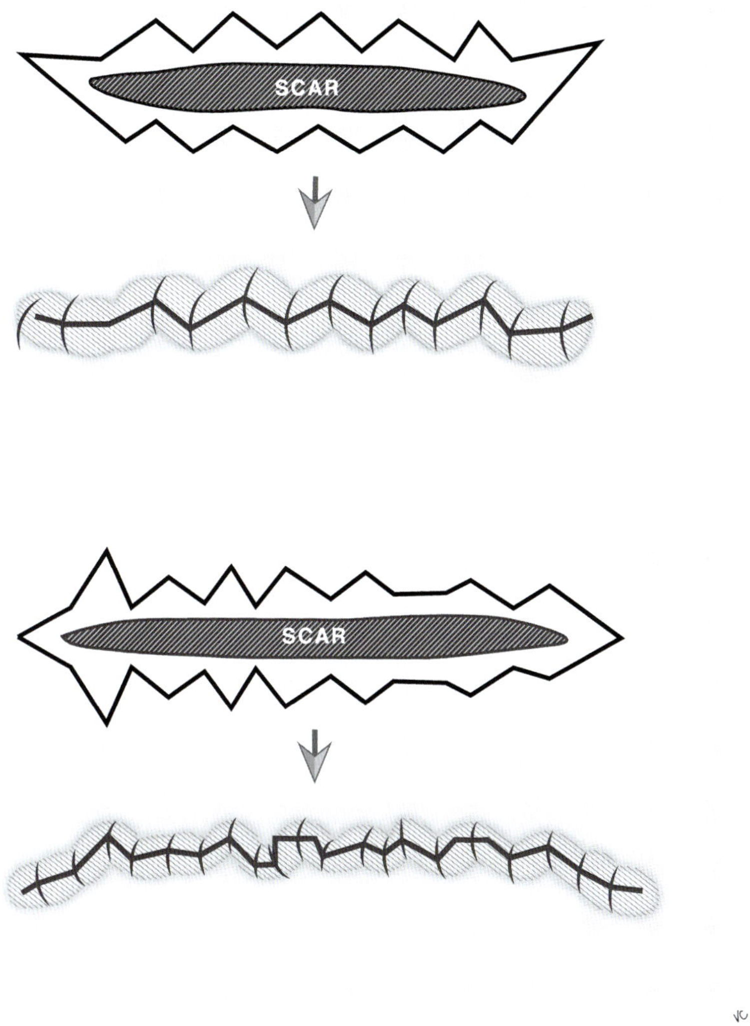

Fig. 16.4 Diagrams of scar excision with w-plasty and geometric broken line closure. The patterns on both sides should match well prior to the scar excision

semicircles to create an even more irregular pattern. Care should be taken to ensure that the pattern on both sides matches well prior to incision, in order to ensure that the edges are well approximated at the end of the procedure.

Though both the W-plasty and GBLC can be used to change the overall orientation of a scar somewhat, other techniques such as the Z-plasty are better suited for this purpose.

Tissue Rearrangement

As tension is the enemy of wound healing, the facial surgeon must be adept at using tissue transposition to minimize the effects of or redirect tension away from a healing incision. Furthermore, these techniques can be used to move a scar into a more cosmetically favorable location, such as the junction between two facial subunits. There are two techniques worth noting: the Z-plasty and the V-Y advancement flap.

The Z-plasty is a versatile technique for spreading tension over a longer incision, while also changing the orientation of the healing wound to further mitigate tensile forces. The classic Z-plasty involves limbs oriented 60° from the original incision, yielding a 75% theoretical gain in length. Each limb should measure equal the central segment. The limb should begin with a small incision directly perpendicular to the central segment before continuing at the desired angle. Doing so allows for better blood flow to the "corners" of the Z-plasty (Fig. 16.5).

Angles other than 60° can be chosen, with more acute angles offering less final length and the opposite being the case with increasing angles up to 90°. While a Z-plasty performed with limbs at 90° can theoretically add 120% to the original length, doing so may come at the cost of introducing new points of tension. In addition to adding length to the incision, Z-plasty also rotates the orientation of the central limb. For a 60° Z-plasty, the central limb will rotate by 90°, while in a 30° Z-plasty, the rotation will be 45°. Other considerations include the fact that large Z-plasties are often unsightly on the face, and the same benefit can largely be achieved by instead performing sequential Z-plasties. Just as with W-plasties, limb lengths of <5 mm are inadvisable, while 10 mm may serve as a rough upper limit for optimal aesthetic outcomes.

Another tissue advancement approach that can be used relieve tension is the V-Y flap. This technique involves a V-shaped incision that can be used to either move the tissue within the V to cover a defect left by scar excision, or can be used to release disfiguring contractures caused by advanced scarring. In both cases, the skin on either side of the V is closed to each other, resulting in a Y-shaped closure. The reverse or Y-V flap may also be used as a single flap or sequential flaps to lengthen a scar. In this case, a Y incision is made, and the V portion is advanced into the base of the Y leaving a V closure (Fig. 16.6).

Both the Z-plasty and the V-Y flap can be used to reorient or move incision lines to more visually camouflaged locations. For example, by adjusting the angle of the Z-plasty limbs—and as a consequence, the final rotation of the central segment—the Z-plasty can be used to align a scar with resting skin tension lines. Alternatively, by designing the segments of the V-Y flap appropriately, the resultant incisions can be positioned at borders between facial subunits, such as at the philtral column or vermilion border.

Use of prefabricated tissue expanders can be employed to increase the area of available tissue that can be mobilized for a flap. This comes with the advantage

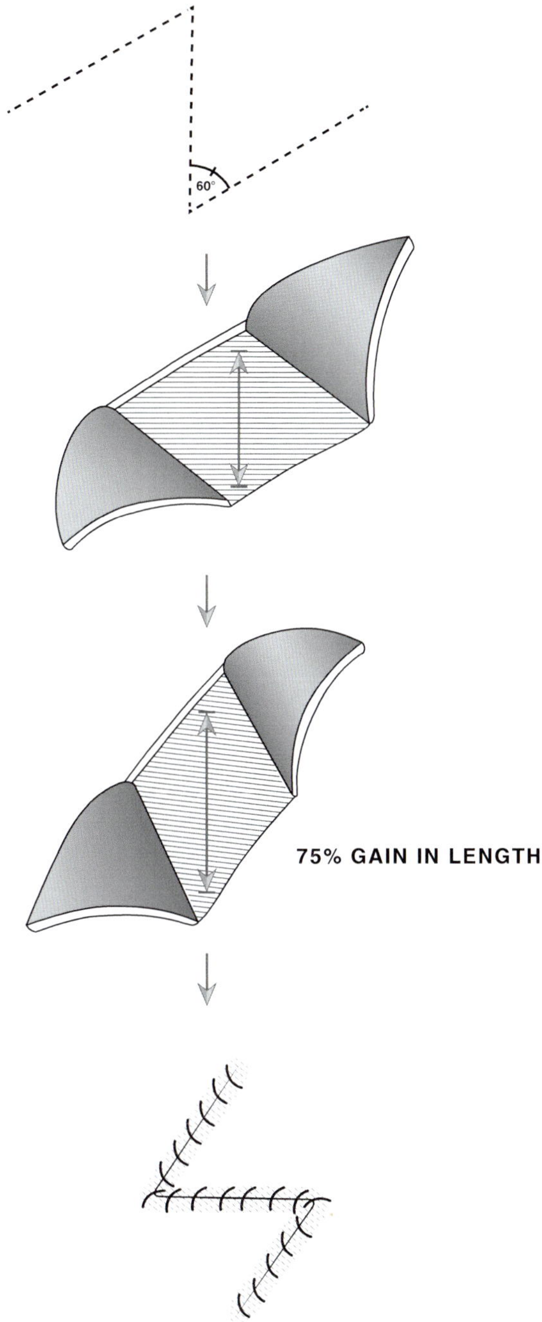

Fig. 16.5 A classic z-plasty with 60° angles and 75% theoretical gain in length. Sequential z-plasties can be used for longer scars

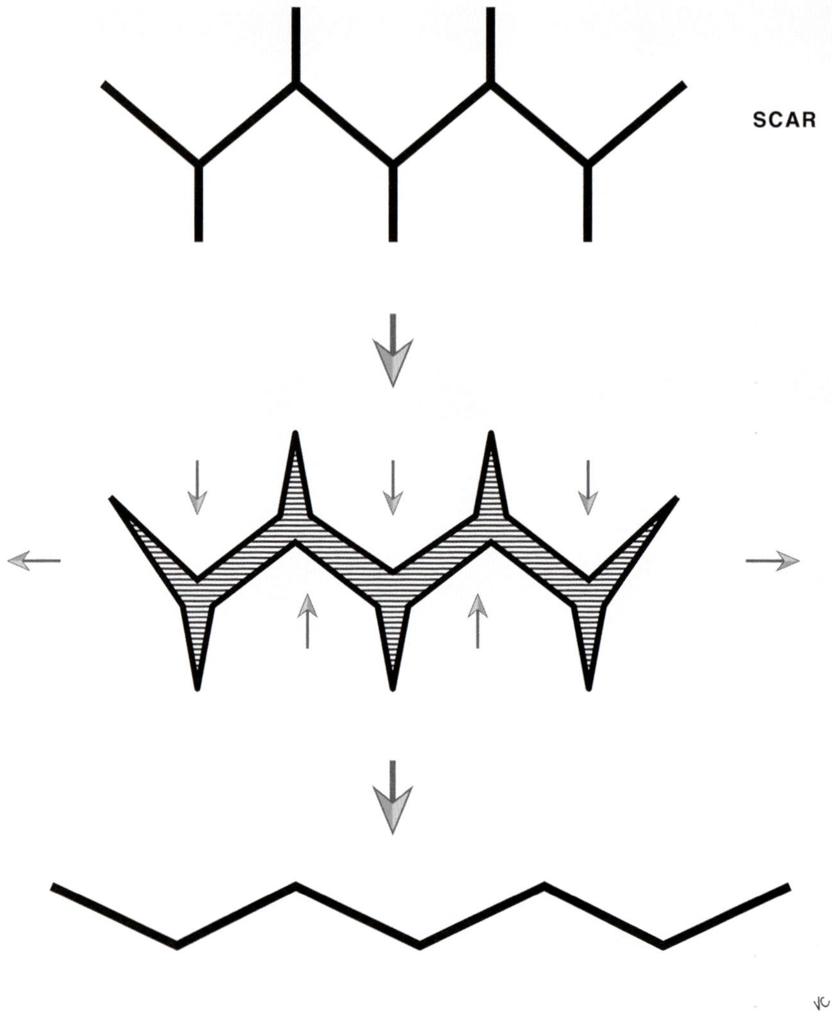

Fig. 16.6 A scar can be lengthened with multiple Y-V flaps as shown above. The Y-V and V-Y flaps are very useful

of being able to use more tissue that matches the native skin in color and texture. To effectively leverage the benefits of tissue expansion, the surgeon must pre-plan the incisions for flap mobilization prior to placing the expander, taking care not to violate vascular pedicles that will be necessary to perfuse the final flap. The skin of the face and forehead offers sufficient opportunities for expansion, but placement of larger expanders should be reserved for the operating room rather than the office due to the significant dissection and undermining that may be necessary.

Patients undergoing tissue expansion also require close follow up both for serial expansions and to monitor for infection or other complications. As the face is a very conspicuous area, patients may struggle psychologically with the obvious deformities that become apparent late in the expansion process. Repeated reassurance is important during this period in helping the patient understand that the end result will be worthwhile.

Skin Grafting

Skin grafting can be used on the face to fill defects ranging from small punch excisions to large burn excisions that cannot be adequately covered by local tissue transfer. Skin grafts on the face can be either full or split thickness, with the understanding that the former allows for better space filling and more aesthetic result while the latter may prove a more practical option in covering broader areas. There are a number of sites on and around the face that can serve as donor sites for full thickness skin grafting: the forehead, preauricular skin, postauricular skin, the neck, and supraclavicular skin. Split thickness grafts are typically obtained from the arm, thigh, or scalp. Of note, skin obtained from above the clavicle tends to color match existing skin better, and is therefore preferred.

The Future of Scar Revision

As science and technology progress, new strategies for scar revision will inevitably be developed. One such emerging therapy is the use of platelet-rich plasma (PRP). Long studied for a potential role in tissue repair and regeneration [58], PRP has recently seen applications in wound healing and scar treatments, including as an adjunct to other therapies such as CO_2 lasers [59]. PRP has shown synergistic benefit in conjunction with fractional CO_2 ablation for acne scarring, both improving skin recovery and final appearance [60], though its benefit as a standalone therapy is unclear. When used in conjunction with microneedling for acne scars, PRP reduces post-procedural edema, though it does not clearly add benefit in terms of aesthetics or patient satisfaction scoring [61]. Studies of PRP injection during cesarean section have demonstrated improved postoperative scarring results [62], but it is unknown how well this translates to facial scarring.

Autologous cell therapy is another area of research focusing on collagen scaffolding and fibroblast matrices that may produce new treatments in the future. Derived from samples of postauricular skin, autologous cultured fibroblasts (LaViv; Fibrocell Technologies) gained FDA approval for aesthetic improvement of prominent nasolabial folds in 2011 and have also shown benefit in management of acne scarring and dermal defects [63]. While use of autologous fibroblast therapy has yet to be studied in scar revision, this may be a new horizon and future application for the technology.

Conclusion

While the materials and techniques continue to evolve, the crux of scar revision remains solving the problems of tensile forces and unnatural wound remodeling. Before undergoing a revision, it is up to the surgeon to identify patients that are appropriate for revision in the office, both from a safety and an outcomes standpoint. For the latter, a frank discussion with patients about the goals of revision is the best way to ensure the highest likelihood of patient satisfaction. Starting with topical therapies and pressure can give the patient a sense of ownership over treating their scars while also allowing the scar time to mature. Should the patient require further treatment, a stepwise approach can begin with minimally invasive procedures and progress to surgical options. As new technology develops, additional strategies may be utilized, but achievable and safe outcomes must remain the priority.

References

1. Barbul A, Efron DT, Kavalukas SL. Wound healing. In: Brunicardi FC, Andersen DK, Billiar TR, et al., editors. Schwartz's principles of surgery. 10th ed. New York, NY: McGraw-Hill Education; 2015. p. 241–73.
2. Stedman's medical dictionary for the health professions and nursing. Illustrated 7th ed. Lippincott Williams & Wilkins; 2011.
3. Brown BC, McKenna SP, Siddhi K, McGrouther DA, Bayat A. The hidden cost of skin scars: quality of life after skin scarring. J Plast Reconstr Aesthet Surg. 2008;61(9):1049–58. https://doi.org/10.1016/j.bjps.2008.03.020.
4. Kwok T, Rao J. A practical approach to classification and treatment of scars. Skin Ther Lett Family Pract. 2011;7(6)
5. More than $16 billion spent on Cosmetic Plastic Surgery: American Society of Plastic Surgeons Releases Report Showing National Average of Cosmetic Surgical Fees in 2016. American Society of Plastic Surgeons News: Press Releases; April 12, 2017.
6. Thomas Hess C. Checklist for factors affecting wound healing. Adv Skin Wound Care. 2011;24(4):192. https://doi.org/10.1097/01.ASW.0000396300.04173.ec.
7. Han J, Jin W, Ho NA, et al. Decursin and decursinol angelate improve wound healing by upregulating transcription of genes encoding extracellular matrix remodeling proteins, inflammatory cytokines, and growth factors in human keratinocytes. Biochem Biophys Res Commun. 2018;499(4):979–84. https://doi.org/10.1016/j.bbrc.2018.04.031.
8. American Society of Plastic Surgeons. 2016 Plastic Surgery Statistics | Average Surgeon Fees; 2016.
9. Eshun K, He Q. Aloe Vera: a valuable ingredient for the food, pharmaceutical and cosmetic industries—a review. Crit Rev Food Sci Nutr. 2004;44(2):91–6. https://doi.org/10.1080/10408690490424694.
10. Spoerke DG, Ekins BR. Aloe Vera—fact or quackery. Vet Hum Toxicol. 1980;22:418–24.
11. Meadows TP. Aloe as a humectant in new skin preparations. Cosmet Toilet. 1980;95(11):51–6.
12. Dat AD, Poon F, Pham KBT, Doust J. *Aloe vera* for treating acute and chronic wounds. Cochrane Database Syst Rev. 2012;2 https://doi.org/10.1002/14651858.CD008762.pub2.
13. Maenthaisong R, Chaiyakunapruk N, Niruntraporn S, Kongkaew C. The efficacy of aloe vera used for burn wound healing: a systematic review. Burns. 2007;33(6):713–8. https://doi.org/10.1016/j.burns.2006.10.384.
14. Ehrlich HP, Tarver H, Hunt TK. Inhibitory effects of vitamin E on collagen synthesis and wound repair. Ann Surg. 1972;175(2):235–40.

15. Jenkins M, Alexander JW, MacMillan BG, Waymack JP, Kopcha R. Failure of topical steroids and vitamin E to reduce postoperative scar formation following reconstructive surgery. J Burn Care Rehabil. 1986;7(4):309–12. https://doi.org/10.1097/00004630-198607000-00002.
16. Khoo TL, Halim AS, Zakaria Z, Mat Saad AZ, Wu LY, Lau HY. A prospective, randomised, double-blinded trial to study the efficacy of topical tocotrienol in the prevention of hypertrophic scars. J Plast Reconstr Aesthet Surg. 2011;64(6):e137–45. https://doi.org/10.1016/j.bjps.2010.08.029.
17. Baumann LS, Spencer J. The effects of topical vitamin E on the cosmetic appearance of scars. Dermatol Surg. 1999;25(4):311–5. https://doi.org/10.1046/j.1524-4725.1999.08223.x.
18. Palmieri B, Gozzi G, Palmieri G. Vitamin E added silicone gel sheets for treatment of hypertrophic scars and keloids. Int J Dermatol. 1995;34(7):506–9. https://doi.org/10.1111/j.1365-4362.1995.tb00628.x.
19. Shin TM, Bordeaux JS. The role of massage in scar management: a literature review. Dermatol Surg. 2012;38(3):414–23. https://doi.org/10.1111/j.1524-4725.2011.02201.x.
20. Kaada B, Torsteinbø O. Increase of plasma beta-endorphins in connective tissue massage. Gen Pharmacol Vasc S. 1989;20(4):487–9.
21. Saulis AS, Mogford JH, Mustoe TA. Effect of mederma on hypertrophic scarring in the rabbit ear model. Plast Reconstr Surg. 2002;110(1):177–83.
22. Cho JW, Cho SY, Lee SR, Lee KS. Onion extract and quercetin induce matrix metalloproteinase-1 in vitro and in vivo. Int J Mol Med. 2010;25(3):347–52. https://doi.org/10.3892/ijmm_00000351.
23. Draelos ZD. The ability of onion extract gel to improve the cosmetic appearance of postsurgical scars. J Cosmet Dermatol. 2008;7(2):101–4. https://doi.org/10.1111/j.1473-2165.2008.00371.x.
24. Draelos ZD, Baumann L, Fleischer AB, Plaum S, Avakian EV, Hardas B. A new proprietary onion extract gel improves the appearance of new scars: a randomized, controlled, blinded-investigator study. J Clin Aesthet Dermatol. 2012;5(6):18–24.
25. Chung VQ, Kelley L, Marra D, Jiang SB. Onion extract gel versus petrolatum emollient on new surgical scars: a prospective double-blinded study. Dermatol Surg. 2006;32(2):193–7. https://doi.org/10.1111/j.1524-4725.2006.32045.x.
26. Perkins K, Davey RB, Wallis KA. Silicone gel: a new treatment for burn scars and contractures. Burns. 1983;9(3):201–4. https://doi.org/10.1016/0305-4179(83)90039-6.
27. O'Brien L, Jones DJ. Silicone gel sheeting for preventing and treating hypertrophic and keloid scars. Cochrane Database Syst Rev. 2013;9 https://doi.org/10.1002/14651858.CD003826.pub3.
28. Wei Y, Wang Y, Zhang M, et al. The application of 3D-printed transparent facemask for facial scar management and its biomechanical rationale. Burns. 2018;44(2):453–61. https://doi.org/10.1016/j.burns.2017.08.006.
29. Berman B, Harrison-Balestra C, Perez OA, Viera M, Villa A, Zell D, Ramirez C. Treatment of keloid scars post-shave excision with imiquimod 5% cream: a prospective, double-blind, placebo-controlled pilot study. J Drugs Dermatol. 2009;8(5):455–8.
30. Patel PJ, Skinner RB. Experience with keloids after excision and application of 5% imiquimod cream. Dermatol Surg. 2006;32(3):462. https://doi.org/10.1002/hbm.20245.
31. Martin-Garcia RF, Busquets AC. Postsurgical Use of Imiquimod 5% Cream in the Prevention of earlobe keloid recurrences: results of an open-label, pilot study. Am Soc Dermatologic Surg. 2005;31(11):1394–8.
32. Stashower ME. Successful treatment of earlobe keloids with imiquimod after tangential shave excision. Dermatol Surg. 2006;32(3):380–6. https://doi.org/10.1111/j.1524-4725.2006.32077.x.
33. Humphrey CD, Thomas JR. Improving scars with minimally invasive and topical treatment. Oper Tech Otolaryngol. 2011;22(1):94–100. https://doi.org/10.1016/j.otot.2010.10.002.
34. Niessen FB, Spauwen PHM, Schalkwijk J, Kon M. On the nature of hypertrophic scars and keloids: a review. Plast Reconstr Surg. 1999;104(5):1435–58.
35. Chowdri NA, Mattoo MMA, Darzi MA. Keloids and hypertrophic scars: results with intra-operative and serial postoperative corticosteroid injection therapy. Aust N Z J Surg. 1999;69(9):655–9. https://doi.org/10.1046/j.1440-1622.1999.01658.x.

36. McCoy BJ, Diegelmann RF, Cohen IK. In vitro inhibition of cell growth, collagen synthesis, and prolyl hydroxylase activity by triamcinolone acetonide. Proc Soc Exp Biol Med. 1980;163(2):216–22.
37. Khansa I, Harrison B, Janis JE. Evidence-based scar management: how to improve results with technique and technology. Plast Reconstr Surg. 2016;138(3):165S–78S. https://doi.org/10.1097/PRS.0000000000002647.
38. Atiyeh BS. Nonsurgical management of hypertrophic scars: evidence-based therapies, standard practices, and emerging methods. Aesthetic Plast Surg. 2007;31(5):468–92. https://doi.org/10.1007/s00266-006-0253-y.
39. Longley DB, Harkin DP, Johnston PG. 5-Fluorouracil: mechanisms of action and clinical strategies. Nat Rev Cancer. 2003;3(5):330–8. https://doi.org/10.1038/nrc1074.
40. Gupta S, Kalra A. Efficacy and safety of intralesional 5-fluorouracil in the treatment of keloids. Dermatology. 2002;204(2):130–2. https://doi.org/10.1159/000051830.
41. Kontochristopoulos G, Stefanaki C, Panagiotopoulos A, et al. Intralesional 5-fluorouracil in the treatment of keloids: an open clinical and histopathologic study. J Am Acad Dermatol. 2005;52(3):474–9. https://doi.org/10.1016/j.jaad.2004.09.018.
42. Payapvipapong K, Niumpradit N, Piriyanand C, Buranaphalin S, Nakakes A. The treatment of keloids and hypertrophic scars with intralesional bleomycin in skin of color. J Cosmet Dermatol. 2015;14(1):83–90. https://doi.org/10.1111/jocd.12132.
43. Har-Shai Y, Sabo E, Rohde E, Hyams M, Assaf C, Zouboulis CC. Intralesional cryosurgery enhances the involution of recalcitrant auricular keloids: a new clinical approach supported by experimental studies. Wound Repair Regen. 2006;14:18–27. https://doi.org/10.1111/j.1743-6109.2005.00084.x.
44. Zouboulis CC, Rosenberger AD, Forster T, Beller G, Kratzsch M, Felsenberg D. Modification of a device and its application for intralesional cryosurgery of old recalcitrant keloids. Arch Dermatol. 2004;140(10):1293–4. https://doi.org/10.1001/archderm.140.10.1293.
45. Namazi MR, Fallahzadeh MK, Schwartz RA. Strategies for prevention of scars: what can we learn from fetal skin? Int J Dermatol. 2011;50(1):85–93. https://doi.org/10.1111/j.1365-4632.2010.04678.x.
46. Coleman SR. Structural fat grafting: more than a permanent filler. Plast Reconstr Surg. 2006;118(3 Suppl):108–20. https://doi.org/10.1097/01.prs.0000234610.81672.e7.
47. Rigotti G, Marchi A, Galiè M, et al. Clinical treatment of radiotherapy tissue damage by lipoaspirate transplant: a healing process mediated by adipose-derived adult stem cells. Plast Reconstr Surg. 2007;119(5):1409–22. https://doi.org/10.1097/01.prs.0000256047.47909.71.
48. Kim M, Kim I, Lee SK, Bang SI, Lim SY. Clinical trial of autologous differentiated adipocytes from stem cells derived from human adipose tissue. Dermatol Surg. 2011;37(6):750–9. https://doi.org/10.1111/j.1524-4725.2011.01765.x.
49. Klinger M, Marazzi M, Vigo D, Torre M. Fat injection for cases of severe burn outcomes: a new perspective of scar remodeling and reduction. Aesthetic Plast Surg. 2008;32(3):465–9. https://doi.org/10.1007/s00266-008-9122-1.
50. Boxrud CA. Adipocyte-derived stem cells for the face. Facial Plast Surg Clin North Am. 2012;20(2):231–4. https://doi.org/10.1016/j.fsc.2012.02.012.
51. Castro DJ, Abergel RP, Meeker C, Dwyer RM, Lesavoy MA, Uitto J. Effects of the Nd:YAG laser on DNA synthesis and collagen production in human skin fibroblast cultures. Ann Plast Surg. 1983;11(3):214–22. https://doi.org/10.1097/00000637-198309000-00007.
52. Sobanko JF, Alster TS. Laser treatment for improvement and minimization of facial scars. Facial Plast Surg Clin North Am. 2011;19(3):527–42. https://doi.org/10.1016/j.fsc.2011.06.006.
53. Alster T, Zaulyanov-Scanlon L. Laser scar revision: a review. Dermatol Surg. 2007;33(2):131–40. https://doi.org/10.1111/j.1524-4725.2006.33030.x.
54. Kuo YR, Jeng SF, Wang FS, et al. Flashlamp pulsed dye laser (PDL) suppression of keloid proliferation through down-regulation of TGF-β1 expression and extracellular matrix expression. Lasers Surg Med. 2004;34(2):104–8. https://doi.org/10.1002/lsm.10206.
55. Reiken SR, Wolfort SF, Berthiaume F, Compton C, Tompkins RG, Yarmush ML. Control of hypertrophic scar growth using selective photothermolysis. Lasers Surg Med. 1997;21(1):7–12. https://doi.org/10.1002/(SICI)1096-9101(1997)21:1<7::AID-LSM2>3.0.CO;2-U.

56. Fitzpatrick RE, Rostan EF, Marchell N. Collagen tightening induced by carbon dioxide laser versus erbium: YAG laser. Lasers Surg Med. 2000;27(5):395–403. https://doi.org/10.1002/1096-9101(2000)27:5<395::AID-LSM1000>3.0.CO;2-4.
57. Mobley SR, Sjogren PP. Soft tissue trauma and scar revision. Facial Plast Surg Clin North Am. 2014;22(4):639–51. https://doi.org/10.1016/j.fsc.2014.07.007.
58. Pierce GF, Mustoe TA, Lingelbach J, et al. Platelet-derived growth factor and transforming growth factor-β enhance tissue repair activities by unique mechanisms. J Cell Biol. 1989;109(1):429–40. https://doi.org/10.1083/jcb.109.1.429.
59. Min S, Yoon JY, Park SY, Moon J, Kwon HH, Suh DH. Combination of platelet rich plasma in fractional carbon dioxide laser treatment increased clinical efficacy of for acne scar by enhancement of collagen production and modulation of laser-induced inflammation. Lasers Surg Med. 2018;50(4):302–10. https://doi.org/10.1002/lsm.22776.
60. Lee JW, Kim BJ, Kim MN, Mun SK. The efficacy of autologous platelet rich plasma combined with ablative carbon dioxide fractional resurfacing for acne scars: a simultaneous split-face trial. Dermatol Surg. 2011;37(7):931–8. https://doi.org/10.1111/j.1524-4725.2011.01999.x.
61. Ibrahim MK, Ibrahim SM, Salem AM. Skin microneedling plus platelet-rich plasma versus skin microneedling alone in the treatment of atrophic post acne scars: a split face comparative study. J Dermatolog Treat. 2018;29(3):281–6. https://doi.org/10.1080/09546634.2017.1365111.
62. Tehranian A, Esfehani-Mehr B, Pirjani R, Rezaei N, Sadat Heidary S, Sepidarkish M. Application of autologous platelet-rich plasma (PRP) on wound healing after caesarean section in high-risk patients. Iran Red Crescent Med J. 2016;18(7) https://doi.org/10.5812/ircmj.34449.
63. Weiss RA, Weiss MA, Beasley KL, Munavalli G. Autologous cultured fibroblast injection for facial contour deformities: a prospective, placebo-controlled, phase III clinical trial. Dermatol Surg. 2007;33(3):263–8. https://doi.org/10.1111/j.1524-4725.2007.33060.x.

Chemical Peels

17

Nicholas A. Nagaki and Elie M. Ferneini

Introduction

There are many factors that contribute to skin aging: weight change, smoking and tobacco use, age related change in sex hormones, and most importantly photoaging. Photoaging is the damage caused to skin at the molecular level by ultraviolet UV radiation. Ultraviolet A and B (UVA and B, respectively) are the primary culprits in skin damage and aging [1].

Chemical peels are agents that are used to cause controlled injury to the skin. Chemical peels differ by the depth of injury to the skin surface from epidermis to deep dermis, classifying from superficial, medium and deep peels. This destruction leads to an exfoliation of these layers and subsequent inflammatory response of wound healing, regeneration and remodeling of the skin layers. The end result of this process is an improved appearance and texture of treated skin.

Chemical peels can be used to treat an array of cutaneous conditions including photoaging (changes in skin texture, fine rhytids, and pigmentation changes), acne vulgaris, actinic or solar keratosis, melasma, and scarring [2–4]. They may be used alone or in combination with other cosmetic procedures for aesthetic enhancement [5–8].

In this chapter we will discuss the classification and mechanism of action of various chemical peels, indications, contraindications, patient selection and counseling, preoperative care, general application principles, postoperative care, complications and complication prevention.

N. A. Nagaki (✉)
University of Connecticut Oral and Maxillofacial Surgery, Farmington, CT, USA
e-mail: nagaki@uchc.edu

E. M. Ferneini
Beau Visage Med Spa, Greater Waterbury OMS, Cheshire, CT, USA

E. M. Ferneini, M. T. Goupil (eds.), *Office-Based Maxillofacial Surgical Procedures*, https://doi.org/10.1007/978-3-030-22371-7_17

Classification of Chemical Peels

Chemical peels are classified according to the depth of the penetration of the epidermis and dermis into superficial, medium, and deep subtypes. The depth of penetration is determined by the concentration, pH/pKa and type of peeling agent used. pKa is an important in chemical peeling, it is defined as the pH at which 50% of the solution is in free acid form. Lower pKa value peels have a stronger exfoliative potential [5, 7].

Superficial

These peels cause their effects on the epidermis and epidermis/dermis interface causing partial or complete necrosis of those layers and associated cell types. They exfoliate the skin from the stratum corneum down to the papillary dermis. Their mechanism of action is causing decreased corneocyte adhesion, epidermolysis and exfoliation, and increased dermal collagen deposition. This leads to thinning of the stratum corneum, increased epidermal thickness and more even melanin distribution [5, 9].

Superficial peels are indicated in the treatment of photoaging, pigmentary disorders, and acne [3, 4, 6, 9]. They are suitable for all Fitzpatrick skin photo-types and may be used on extra-facial skin such as the upper extremities, neck, and chest. Superficial peeling agents include the alpha-hydroxy acids (AHAs) such as glycolic acids, the beta-hydroxy acids (BHAs) including salicylic acid, the beta-lipohydroxy acids (LHAs), and the tretinoins. Glycolic acid is the most commonly used of the superficial peeling agents [5, 10].

Alpha-Hydroxy Acids

The chemical structure of the AHA is a carboxylic acid with a hydroxyl group at the alpha position of the carboxyl group. They are derived from fruit acids such as malic acid (apples) tartaric acid (grapes), citric acid (lemons and oranges), glycolic acid (sugar cane), and lactic acid (milk). At low concentrations AHAs cause decreased corneocyte adhesions, at high concentrations they promote epidermolysis. AHAs require a neutralizing agent to terminate their action; these agents include water, sodium bicarbonate, sodium hydroxide, or ammonium salt solutions. AHAs do not induce a frosting. Glycolic acid is the most commonly used AHA and has a pKa of 3.83 and is soluble in water [5, 7, 10].

Beta-Hydroxy Acids

Salicylic acid is the most commonly used BHA. It is derived from sweet birch, wintergreen leaves and willow tree bark. Its chemical structure has a hydroxyl group at the second carbon atom position. It has a pKa of 2.97 and is poorly soluble in water. Salicylic acid causes disruption of intercellular lipids covalently linked to the cornified keratinocytes. This causes desquamation of the stratum corneum and subsequent activation of basal keratinocytes and fibroblasts. They do not have a frosting pattern. They do not require neutralization. They are used in comedonal and inflammatory acne as well as in oilier skin types [5, 7].

Beta-Lipohydroxy Acids

LHAs is a lipophilic derivative of salicylic acid with an 8-carbon acyl fatty chain that is attached to the fifth carbon of the benzene ring. LHA targets carneodesmosome protein to separate corneocytes uniformly. The increased lipophilicity means it is more targeted to the epidermis and sebaceous follicle and a greater keratolytic effect than salicylic acid. LHA are unique in that they have been found to have antifungal, antibacterial, and anti-inflammatory properties in addition to their peeling properties. They are preferentially used in those patient populations with a predisposition to develop post-inflammatory hyperpigmentation. They do not require neutralization [5]. LHA has a pH similar to normal skin which has proven to make it more tolerable [7].

Medium

Medium peels are effective in treating fine lines and wrinkles, pigmentary disorders, and superficial atrophic scars. They are contraindicated in melasma as they can produce post-inflammatory hyperpigmentation and worsen the primary condition [4]. Trichloroacetic acid (TCA) is used for medium peels, it has a pKa of 0.26 and is hydrophilic. TCA causes precipitation of epidermal proteins which leads to the destruction of the upper dermis. TCA does cause frosting after application, frosting is defined as whitening of the skin due to protein coagulation [5–7, 11].

Deep

Deep chemical peels are used for severe photoaging, pigmentary disorders, and scars. Deep peels most effectively induce collagen formation due to their deeper penetration into the mid-reticular dermis leading to restoration of the dermal architecture to its native state. The active components of deep peels are phenols and croton oils. Deep peels are very painful and typical require general anesthesia or deep sedation [6].

Phenol is an aromatic hydrocarbon derived from coal tar with a pKa of 9.99. Its effect depends on the phenol concentration, at higher concentrations (>80%) it causes rapid and irreversible denaturation and coagulation of epidermal keratin and proteins which results in a barrier that prevents penetration into the deep dermis. At diluted concentrations around 50% it acts as a keratolytic agent disrupting sulfur bridges allowing the phenol to penetrate further into the dermis and allowing for greater destruction and systemic absorption. Systemic absorption cause leaves to severe adverse effects including cardiac arrhythmias, renal failure, and hepatotoxicity. Cardiac monitoring is required [5, 6].

Croton oil is a vesicant derived from the seed of the croton tiglium plant that promotes deeper penetration and absorption of phenol. It is used in many peel combination variants to promote phenol effect [5, 6].

Patient Selection and Counseling

History

Just like any other office visit when a patient comes in for a consultation for a surgical procedure you should start with a chief complaint. A conversation with a patient regarding their motivation for chemical peeling as well as what results they expect the treatment will provide them. This will provide you valuable information on both their goals and expectations so that you can properly guide them in treatment.

It is also very importation to obtain a thorough medical history. History of cardiac, hepatic, or renal disease, diabetes mellitus, immune deficiency or suppression or nutritional deficiency places a patient at increased risk of toxicity, poor/delayed wound healing, and infection. Herpes simplex infection, abnormal scarring or keloid formation, photosensitivity, and inflammatory hyperpigmentation, these conditions can increase the likelihood of post-peel complications. It is also important to know of a patient's history of any previous resurfacing or facial surgery and their body's response to these treatments.

It is important to know if the patient has any other dermatologic conditions including eczema, psoriasis, vitiligo, rosacea, and seborrheic dermatitis; these conditions can be exacerbated by chemical peels [5, 12].

All medications, supplements and over the counter/prescription skin treatments also need to be reviewed. Any use of isotretinoin in the last 6–12 months increased the risk of delayed re-epithelialization and scarring with medium-depth and deep chemical peels [11]. The use of photosensitizing medications including hormonal agents and OCPs increase the risk of post-peel hyperpigmentation [5, 12].

An assessment of the patients UV exposure time through their lifestyle and work activities should also be considered [8, 12]. As well as the patients smoking status is also important, and cessation for 1 week or more before and 6 months after each procedure is recommended [5].

Patient Examination

Begin with an assessment of skin color using the Fitzpatrick skin photo-type scale. The degree of photoaging should also be assessed. A close exam of the skin is accomplished to determine the presence of pilosebaceous units, sebaceous gland activity, skin thickness and health, laxity of periorbital skin, preexisting inflammatory changes and hypertrophic or keloid scarring [5, 8, 12].

Using photography as a part of your patient assessment is very important [5, 8].

Patient Selection

As discussed earlier superficial peels have favorable results in all Fitzpatrick skin photo-types. Medium and deep chemical peels work ideally in fair complexion females. Drier skin types, fine rhytids, and minimal gross redundancy are also favorable characteristics [2]. Fitzpatrick III–IV photo-types have a greater risk for developing pigmentary dyschromia and scarring. Men typically have thicker, coarser, more oleaginous skin which makes it difficult to predict how well the peel will penetrate the skin [5–8, 12].

Pre-peel Care

Priming the skin encompasses the pretreatment and preparation activities that help to prepare the skin for peeling. The goal is to thin the stratum corneum, enhance the penetration of the active peel agent, and improve post-peel heeling [5]. When performed correctly they enhance patient compliance, detect intolerances and reduce risk of peel complications. They can also provide you the opportunity to identify patient who are non-adherent with pretreatment regimens, making them less suitable for chemical peeling [5].

The pretreatment of the skin should begin at least 2–4 weeks prior and stopped 3–5 days prior to chemical peeling [8]. Patients should be instructed to limit their UV exposure and apply broad-spectrum sunscreen with SPF 50 or greater with UVA and UVB coverage daily. Patients should start applying sunscreen at least 3 months prior to any peel and should be encouraged to continue applying indefinitely after treatment, as we now know UV photodamage is one of the main cuprite for photoaging [5].

Tretinoin cream (0.025–0.05%) should be applied daily for at least 2 weeks prior to chemical peel. Tretinoin decreases epidermal adhesion leading to thinning of the stratum corneum. This thinning leads to more predictable and deeper penetration of the peeling agent. Tretinoin also accelerates epithelial proliferation, which improves post-peel re-epithelialization.

Hydroquinone 2–4% cream is a phenolic compound used to treat dyschromia and reduces the risk of post-inflammatory hyperpigmentation. It is a bleaching agent, which reversibly inhibiting tyrosinase and selectively damages melanocytes and melanosomes by the formation of free radicals. Adverse effects include allergic and irritant contact dermatitis as well as ochronosis. In patients who are high risk for post-inflammatory hyperpigmentation hydroquinone cream should be started 2 weeks pre-peel and restarted 1–2 weeks post-peel [5].

Patients should also avoid waxing, electrolysis, and dermabrasion for a minimum of 3–4 weeks prior to chemical peeling [8]. Those patients with a history of herpes simplex virus should receive antiviral therapy prior to medium and deep peels.

The day of and the day prior to treatment the patient should wash their skin with a non-residue soap and refrain from using makeup and moisturizers. On the day of the procedure the patient should not wear contacts or jewelry. Skin should be prepared with acetone, triclosan, or isopropyl alcohol to removed makeup, oil, loose keratin, and other debris [5].

Test spotting is a procedure than can also help in assessing patient reaction to medium and deep peeling agents. It involves application of these chemical agents to an area close to the planned peeled areas that will be inconspicuous if there is a poor reaction. These areas include lateral temple, anterior hairline and pre-auricular region [5]. Test spotting aids both the provider and patient with valuable information on peel efficacy, healing time, pigmentary response and post-peel complications. Disadvantages include delay of treatment, misrepresentation of results, and persistence of the test spot until the definitive treatment occurs.

Procedure

Setup

Chemical peeling should be performed in the proper setting, with adequate lighting and ventilation as well as accept to emergency resuscitation equipment. Your assistant should be prepared to help maintain patient position and equipment, clear/wipe away tears from the medial canthal regions to prevent the peeling agent from contacting the eye. The patient should be placed on appropriate monitors and someone should monitor the patient at all times.

The peeling agent should be placed into a clearly labeled glass receptacle or prepared to the manufacturer's specifications away from the patient to avoid accidental spills. To this note, the receptacle should never pass over the patient. Any crystals that have precipitated out should be removed as they can increase the peel concentrations. Neutralizing agents and emergency eye irrigation solution (water, saline, or glycerine) must be readily available [5, 8, 12, 13].

Positioning/Preparation

The patient should be supine with the head elevated with a pillow to approximately 45° and a towel placed around their neck. The patient should be instructed to keep their eyes closed throughout the procedure and given proper eye shielding when appropriate. The hair should be pulled back out of the peel treatment area and secured with a band or surgical cap. Petroleum jelly or zinc oxide paste may be applied to the lateral canthi, nasal alar grooves, nasolabial folds, lips, and oral commissures to prevent pooling of the peeling agent in these areas [5, 12].

Application

How you apply the agents depends on the peeling agent being used. Liquid agents can be applied with a brush, cotton tip applicator or cotton or gauze swab. Wooden spatula can be used to apply more viscous gel agents.

The peel application should first be applied to areas with thicker skin: the forehead, malar areas, nose, and chin; this should be followed by application to thinner skin areas: perioral and periorbital skin [5, 12]. The peeling agent should be applied in an upward direction with firm even strokes and extending beyond the vermillion border into the oral commissure. Care should be taken to ovoid overlapping strokes and missing areas. Near the edges of the peel area should be feathered to help avoid sharp demarcation borders. Rhytids should be stretched out when applying peel to avoid pooling in these areas [5].

Postoperative Care

Good postoperative care helps to ensure good post-peel recovery of the skin and helps to prevent complications. As with any procedure the patient should be given written instructions on how to care for their skin after a peel and what to expect in the days follow a peel. Patients should be instructed to wash their face with a non-soap cleanser and avoid rubbing, scrubbing, scratching or picking at their skin. A non-scented, non-dyed lotion or emollient should be applied to the skin regularly until the peeling process is complete [5, 8, 12].

If crusting occurs, topical antibiotics can be prescribed. Makeup application should not occur until after the skin has re-epithelialized. Sun and UV avoidance and daily application of sunscreen should be encouraged [5].

Complications

Though chemical peels are relatively safe they are not without risk of complication. The first step in avoidance of complication is in appropriate patient selection, education and counseling. Selecting the right peeling agent for the circumstances as well as pre-peel skin prep and post-peel skin care can help in minimizing the risk of complications. Despite these measures to provide safe care adverse effects may still occur following a chemical peel and vary according to depth.

Some minor complications that may present within minutes to hours include irritation, burning, erythema, pruritus, edema, and blistering (Fig. 17.1). Minor complications that may occur days to weeks post-peel include development of acneiform eruptions, infection, persistent erythema, demarcation lines, and milia (Fig. 17.2). Pigmentary changes, textural changes, scarring, and increased pigmentation of nevi may also occur [5, 8, 12].

More major complications, though rare, can occur. These include local and systemic complications including allergic reactions, laryngeal edema, toxic shock syndrome, cardiotoxicity, salicylism, acute kidney injury, lower lip ectropion, corneal damage, significant scarring, and dyspigmentation [5, 8, 12, 14].

Complications are more common in darker skinner patients and with medium and deep peels as compared to superficial peels [8, 11, 12, 15].

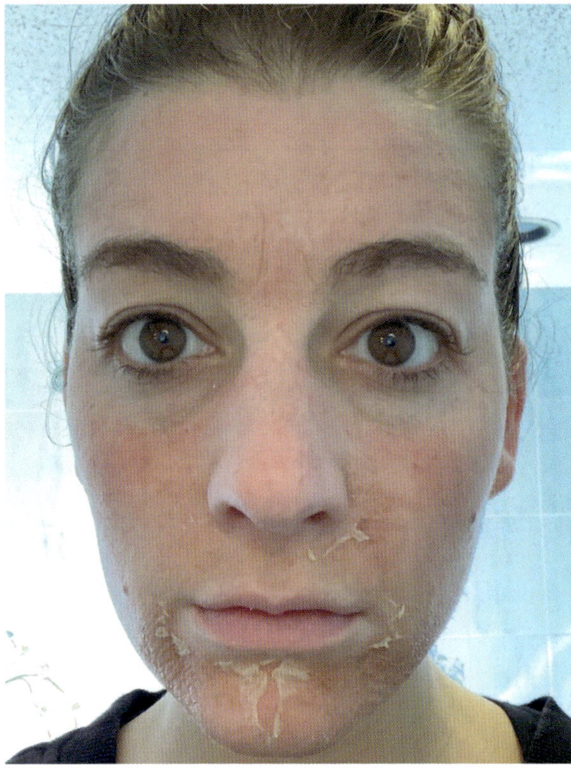

Fig. 17.1 Patient post-peel day 3. Notice some expected erythema and edema

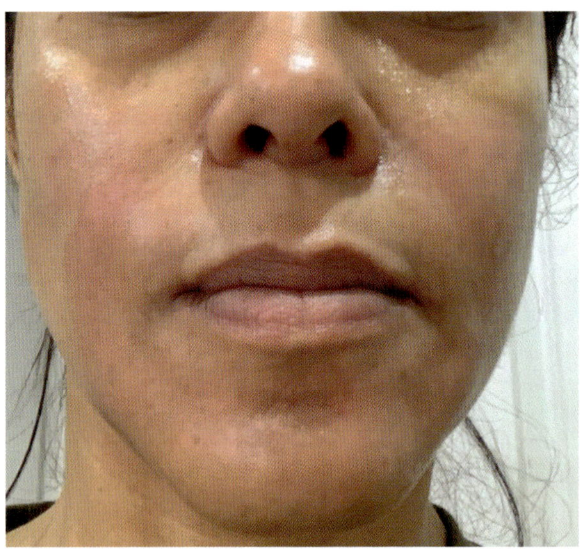

Fig. 17.2 Persistent erythema 2 weeks post-peel. The erythema persisted up to 4 weeks

Conclusion

Chemical peeling is a relatively safe procedure that can be performed in the outpatient setting that is both simple and cost-effective. In well-trained hands with the proper provider and patient education and selection complications are few and can be avoided and treated.

References

1. Commander SJ, Chang D, Fakhro A, Nigro MG, Lee EI. Noninvasive facial rejuvenation. Part 1: patient-directed. Semin Plast Surg. 2016;30(3):129–33.
2. Baker TJ. The ablation of rhitides by chemical means. A preliminary report. J Fla Med Assoc. 1961;48:451–4.
3. Castillo DE, Keri JE. Chemical peels in the treatment of acne: patient selection and perspectives. Clin Cosmet Investig Dermatol. 2018;11:365–72. https://doi.org/10.2147/CCID.S137788.
4. Sarkar R, Bansal S, Garg VK. Chemical peels for melasma in dark-skinned patients. J Cutan Aesthet Surg. 2012;5(4):247–53.
5. O'Connor AA, Lowe PM, Shumack S, Lim AC. Chemical peels: a review of current practice. Australas J Dermatol. 2018;59:171–81. https://doi.org/10.1111/ajd.12715.
6. Meaike JD, Agrawal N, Chang D, Lee EI, Nigro MG. Noninvasive facial rejuvenation. Part 3: physician-directed-lasers, chemical peels, and other noninvasive modalities. Semin Plast Surg. 2016;30(3):143–50.
7. Rendon MI, Berson DS, Cohen JL, Roberts WE, Starker I, Wang B. Evidence and considerations in the application of chemical peels in skin disorders and aesthetic resurfacing. J Clin Aesthet Dermatol. 2010;3(7):32–43.
8. Anitha B. Prevention of complications in chemical peeling. J Cutan Aesthet Surg. 2010;3(3):186–8.
9. Berson DS, Cohen JL, Rendon MI, et al. Clinical role and application of superficial chemical peels in today's practice. J Drugs Dermatol. 2009;8:803–11.
10. Sharad J. Glycolic acid peel therapy—a current review. Clin Cosmet Investig Dermatol. 2013;6:281–8.
11. Camacho FM. Medium-depth and deep chemical peels. J Cosmet Dermatol. 2005;4:117–28.
12. Khunger N, Force IT. Standard guidelines of care for chemical peels. Indian J Dermatol Venereol Leprol. 2008;74(Suppl):S5–12.
13. Soleymani T, Lanoue J, Rahman ZA. Practical approach to chemical peels: a review of fundamentals and step-by-step algorithmic protocol for treatment. J Clin Aesthet Dermatol. 2018;11(8):21–8.
14. Eller JJ, Wolff S. Skin peeling and scarification: in the treatment of pitted scars, pigmentations and certain facial blemishes. JAMA. 1941;116:934–8.
15. Nikalji N, Godse K, Sakhiya J, et al. Complications of medium depth and deep chemical peels. J Cutan Aesthet Surg. 2012;5:254–60.

Laser Skin Resurfacing

18

L. Angelo Cuzalina and Craig H. Rhyne

Skin Anatomy and Physiology

An organ is defined as a system having two or more primary tissues that serve differing functions and work together. The integumentary system or skin is the largest human organ. Its tissue functions cooperate to serve the purposes of human skin: protection from elements, pathogenic organisms, abrasion, radiation, heat, cold, dehydration, and pain and injury avoidance in conjunction with other organ systems. Also, the skin produces and stores vitamin-D, regulates temperature, communicates to other humans, and aids in excretion. Lastly, the skin is subject to various diseases and gives signs to underlying systemic diseases.

The layers of skin include the epithelial tissue epidermis (stratum corneum, stratum granulosum, stratum spinosum, and stratum basale or germinativum), the connective tissue dermis (which contains the muscle tissue arrector pili muscles), the nerve tissues motor and sensory nerves, sebaceous glands—hair (pilo-sebaceous unit), sweat glands, and blood vessels (see Fig. 18.1).

Facial skin is composed of more repeating epithelial proliferative units (EPU) per given surface area. These are the sebaceous gland, sweat gland duct, and hair shaft epithelial linings that can quickly re-epithelialize the face after ablation of the epidermis.

L. A. Cuzalina
OSU Medical School/Surgical Residency Program, Tulsa, OK, USA
e-mail: angelo@tulsasurgicalarts.com

C. H. Rhyne (✉)
United States Air Force, Alamo Heights, TX, USA

E. M. Ferneini, M. T. Goupil (eds.), *Office-Based Maxillofacial Surgical Procedures*, https://doi.org/10.1007/978-3-030-22371-7_18

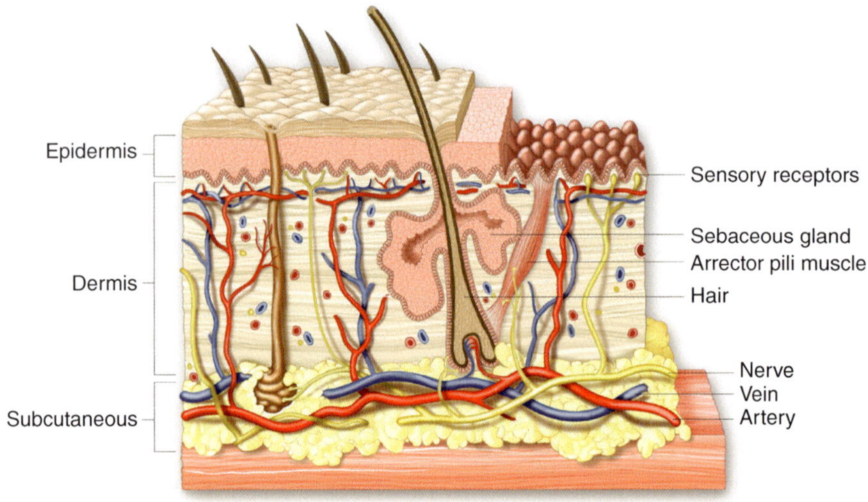

Fig. 18.1 Components of skin

Patient Selection

In the patient interview, consultation, and examination, one must identify patients who can benefit from laser skin resurfacing and identify risks to patient based on skin phototype, past medical history, social history—including tobacco use, skin care routine, current level of solar damage, and sun exposure hygiene.

In 1975 Dr. Thomas B. Fitzpatrick, an American Dermatologist, developed a classification of skin type based on reaction to ultraviolet radiation exposure [1]. The Fitzpatrick Phototyping Scale was a simplification of an early-described classification scale. It is often associated with hair and eye color but was not related to these features other than as a correlation (see Table 18.1)

Photodamage is the result of exposure to ultraviolet radiation, regardless of Fitzpatrick Type. First described and classified by American Dermatologist, Richard G. Glogau, the scale can be used as a good predictor of benefit from laser resurfacing [2] (see Table 18.2).

Laser skin resurfacing of the face is a great adjunctive procedure or used as a lone procedure to produce great results if properly planned and executed but should not be considered unless the patient is prepared to begin and continue facial skin care. This includes cleaning, moisturizing, and use of sunscreen.

Lasers and Laser Safety

The word laser began as an acronym—LASER, standing for: "Light Amplification by Stimulated Emission of Radiation." The laser was designed and built in 1960 by Hughes Research Laboratories, the research arm of Hughes Aircraft, owned by Howard Hughes.

Table 18.1 Fitzpatrick phototyping scale

Fitzpatrick phototyping	Reaction to ultraviolet (UV) light exposure
I	Always burns easily and never tans (pale skin with freckles)
II	Usually burns and minimally tans
III	Medium burns and uniformly tans
IV	Minimal burns and tans well (moderate brown skin)
V	Rarely burns and always tans easily (dark brown skin)
VI	Never burns (very darkly pigmented brown skin)

Hair and eye color often correlate, but can mislead and should not be used to describe Fitzpatrick Type

Table 18.2 Glogau photoaging scale

Glogau photoaging scale	Typical age (YEARS)	Description
Mild	28–35	Mild wrinkles in animation only, no keratosis evidence
Moderate	35–50	Minimal wrinkles, complexion changes, early keratosis
Advanced	50–60	Static wrinkles, discolorations, telangiectasia and keratosis
Severe	60–75	Deep wrinkles, advanced loss of support, possible cancers

All lasers work for skin resurfacing by photothermolysis. This process means that the laser is absorbed by a specific component of skin or color of tissue type. The absorbed energy is converted to heat and the heat creates tissue damage or frank removal (ablation) of tissue. Too much tissue damage can cause unfavorable results, and so therefore the optimum amount and focus of damage is imperative.

Lasers are best summarized by their type of technology. There are non-ablative and ablative lasers. There are also fractional and non-fractional lasers in the ablative classification (see Fig. 18.2).

Non-ablative lasers have a shorter wavelength and target specific colors or chromophores that absorb that specific wavelength. For instance, one can target vascular lesions by focusing on the color red. For the purpose of this chapter, we are focused primarily on ablative lasers that function at longer wavelengths—specifically, carbon dioxide lasers (Fig. 18.3).

Non-fractional, ablative lasers target water as the chromophore and simply remove a section of skin with each treatment. These preceded the use of fractional lasers but are still used by some providers today. Again, for the purpose of this chapter, we will focus primarily on fractional, ablative lasers.

A fractional ablative laser functions by heating and vaporizing a small column of tissue at rapidly patterned increments. These columns are referred to as microthermal treatment zones (MTZ). These MTZs are able to penetrate more deeply than a non-fractional ablative laser without extensive collateral thermal tissue damage. Therefore, the results of skin resurfacing can be as good as or better than with a fractional ablative laser while offering decreased risk of complications [3].

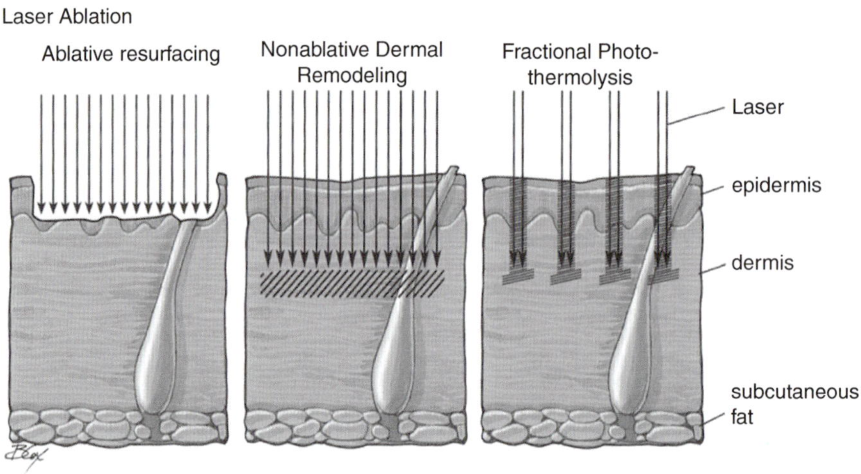

Fig. 18.2 Type of laser determines depth of beam penetration

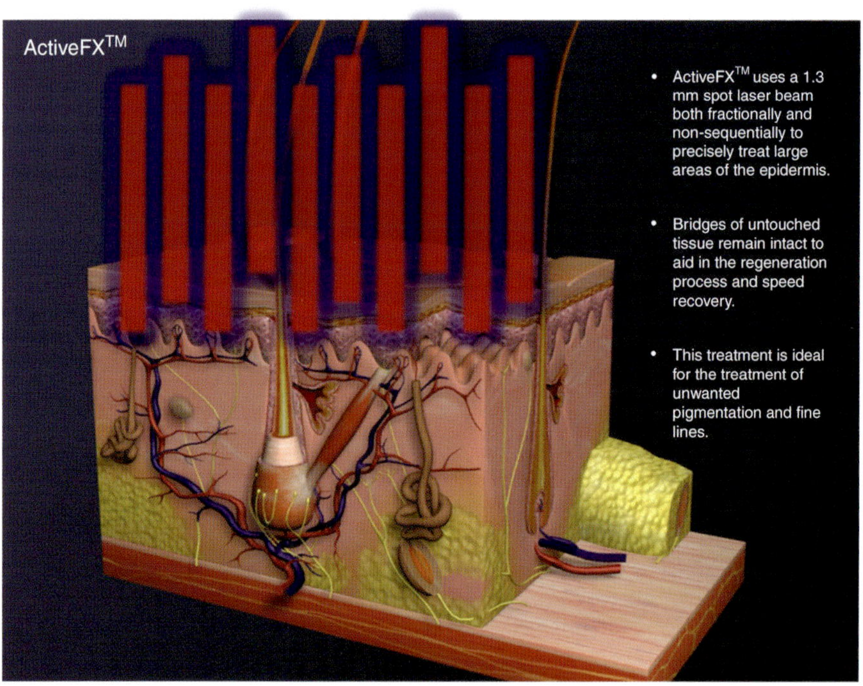

Fig. 18.3 ActiveFX™ laser beam profile

Laser safety is a priority when endeavoring to offer laser skin resurfacing to patients. The provider, staff, and patient are all at risk. The laser or lasers must be calibrated, maintained properly, tested, documented and it helps to assign a staff member as the Laser Safety Officer. Laser eye shields are mandatory for the patient when laser resurfacing a patient's face (see Fig. 18.4).

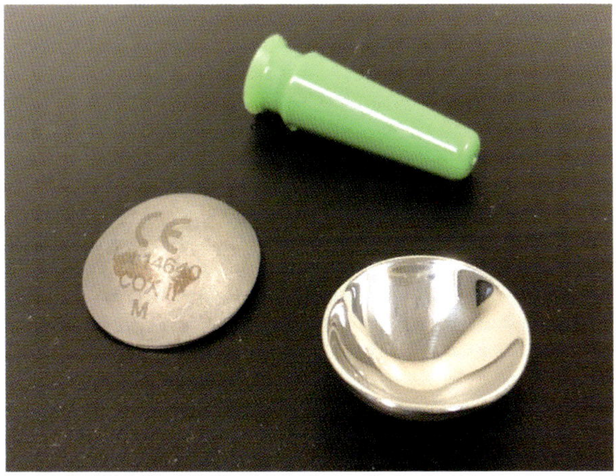

Fig. 18.4 Examples of protective eye shields for undergoing laser resurfacing

In addition to the patient's eye protection, all persons in the treatment area should use laser protective eyewear. A sign must be posted on the closed door indicating the wavelength of the laser in use. Vacuum and filtration should be used for the smoke flume created from the thermal ablation as this contains potentially hazardous particles. A carbon dioxide laser can be an ignition source for concentrated oxygen and should therefore not be used with closed drapes and around a non-laser safe airway. The concentration of oxygen delivered to the patient should ideally be below 30%. Other flammable items should be removed or not used all together prior to beginning laser skin resurfacing.

Skin Preparation

Prior to a laser skin resurfacing of the face, a preparation protocol is recommended. This is especially true of Fitzpatrick Phototype patients IV–VI, who are more likely to have hyperpigmentation issues in the recovery phase or permanent alteration in skin tone.

Indeed, the goal is for patients to have a rapid recovery with decreased risks of both short-term and long-term complications. The use of retinoids helps prepare the facial skin for a more rapid and predictable re-epithelialization, and therefore quick healing. We prefer 0.025–0.05% tretinoin topical cream or gel used for a period of 6 weeks and discontinued 3–5 days prior to laser use. It can be reintroduced after complete healing and after the skin is less sensitive to irritation.

With darker skin phototypes, the use of 4% hydroquinone cream or gel for a period of six weeks prior to the procedure is appropriate and can help minimize the risk of hyperpigmentation. More often than not, we prescribe a compounded or combined preparation of tretinoin, hydroquinone and sometimes including fluocinolone, especially if there is post-laser hyperpigmentation.

In all patients, regardless of history, it is recommended to use an oral antiviral to minimize the risk of a viral outbreak on the facial skin [4]. Both acyclovir and valacyclovir are reasonable options.

Procedures and Laser Settings

The fractional ablative laser that we use exclusively and will write about is the Lumenis Ultra-Pulse. We have no disclaimers or financial interests in this product.

The Lumenis UltraPulse has a few different available attachments and operation modes to allow for superficial, deep, blended and scar specific laser penetrations. ActiveFX is the brand's superficial ablative workhorse. It is the most commonly utilized mode in our practice. The manufacturer publishes recommended guidelines for settings and treatment parameters on the various modes and handpieces [5].

The settings for a Lumenis UltraPulse carbon dioxide laser allow for manipulation of energy (mJ), power (W), fluence (J/cm^2), scan size (mm), density, frequency (Hz), and repeat delay (/s) (see Fig. 18.5)

Our favored settings for an ActiveFX set up for a patient with moderate photodamage might be: 80–125 mJ energy, 6–7 mm scan size, 2–3 density, 100–150 Hz frequency, and 0.3–1.5 s repeat delay.

As the energy is increased, we typically decrease frequency, and conversely if we increase frequency, we will typically decrease energy. The depth of the ablation is directly related to the increase or decrease of these settings. Knowing the settings of your particular laser is imperative to achieve the desired result.

It is important to "feather" and blend the resurfacing at the edges and onto the neck skin. If ablative laser skin resurfacing is used concurrently with another

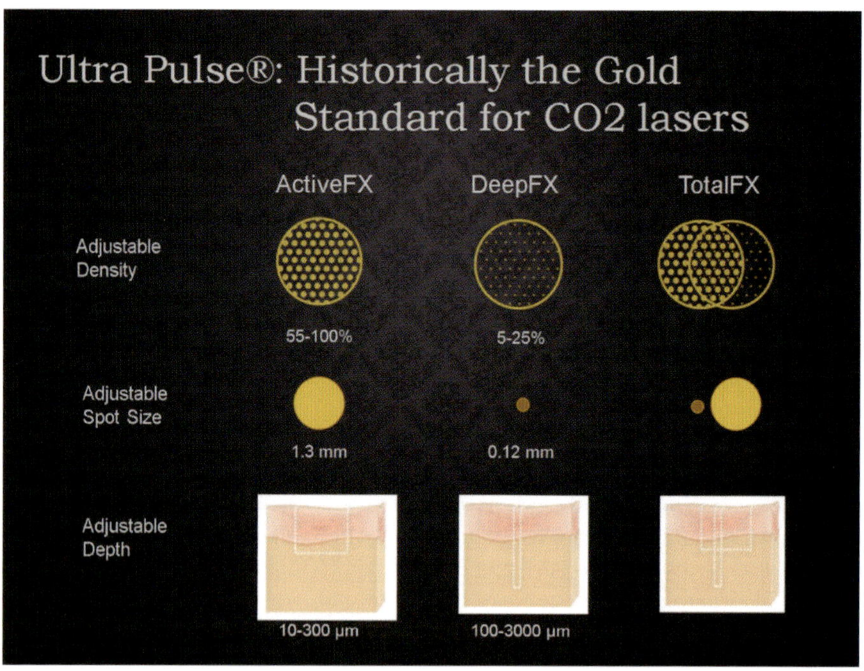

Fig. 18.5 Recommended laser settings

Table 18.3 Laser resurfacing complications

Complications associated with laser skin resurfacing
Pain
Erythema
Edema
Contact dermatitis
Infection (viral, fungal, bacterial)
Milia
Hyperpigmentation
Hypopigmentation
Ocular injury
Ectropion
Scarring
Need for more surgery

procedure such as facelifting, it is advisable to use lower settings blend to these lower settings as not to injury to deeper layers of skin into the dermis thereby compromising blood flow.

Complications and Avoidance

Complications seen with laser resurfacing can be categorized into short term and long term. They are essentially the same as seen with non-laser resurfacing techniques. As with any surgery, pain, swelling, infection, damage to adjacent areas, need for more surgery, and to a limited extent—bleeding are risks.

Specific to laser skin resurfacing, we expect patients to the following short-term complications: pain, erythema, and edema. Occasionally, we see transient pigmentation changes. Other short-term complications include contact dermatitis, infection (viral, fungal and bacterial), and milia. Long-term complications include dyspigmentation, scarring, ectropion, ocular injury, and need for more surgery. Any of these cause a breakdown of the doctor-patient relationship (see Table 18.3).

To best avoid or minimize these complications, use appropriate laser safety and settings, prepare the skin and use postoperative care. Both informed consent and informed refusal should be discussed and documented as with any elective procedure.

Recovery and Post-laser Care

Skin protection and moisturizing are key to optimal recovery. We recommend a petrolatum-based ointment preparation, such as Aquaphor Healing Ointment and often use a lidocaine cream or ointment as well, for the patient's comfort.

Occasionally, we will use platelet-rich plasma on the laser treated skin to help introduce growth factors and speed recovery [6].

Prescriptions are given to the patient with postoperative recovery instructions and include an antibiotic, an antiviral, analgesics, and ointment. Care instructions

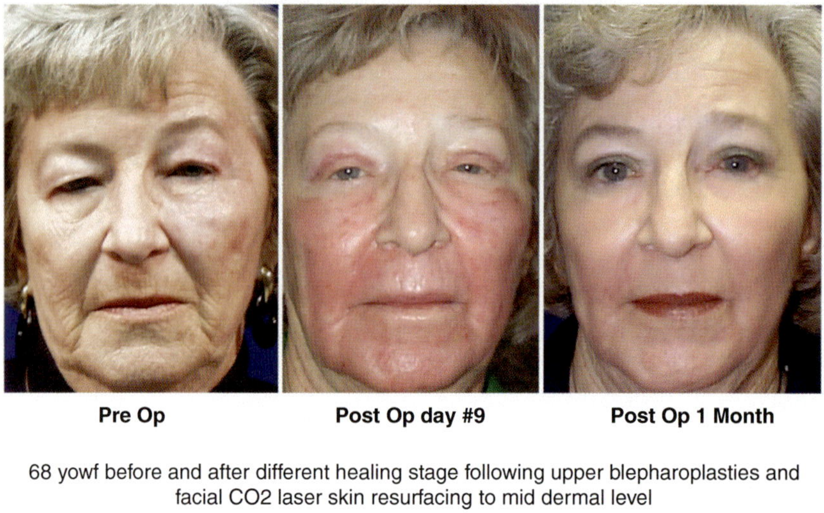

Fig. 18.6 Example of laser resurfacing

include gentle cleaning with a mild soap and water or a dilute vinegar solution. Afterward, it should be expecting that the skin will peel and be replaced by new epithelium. After complete re-epithelium, it is important to have the patient reintroduce a skin care regiment including sunscreen. Ultraviolet exposure can induce dyspigmentation and scarring.

Sometimes, it will be necessary for patients to use a steroid to help reduce inflammation. Steroids should be used judiciously and in a very limited fashion, as they can reduce some of the beneficial effects of laser skin resurfacing.

The timeframe of healing varies by patient, depth of laser penetration and degree of ablation. Generally, patients who use makeup can begin reusing to cover the pink skin by the end of two weeks. Again, a sunscreen should be used as part of that routine (see Fig. 18.6).

Lifetime Skincare

All patients should be advised on proper skincare to "protect their investment" and to optimize their results. Of course, sunscreen is a necessity, but proper cleansing and an effective moisturizer must be used by men and women alike.

Additionally, retinoids, keratolytics (mild peeling agents), skin-lightening agents, vitamins, and antioxidants should be used routinely and offering or referring to a skin-care specialist should be part of any Laser Skin Resurfacing provider's armamentarium.

Before and After Case Presentation

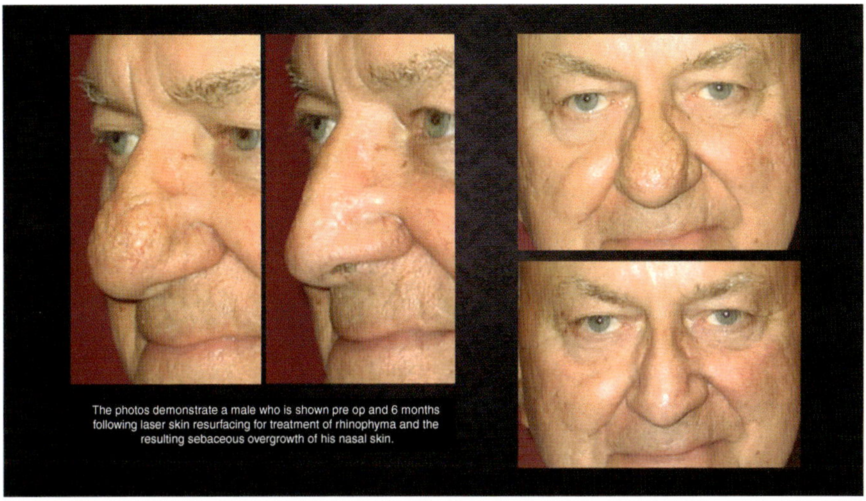

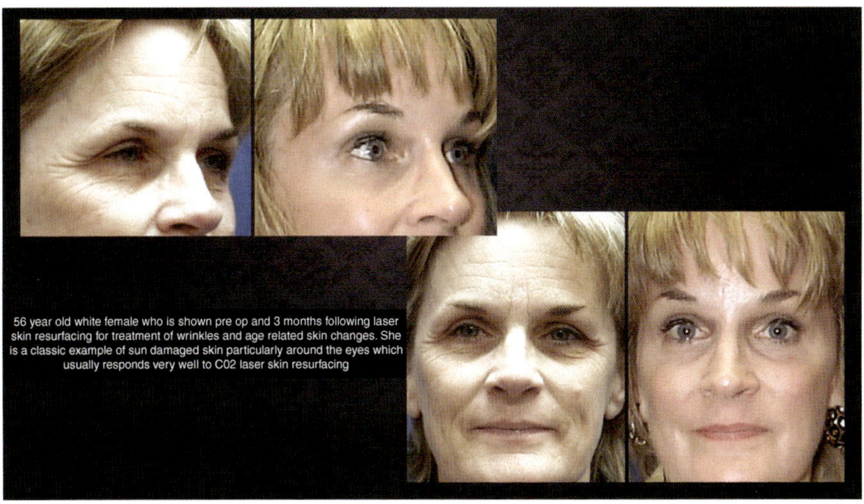

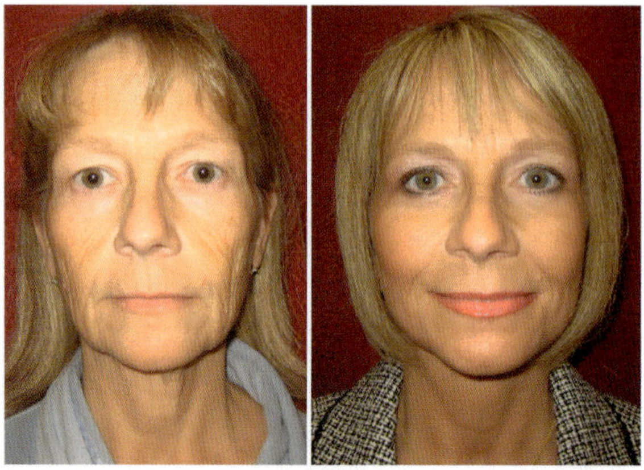

Before & 7 months after lower facelift, chin & cheek implants and laser skin resurfacing

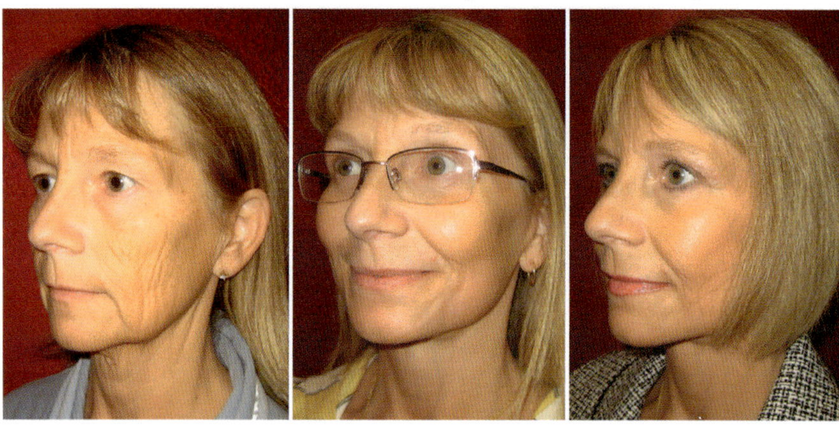

6 months post op with glasses *7 months post op without glasses & new haircut*

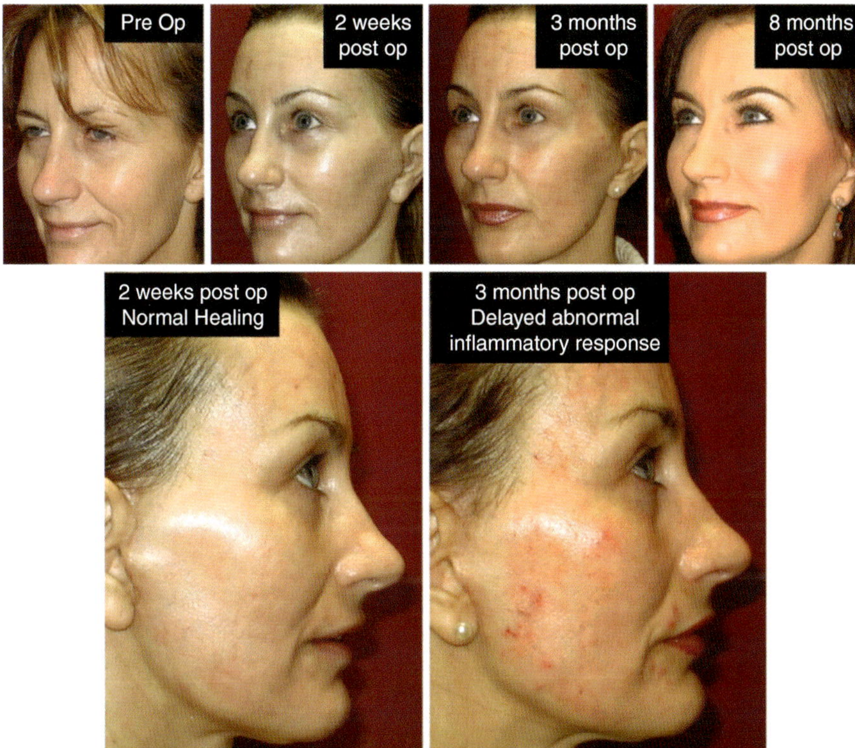

The series of photographs demonstrate a patient who had normal healing following lase skin resurfacing for a few weeks post operatively followed by an abnormal post inflammatory response treated by removing all potentially irritating topicals and use of very bland moisturizers and a short course of Doxycycline to also decrease any immunologic or low grade bacterial component. Cultures were all negative.

References

1. Fitzpatrick TB. Soleil et peau [Sun and skin]. J de Médecine Esthétique. 1975;(2):33–4. (in French)
2. Glogau RG. Aesthetic and anatomic analysis of the aging skin. Semin Cutan Med Surg. 1996;15:134.
3. Manstein D, Herron GS, Sink RK, Tanner H, Anderson RR. Fractional photothermolysis: a new concept for cutaneous remodeling using microscopic patterns of thermal injury. Lasers Surg Med. 2004;34:426–38.
4. Mirmanesh M, Borab Z, Gantz M, Maguina P. Peri-procedure laser scar therapy protocol: a pilot survey of plastic surgeons' practices. Aesthetic Plast Surg. 2017 Jun;41(3):689–94.
5. Clementoni MT, Galimberti M, Tourlaki A, Catenacci M, Lavagno R, Bencini PL. Random fractional ultrapulsed CO2 resurfacing of photodamaged facial skin: long-term evaluation. Lasers Med Sci. 2013 Feb;28(2):643–50.
6. Hsiao FC, Bock GN, Eisen DB. Recent advances in fractional laser resurfacing: new paradigm in optimal parameters and post-treatment wound care. Adv Wound Care (New Rochelle). 2012;1(5):207–12.

Dermabrasion

19

Damon McIntire, Frank Paletta, and Douglas Johnson

Introduction

Dermabrasion is a widely used method for skin resurfacing [1], which is frequently employed for revision of unsightly scars [2], facial rejuvenation [3], or in the treatment of conditions such as rhinophyma [4], or benign growths [5]. There are a multitude of treatment options available within the wide realm of skin resurfacing, including chemical peels and CO_2 laser resurfacing, and in lay terminology these treatments can frequently be misidentified as dermabrasion. Within this chapter we will define dermabrasion as procedural mechanical resurfacing. Mechanical abrasion involves the use of a handheld, powered tool such as a wire brush or a diamond fraise in order to remove the outer layer of the skin, the epidermis, as well as a less significant portion of the underlying dermis [1]. The mechanism of dermabrasion is rooted in the manipulation of physiologic wound healing. In short, the process is intended to remove unhealthy or otherwise undesirable tissue, create a partial-thickness wound, and allow the opportunity for replacement with healthier dermis and epidermis through the stimulation of dermal fibroblasts.

As with any procedure, a thorough understanding of appropriate patient selection, pre-procedure setup for maximization of results, and postoperative care is at least as important as knowledge and application of technique. Within this chapter we will discuss indications for dermabrasion, patient selection, pre-procedural

D. McIntire · F. Paletta (✉)
Warren Alpert Medical School of Brown University, Providence, RI, USA
e-mail: damon_mcintire@alumni.brown.edu

D. Johnson
University of Florida Shands Jacksonville, Jacksonville, FL, USA
e-mail: dlj@floridafacedoc.com

E. M. Ferneini, M. T. Goupil (eds.), *Office-Based Maxillofacial Surgical Procedures*, https://doi.org/10.1007/978-3-030-22371-7_19

considerations, procedural technique, and post-procedure care. In addition, we will examine how to avoid and manage complications of the procedure and finally review two case examples.

Indications

The most common indication for mechanical dermabrasion is scar revision in the setting of previous traumatic injury, surgical intervention, or acne scarring [2]. Other conditions, such as wrinkled or sun-damaged skin, may also be treated by dermabrasion in well-selected patients [3]. Rhinophyma has been shown to have an excellent response to cold resurfacing via dermabrasion [4]. Benign growths with an epithelial origin may be fully treated by mechanical dermabrasion whereas growths with dermal components may be improved but will inevitably recur due to subtotal resection [5].

Patient Selection

Before performing any procedural intervention, it is of utmost importance to perform a careful, targeted review of medications and past medical and surgical history. Current use of isotretinoin (frequently employed in the treatment of severe acne) is an absolute contraindication to use of dermabrasion as it has been linked to impaired wound healing and subsequent keloid formation or hypertrophic scarring. Patients currently using isotretinoin that are interested in mechanical dermabrasion should stop the medication 6–12 months before undergoing the procedure [1].

Although anticoagulation is not an absolute contraindication to dermabrasion, before treating any patient taking warfarin, aspirin, or any other "blood-thinning" medication including herbal supplements, there should be a frank discussion of the risks and benefits of the procedure in the setting of increased risk of bleeding, especially if performing dermabrasion over a large area (i.e., full-face dermabrasion for facial rejuvenation). If medically appropriate, anticoagulation should be stopped approximately two weeks before procedural intervention [1].

There has been some evidence linking use of exogenous hormones like oral contraceptives or estrogen to increased risk of post-procedure hyperpigmentation. Before performing any intervention, it is important to counsel patients to this risk, and, if amenable, patients may elect to halt hormones before the procedure in order to decrease the risk of complications [3].

It is vital to inquire about history of keloid formation or hypertrophic scarring in the patient or patient's family. It can be useful to inspect keloid-prone areas like the earlobes and sternum if the patient is unsure. If the patient is susceptible to keloids and the practitioner feels comfortable proceeding, it may be prudent to test a small area to assess the patient's reaction to the intervention before proceeding to a larger area of dermabrasion.

Patients with disorders of collagen formation may have a suboptimal response to dermabrasion and poor results. In addition, patients with diabetes mellitus or who are immunosuppressed are likely to experience delayed wound healing with higher risk of hypertrophic scarring. Patients with these disorders should be counseled before intervention so that they have appropriate expectations.

Patients with a history of infection with herpes simplex virus or "cold sores" should begin prophylaxis with acyclovir prior to intervention. In any patient who displays active herpetic lesions, dermabrasion should be postponed until after complete resolution [1]. For the protection of the practitioner and assistants, it is important to inquire about history of, or exposure to, bloodborne infectious diseases such as HIV or hepatitis C which could be transferred via aerosolized blood or tissue during the procedure [2].

A brief review of surgical history is always appropriate prior to performing any procedure, especially as it may give the practitioner the opportunity to assess the patient's previous scarring response. Specifically, any patient who has a history of surgery with extensive skin undermining in the area to be abraded (i.e., face lift procedure) has a much higher risk of skin necrosis due to compromised vascular supply. Procedural intervention should be delayed in these patients for 6 months after surgery.

Optimal timing for dermabrasion for the purpose of scar revision is between 8 and 12 weeks post-injury if possible. Scars of older age may be improved but will likely not be eradicated. It is important to counsel patients to this effect [6].

Pre-procedure Considerations

Improper setup can turn a normally quick, easy, and rewarding procedure into a drawn-out, agonizing, and frustrating experience. If performing a moderate to high volume of dermabrasion procedures, a practitioner should have a standardized setup with which assistants or other ancillary staffs are well acquainted. Items vital to procedure success include the handheld dermabrader with or without a foot pedal, the diamond fraise or wire brush, eye protection and face masks for the practitioner and assistant, local anesthesia (i.e., 1% lidocaine with epinephrine 1:100,000), antiseptic prep solution (i.e., 4% chlorhexidine), and saline- or epinephrine-soaked gauze.

Diamond fraises come in a variety of shapes, sizes, and degrees of coarseness. Choosing the correct fraise for the task is an important consideration in preparation for the procedure. Smaller tips are useful in tight areas or areas of increased caution (i.e., around the lips and eyes). More experienced practitioners may prefer coarser tips that can abrade more effectively with less passes. Newer users may prefer to use less coarse tips and perform more passes until they feel comfortable in order to avoid excessive dermabrasion. If using a less coarse fraise, be aware that over the course of many passes the tip may heat up and cause thermal damage to the skin which can result in delayed healing.

The patient should be placed in the supine position. If performing dermabrasion near hair bearing areas, it is vital to tie or tape hair away from field so as to avoid hair avulsion. If performing dermabrasion over a small area (i.e., scar revision or removal of a confined area of fine rhytids) local anesthesia with or without an anxiolytic is appropriate. For full face dermabrasion in the setting of generalized acne pitting, or extensive facial rhytids, intravenous sedation or general anesthesia is usually necessary [3].

Pretreating the area to be abraded with an ice pack for 20–30 min or with refrigerant spray is useful for hemostasis as well as anesthesia and should be used if available. Some practitioners may choose to stain the area with gentian violet as well. This ink remains confined to the epidermis and can be useful, especially for new practitioners, in knowing when to cease abrasion of a particular spot. Local anesthesia should be infiltrated in order to improve tolerability of the procedure and to act as a tumescent providing increased turgor during the intervention. Finally, the area should be prepped in the usual fashion with the antiseptic agent of the practitioner's choice.

Procedural Technique

The dermabrader unit should be held like a pencil or with four fingers wrapped around the body of the device with the practitioner's thumb directed towards the abrading end. Using the nondominant hand, stretch the skin in order to create a uniform surface. If the staff is available, use of an assistant should be considered to help keep the skin taut, especially when abrading larger areas.

The most important technical factors for consideration during the procedure are the amount of pressure placed on the abrader and the rotation speed of the diamond fraise or wire brush. In general, a rotation speed in the range of 12,000–15,000 rpm is recommended. During the procedure, pull the dermabrader in clean strokes perpendicular to the direction of rotation of the abrader. The rotating piece should be kept parallel to the surface of the skin and it is vitally important to always keep the abrader moving at all times when in contact with the tissue.

In order to maximize visibility, it is important to minimize anything that can obscure the field in which you are working (i.e., blood or tissue debris). Begin the procedure in dependent regions and work against gravity. Try to minimize the use of gauze between passes as it can be caught in the abrader which will not only halt the procedure, but potentially ruin the device.

If performing dermabrasion for the purpose of scar revision, the first pass with the abrader should be performed at 45° to the long axis of the scar. Otherwise choose a direction that seems natural. Each subsequent pass should be performed perpendicular to the direction of the previous pass. Exercise caution over bony prominences (i.e., the mandible and the malar eminence) as it can be easy to apply excess pressure and abrade too deeply, causing hypertrophic scar formation. Use extreme caution in the periorbital and perioral regions, as eyelids and vermilion may get caught in the abrader. In addition, important structures lie deep with thin overlying tissue in these areas, especially around the eye.

Halt the procedure once there is diffuse pinpoint bleeding present throughout the area of interest as this indicates the epidermis has been removed, or if using gentian violet staining, once no stain remains. At the periphery of the designated area, feather with light pressure to improve the transition between the abraded and non-abraded zones as well as minimize pigment contrast.

Finally, hemostasis may be achieved through pressure application over the area with saline- or epinephrine-soaked gauze by the practitioner, the assistant, or the patient. Once there is adequate hemostasis, the area should be treated with petroleum ointment and covered with sterile or petrolatum-impregnated gauze.

Post-procedure Care

For successful dermabrasion, wound care is of utmost importance. Appropriate wound healing occurs most frequently in a moist environment, which can be achieved through either an open or closed regimen. When following an open regimen, instruct the patient to cleanse the abraded area with saline-soaked gauze four to five times per day and apply petroleum ointment. A closed regimen involves covering the area with petrolatum-impregnated gauze and cleaning and replacing the gauze daily for three to five days, after which time the patient may transition to an open regimen. It is very important that the patient keeps the wound clean especially over the next 10–14 days during which healing and reepithelialization occurs.

The patient is allowed to shower whenever they feel comfortable. Instruct them to not scrub the abraded areas, although they may use fingertips to clean the area, and allow water to run over the abraded areas.

Frequently, when performing dermabrasion on the face, patients may feel inclined to use make-up to cover the abraded areas, especially if there is significant post-procedure erythema. Make clear to the patient that they are not to use any sort of makeup on the area until it has fully healed to the satisfaction of the practitioner, typically beyond 2 weeks.

It is very important for the patient to avoid sun exposure, this includes wearing a hat and applying sun screen whenever the patient is outside for the next 6–12 months.

Complications

The most dreaded complications of dermabrasion, especially when not being performed for the purposes of scar revision, are hypertrophic scarring and keloid formation. Both of these complications are caused by excess dermabrasion with entry into the deep dermis. This is easily avoidable through the use of pre-procedure staining with gentian violet or halting the procedure once pinpoint bleeding is seen.

A relatively common condition associated with dermabrasion is the formation of milia, which usually last no longer than 2–3 weeks. Although self-limited, they can be bothersome to the patient and may be removed through in the office with a # 11 blade or needle. It is important to remove the core of the milia to prevent recurrence [3].

Permanent hypopigmentation may occur after dermabrasion and is due to destruction of melanocytes that reside within the dermis. Like scarring, this is caused by excessively deep dermabrasion. Hypopigmentation is most common in darker skinned individuals and in the majority of cases will resolve after 6–10 weeks. However, if permanent hypopigmentation occurs it may be aided by laser-assisted chemabrasion, but the best practice is to avoid it in the first place.

Post-procedure erythema is very common and cannot strictly be termed a complication, as it is simply a side effect. Most cases resolve early on but can last up to 8–12 weeks. If erythema lasts longer than this time period, or is excessively bothersome to the patient, topical or systemic steroids can be employed depending on the size of the erythematous area.

Post-procedure infections, whether bacterial, fungal or herpetic, though rare, can occur. Pre- and postoperative coverage with antibiotics is not evidence-based but does appear to be the standard of most clinicians. As discussed previously, with any resurfacing procedure a viral coverage is indicated pre-procedure and continued until reepithelialization occurs. If one suspects an infection, a culture and sensitivity and/or smear should be performed and treated with the appropriate medication. Having the patient clean their hands before wound care is important as well as keeping the healing wound clean throughout the healing process.

Case Examples

The first patient is a 70-year-old male with rhinophyma who complained of the appearance of his nose (Fig. 19.1). He underwent an in-office procedure utilizing cold gross excision for the larger masses and dermabrasion for further excision, as

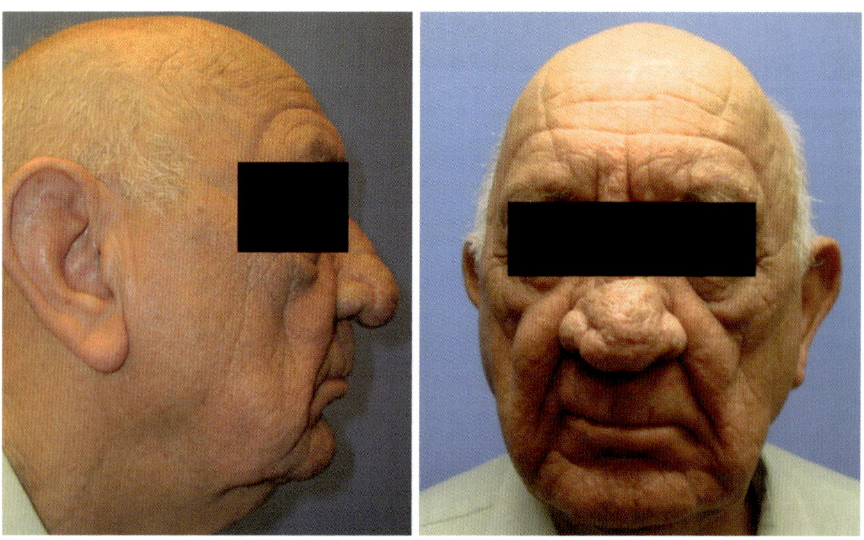

Fig. 19.1 Patient 1 at time of presentation

well as final contouring and blending. He was given intravenous propofol and midazolam for sedation for the duration of the procedure. In addition, 1% lidocaine with 1:100,000 epinephrine was used for local anesthesia and tumescence. Post-procedure sulfamethoxazole-trimethroprim was prescribed for antibiotic prophylaxis and he was given instructions to apply Aquaphor and mupirocin to his nose while it healed. Reepithelialization was 90% complete at his two-week follow-up visit, and he was instructed to begin using sunscreen whenever going outside. At two months, he complained of persistent erythema of the dermabraded area, especially at the nasal tip, and was prescribed 5% topical triamcinolone for 1 month (Fig. 19.2). This resolved the erythema, and he was extremely satisfied with his final result (Fig. 19.3).

The second patient is a 66-year-old male with rhinophyma who complained of not only the negative aesthetic and social consequences of the condition, but also noted nasal obstruction caused by the protuberant mass (Fig. 19.4). He was also treated with in-office cold excision and dermabrasion under intravenous sedation. At the end of the procedure, epinephrine-soaked gauze was used to attain hemostasis and the dermabraded area was covered with topical bacitracin ointment and a petrolatum-impregnated dressing. After the procedure he was prescribed doxycycline (which he had been taking at the behest of his dermatologist) for antibiotic prophylaxis and was instructed to keep the area moist with Aquaphor. After having sufficiently healed from his procedure (Fig. 19.5), he returned to his dermatologist and was prescribed metronidazole and tretinoin creams which he began at 6 months post-procedure. He expressed extreme satisfaction with his breathing function after the procedure and has been able to return to an active social life as he is no longer concerned with the cosmetic appearance of his nose (Fig. 19.6).

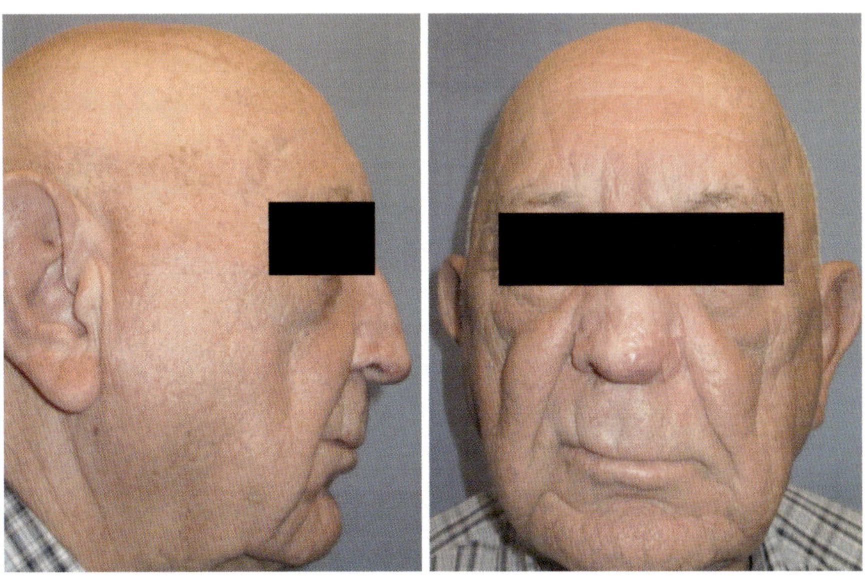

Fig. 19.2 Patient 1 at 6 months follow-up

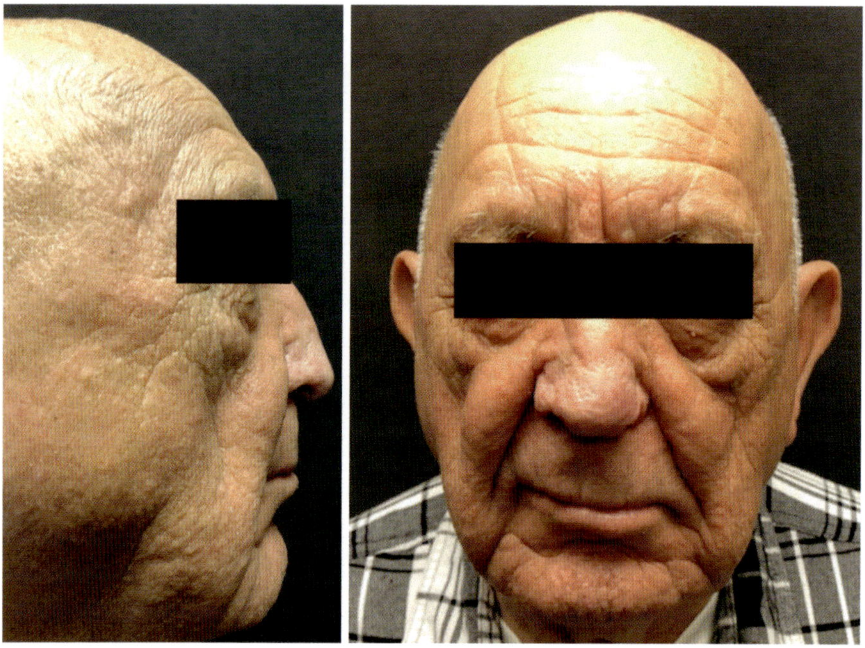

Fig. 19.3 Patient 1 at 3 years follow-up

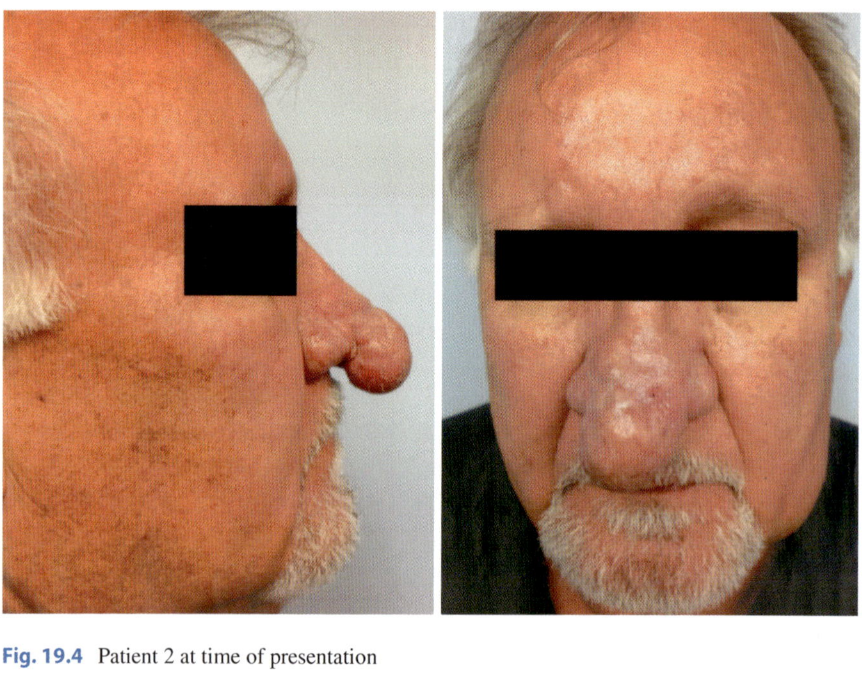

Fig. 19.4 Patient 2 at time of presentation

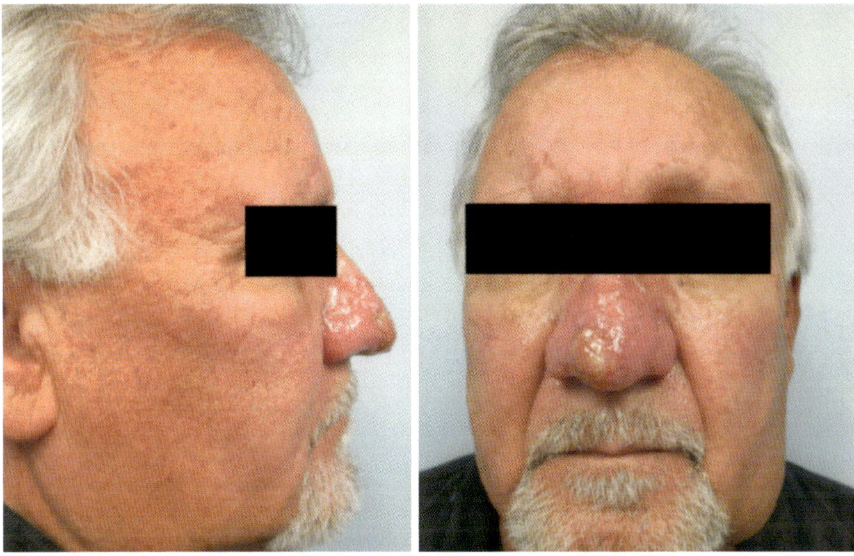

Fig. 19.5 Patient 2 at 2 months follow-up

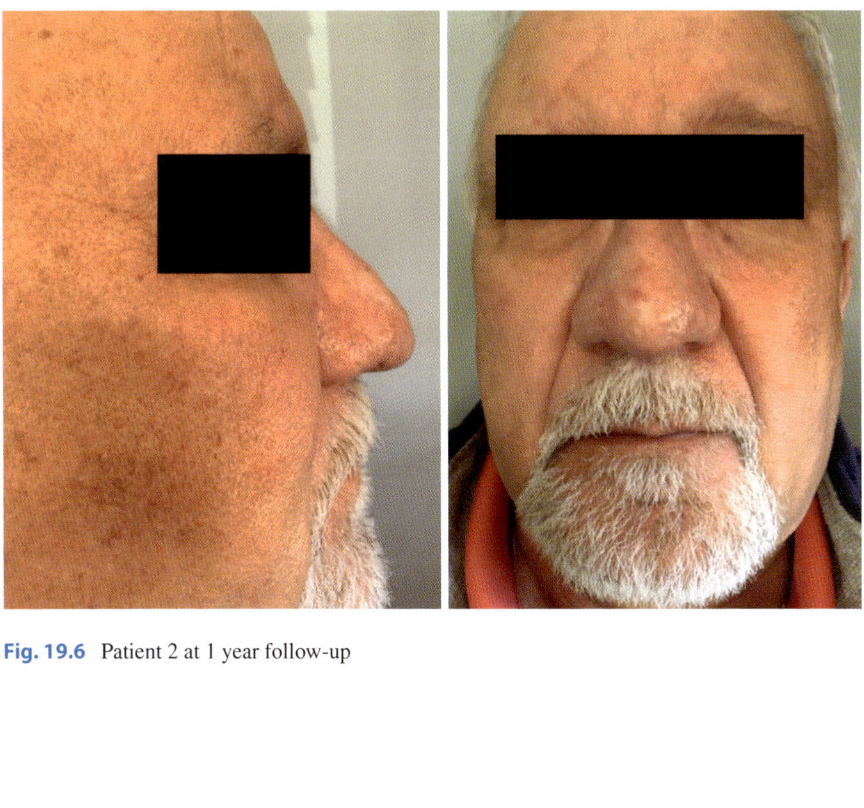

Fig. 19.6 Patient 2 at 1 year follow-up

Conclusions

Dermabrasion is a rewarding procedure that can be easily performed in the office setting with careful preparation and staffing. This technique can be used to treat a wide variety of patients and conditions with the knowledge of appropriate indications and conscientious patient selection. It is vitally important to emphasize post-procedure wound care to patients for maximum benefit from the procedure. When performed correctly dermabrasion can produce excellent results with high levels of patient satisfaction.

References

1. Surowitz JB, Shockley WW. Enhancement of facial scars with dermabrasion. Facial Plast Surg Clin North Am. 2011;19(3):517–25.
2. Zisser M, Kaplan B, Moy RL. Surgical pearl: manual dermabrasion. J Am Acad Dermatol. 1995;33(1):105–6.
3. Farrior RT. Dermabrasion in facial surgery. Laryngoscope. 1985;95(5):534–45.
4. Ferneini EM, Banki M, Paletta F, Ferneini CM. Surgical management of rhinophyma: a case report and review of literature. Conn Med. 2014;78(3):159–60.
5. Lawrence N, Mandy S, Yarborough J, Alt T. History of dermabrasion. Dermatol Surg. 2000;26(2):95–101.
6. Katz BE, Oca AG. A controlled study of the effectiveness of spot dermabrasion ('scarabrasion') on the appearance of surgical scars. J Am Acad Dermatol. 1991;24(3):462–6.

Neuromodulators

20

Matthew J. Goldschmidt and Justin Clemow

Introduction

One of the greatest cosmetic concerns among patients is the aging face and facial rhytids. The aging process is affected in several ways by both intrinsic and extrinsic variables. Intrinsic factors include genetics, loss of soft tissue volume, skeletal changes affecting the foundation of the face, and muscle activity/overactivity of the muscles of facial expression. Extrinsic factors include photodamage (sun tanning and tanning salons), gravity, alcohol consumption, and smoking. Many of the variables can be treated, but typically require multiple modalities and often require staging for optimal results. Treating wrinkled skin requires not only resurfacing the skin (i.e., chemical peels, lasers, Intense Pulse Light, Broad Band Light, dermabrasion), but also addressing the underlying tissues including the muscles of facial expression.

Facial rhytids are one of the most common complaints that are treated with regard to aging. The activity of the muscles of facial expression may contribute to deep furrowing of the skin both in dynamic appearances as well as static. Consequently, the treatment of facial rhytids with Botulinum toxin type A (BTX-A) is the most frequent minimally invasive procedure performed each year in the United States. An estimated 7.4 million BTX-A procedures were performed in 2018. This procedure continues to grow in popularity and has risen over 800% since the year 2000 [1]. This is over 4 times more popular than all of the cosmetic surgeries performed in a year combined!

M. J. Goldschmidt (✉)
The Cosmetic Surgery Center, Independence, OH, USA
e-mail: mattgoldschmidt@mac.com

J. Clemow
Case Western Reserve School of Dental Medicine, Metrohealth Medical Center, Cleveland, OH, USA
e-mail: jclemow@metrohealth.org

E. M. Ferneini, M. T. Goupil (eds.), *Office-Based Maxillofacial Surgical Procedures*, https://doi.org/10.1007/978-3-030-22371-7_20

Botulinum toxin was initially approved in the United States by the FDA in 1989 for the treatment of ophthalmological conditions including strabismus and blepharospasm [2–4]. Subsequent to these indications, it was later discovered that concomitantly, patients had improvement of facial rhytids in the glabellar region [5, 6]. In 2002, BTX-A was approved for the temporary improvement in the appearance of moderate to severe glabellar lines in adults. As of writing this chapter, the specific indications for the cosmetic use per the FDA and manufacturers include the treatment of rhytids in the glabellar, forehead, and lateral canthal regions [7]. Dysport (AbobotulinumtoxinA) and Xeomin (incobotulinumtoxinA) are approved for the treatment of moderate to severe glabellar lines [8, 9]. Botox® owns 65% of the market share (versus Dysport and Xeomin) and this represents 3.17 billion dollars in annual revenue for Allergan [10].

Pharmacology of Botulinum Toxin

There are seven different exotoxins produced by the bacteria, *Clostridium botulinum*. The most commonly used toxins are types A and B (the others are labeled C through H). Type A is in fact the most potent of the various toxins and is the most common cosmetic botulinum toxin used today. Type A toxin is composed of a heavy chain (100 kDa) and a light chain (50 kDA). The mechanism of action has been elucidated by Huang et al. [11]. The heavy chain binds to the membrane of the neuron. Upon binding to the membrane, the toxin is moved intracellularly via endocytosis. The light chain then degrades a protein (SNAP-25) that prevents acetylcholine, stored intravesicularly, from binding to the nerve cell's membrane, and thus being released into the synaptic cleft or gap. The affected nerve is rendered dysfunctional and a flaccid paralysis of the muscle results. Type B Botulinum Toxin works in a similar fashion but affects a different cellular protein, similar to SNAP-25. Most patients will notice the clinical effects of BTX-A a few days after treatment, but the full clinical affect may take up to 10–14 days.

The nerve cell begins to recover several weeks after treatment. The exact mechanism of recovery has still not been elucidated [12]. In the interim, the presynaptic membrane sends out new dendritic processes that establish a new synaptic terminal. The new processes are able to release acetylcholine and affect the motor end plate until the original neurons regain their actual function. Accordingly, the clinical affect ends when the original neurons have regained their function. For most patients, the resulting affect will last roughly 3 months. Some patients who undergo years of BTX-A treatment may derive longer affects but this is certainly not consistent nor the anticipated result of repeated therapy [11]. BTX-B lasts less than BTX-A and most patients will have a duration of action around 6–8 weeks.

BTX-A and BTX-B Production

There are three main corporations that produce BTX-A in the United States: Merz (Xeomin), Galderma/Medicis/Tercica (Dysport), and Allergan Botox. Xeomin is supplied in either 50 or 100 unit vials. Dysport (abobotulinum toxin) is supplied in either 300 or 500 unit vials. In addition, 125 mcg of albumin and 2.5 mg of lactose are compounded with the botulinum toxin and may cause sensitivity in patient allergic to milk protein. Botox is supplied in either 50 or 100 unit vials. There are 0.25 mg of human albumin and 0.45 mg of sodium chloride in each 50 unit vial (there is 0.5 mg and 0.9 mg, respectively, in a 100 unit vial). All three of these products are derived from the fermentation of Hall strain *Clostridium botulinum* serotype A. The preparation and assay method for each of these products is unique. Thus, the potency of each product is difficult to compare to identify relative strengths of each toxin. Xeomin is the only preparation that does not include or compound any additional proteins when it is supplied. The significance of the lack of the accessory proteins (or presence) is not known.

Myobloc (rimabotulinumtoxin) is manufactured by Solstice Neurosciences, Inc. and is supplied in 3.5-mL glass vials. Each single-use vial of formulated Myobloc contains 5000 Units of botulinum toxin type B per milliliter in 0.05% human serum albumin, 0.01 M sodium succinate, and 0.1 M sodium chloride at approximately pH 5.6. The neurotoxin is produced by fermentation of *Clostridium botulinum* type B (Bean strain) [13].

There are several other formulations that are currently in FDA trials that promise increased longevity of the medications. These formulations have not been made available to the public nor have the details regarding their clinical profile or pharmacodynamics, etc. been revealed.

Dilution Technique

Allergan specifies that Botox should be reconstituted with 2.5 mL of preservative-free saline. This yields 4 units of BTX-A per 0.1cc. Dysport and Xeomin do not recommend a specific dilution but does recommend reconstituting the product with preservative-free saline as well. All manufacturers recommend single patient usage, administration within 24 h, and storage between 2 and 8 °C. Off label reconstitution may include addition of local anesthetic (most commonly lidocaine), epinephrine to reduce bruising, and sodium bicarbonate to reduce the discomfort of the injection. One study suggested increase longevity when lidocaine with epinephrine was used in part to reconstitute BTX-A [14].

Indications/Contraindications/Adverse Events

Botox is indicated for the temporary improvement of moderate to severe glabellar lines from the procerus and corrugator muscles, forehead lines from the frontalis muscle, and lateral canthal lines ("crow's feet") associated with the orbicularis oculi muscle. 7 Dysport and Xeomin have indications for the treatment of glabellar lines only [8, 9].

Non-cosmetic indications of Botox include cervical dystonia in adults to decrease the severity of abnormal head position and neck pain. It is also indicated in patients with strabismus, blepharospasm, headache, and Bell's Palsy. Botox is also used in the treatment of axillary hyperhidrosis. Dysport is indicated for the treatment of lower limb spasticity and cervical dystonia. Xeomin has additional indications for upper limb spasticity and blepharospasm in patients previously treated with Botox. Myobloc has indications for the treatment of cervical dystonia as well [7–9, 11]. There are other known uses of these products including hypersecretory syndromes, back pain, and writer's cramp.

The use of BTX-A for cosmetic purposes is not limited to the strict adherence to the indications listed above. Many practitioners regularly treat all the muscles of facial expression and are proficient in obtaining consistent results for facial rejuvenation. This is considered an "off-label" use of this drug.

Adverse Effects of BTX-A Treatment

The most common adverse effects reported by the manufacturers include the following: headache (9%), nasopharyngitis (4%), eyelid ptosis (3%), brow ptosis (2%), facial pain (1%), eyelid edema (1%), muscular weakness—including spread to adjacent sites (1%), injection site pain (less than 1%), hematoma (less than 1%), infection (less than 1%), nausea (less than 1%), syncope (less than 1%), sinusitis (less than 1%), rhinitis (less than 1%), and upper respiratory infection (less than 1%) [7–9, 11].

A firm understanding of the facial anatomy and proper injection technique will aid in avoiding some of these problematic consequences, especially affecting adjacent muscles. The use of devices that help visualize the venous anatomy may also help reduce intravenous injection and trauma to those same vessels. This helps reduce the risk of hematoma and subsequent ecchymosis. Also, having patients avoid anti-inflammatory medications and anticoagulants also reduce the risk of these phenomena. Arnica Montana and Bromelain can also be used in the peri-procedure period to further reduce the risk as well [15, 16].

Injection Technique

Dosing

The various formulations of BTX-A by the manufacturers preclude the ability to standardize dosing between the proprietary drugs. Each BTX-A formulation must be considered individually when used to achieve optimal outcomes. Trying to convert units of BTX-A between the corporations should be avoided (e.g., 3 units of product X equals 1 unit of product Y). In addition, there are several variables that need to be considered when treating patients. First, men may have greater muscle mass and consequently, may require higher doses to achieve a similar effect versus female patients. Second, the facial musculature may have significant variability between patients and each patient should be evaluated for proper dosage. Third, the degree of paralysis requested by patients may be variable. Some patients prefer absolute immobilization of various muscle groups (especially the forehead), while others would like to "soften the wrinkles" and may benefit from lower doses to preserve various facial expressions.

Anatomic Sites and General Dosage Ranges

The glabellar region is the only site approved by the FDA for all three manufacturers of BTX-A. The glabellar muscle groups (corrugators, procerus, depressor supercilii, and orbicularis oculi) create the vertical and horizontal furrows in this region. Allergan recommends the use of 20 units with 5 injection points (4 units per site) injected as follows: 2 injections into each corrugator muscle (paired muscle group) and 1 injection into the procerus. Dysport should be injected in a similar fashion using 10 units per site for a total of 50 units. Xeomin is injected in a similar manner as Botox [7–9, 11].

In all cases, it is recommended to inject at least 1 cm away for the supraorbital rim and to inject perpendicularly to the muscles treated.

The frontalis muscle is the primary brow elevator and is solely responsible for the horizontal furrows across the forehead. The recommended dose to reduce the activity of this muscle is 20 units. In a similar fashion to the treatment of the glabellar region, the frontalis should be injected in 5 sites (4 units per injection site). When injecting above the eyebrow, it is important to stay at least 2 cm cephalad to the eyebrow to reduce the risk of brow ptosis. In the author's (MG) personal experience, using lower doses (1 unit per injection site) and more sites (8–10 sites) tends to produce a more uniform effect and also reduces the risk of brow ptosis.

The crow's feet region or lateral canthal rhytids, are the result of contraction of the orbicularis oculi muscles. Squinting or smiling cause the orbicularis oculi to constrict in a sphincter-like fashion. This results in horizontal rhytids that extend in a radial fashion laterally from the lateral canthal region. Allergan recommends 3 injection sites (4 units per injection, 12 units total per side) staying at least 1 cm away from the orbital rim to reduce the risk of intra-orbital migration affecting the extra-ocular muscles (lateral rectus and inferior oblique muscles). Diplopia may result from intra-orbital migration if these muscles were affected. In addition, injecting too much along the inferomedial aspect of the orbicularis may result in cheek ptosis as this aids in cheek elevation. Patients with laxity of the lower eyelid may experience ectropion or lower lid retraction. Patients with some orbital fat prolapse may exhibit worsening of their condition if the orbicularis oculi is weakened and loses some of its tone.

Chemical Brow Lift or Brow Elevation

Conceptually, brow elevation is achievable when segments of the orbicularis oculi and glabellar region are chemically denervated. Weakening the central portion of the frontalis may also result in increased activity in the frontalis directly cephalad to the brows. This can also be an untoward effect some patients may not like especially if it is unilateral ("Mr. Spock" appearance). By injecting the glabellar region and affecting the medial brow depressors (procerus, corrugators, medial orbicularis oculi) along with the central aspect of the frontalis will allow the medial brow to elevate. Patients who depress their brows (laterally) when they smile may also be injected in the lateral canthal region. Injections towards the tail of the brow in this situation will allow the lateral portion of the brow to elevate. In all of these scenarios, injecting the frontalis over the brow region should be avoided so as not to negate the effects of reducing the brow depressors. Additionally, injection in the eyebrow itself should be done cautiously to help relax the orbicularis oculi in this region. Injecting deep in this region can lead to brow and eyelid ptosis and only 0.5 to 1 unit should be injected in a couple of sites along the brow.

Bunny Lines

The nasalis muscle runs transversely across the nasal dorsum. When activated it leads to diagonal furrows along the lateral aspect of the dorsum. Superiorly to this muscle is the procerus and when this muscle is activated it leads to more horizontal furrows. These are two distinct anatomic sites and as such need to be treated independently. When the nasalis muscle is injected, it should be done superficially and along the maxillary process of the nasal bones. Injections deep and along the maxilla could result in inadvertent injection of the angular artery or hematoma. This also helps prevent BTX-A affecting the levator labii oris and the levator labii alaeque which could result in the upper lip drooping or an asymmetric smile [5].

Mentalis

Patients with strong or hypertrophied mentalis muscles may exhibit unattractive dimpling of the chin, especially in combination with loss of subcutaneous tissue (*peau d' orange)*. Sometimes the activity can also lead to noticeable horizontal furrow across the same region. 5–10 units of Botox may be injected (20–30 units of Dysport) into the superficial aspect of the mentalis. Caution should be taken to not over-inject, inject too superiorly, or inject deeply as this could possibly affect the lower lip and oral competency. Some patients may present with hypertrophied mentalis muscles, retrognathia, and oral incompetence and should not be treated with BTX-A in the chin region. Injecting towards the midline will also reduce the possibility of injecting the depressor labii and/orbicularis oris as this can lead to drooling, drooping of the lower lip, and/or an asymmetric smile.

Platysmal Bands

Platysmal bands can be seen in the aging neck and may be seen as a residual effect after rhytidectomy. They can be easily treated with BTX-A. The patient can easily exhibit the bands by clenching their teeth and showing the lower anterior teeth. Patients with skin laxity are better candidates for neck lift with platysmaplasty. Patients with significant laxity of skin will have modest results and likely be displeased. The bands are injected just below the inferior border of the mandible and injected every centimeter along the band. Typically, 20 units of Botox may be used to treat this anatomic region. The best way to inject the band is to grasp the band with the non-injecting thumb and index finger to isolate the muscle band. Over-injection in the neck and diffusion to the strap muscles can lead to significant problems including postural issues/neck weakness, dysphagia, and dysphonia.

Depressor Anguli Oris

One of the most common complaints patients present with is the downward corner of the mouth or marionette line. The depressor anguli oris (DAO) is the primary muscle responsible for this appearance along with frowning. The DAO can be injected near its origin on the mandible. 2–5 units can be injected either at 1 or 2 sites. Cephalad injections that encroach on the lower lip and orbicularis oris may result in drooling or asymmetric smile. Patients with injuries to the marginal mandibular nerve may benefit from injecting this muscle on the contralateral side to help improve symmetry. Patients with oral incompetency may also see benefit with injection of the DAO on the affected side to elevate the lower lip and commissural region. The addition of a filler (Hyaluronic acid) to this region may also help support the lower lip and further improve the aesthetics of this area.

Upper Lip/Peri-Oral Rhytids

The actions of the orbicularis oris may result in dynamic furrows or rhytids in the peri-oral region. The orbicularis oris may be injected in a superficial fashion with 2–4 units of BTX-A in multiple sites (0.5 units or 1 unit per site). Most patients will also benefit from concomitant injection of filler (Hyaluronic acid) to restore volume and improve the rhytids in these areas. Several injection sites should be used either at the vermillion border or just above. Injecting the upper lip towards the base of the nose may result in lengthening of the upper lip. This may be intentional for patients with vertical maxillary excess ("gummy smile"). Asymmetric lip position may also result if disproportionate amounts of BTX-A is used in the upper lip. Over-injection can affect speech, facial expressions, speech, eating, drinking, and playing wind instruments.

Posttreatment Instructions

After treatment, patients are instructed to avoid heavy exertion/lifting, apply cold compresses for reduction of bruising/swelling/discomfort, and avoid rubbing or massaging the treated areas. In addition, some providers instruct their patients to perform exercises to help the BTX-A "work into the muscles." Some providers also tell their patients to avoid airline travel and not to bend for up to 24 h after treatment. None of these instructions have been shown to alter the outcomes or longevity of the desired effects of BTX-A. It is generally believed that after 90 min, the toxin has bound to its receptor sites and will not be significantly altered at this time. The author instructs patients they should avoid exercise and laborious activity for the first 2 h after treatment and use Tylenol as some may experience a headache post treatment.

Longevity of Effect

The duration of effect has several variables that must be considered in the discussion of longevity of effect. Allergan reports that the duration of effect for 20 units of Botox on glabellar lines is approximately 3–4 months. Galderma states a similar duration (up to 4 months) for 50 units of Dysport in the glabellar region. The package insert for Xeomin states 20 units should be administered no more frequently than every 3 months [7–9]. Generally speaking, this seems to be the standard duration of action for most anatomic regions. With that said, this effect may vary based on dosage, muscle density, degree of facial animation, anatomic site, age, and anatomic variations. Many patients will return prior to the 3-month interval to reduce the possibility of the effect completely "wearing off." The maximum dose per Allergan is 400 units within 3 months [7].

Patient Evaluation

A patient interview must include an accurate medical history as well as a meticulous physical exam. The medical history will illicit any information regarding muscle-related disorders (e.g., myasthenia gravis, motor neuron diseases, amyotrophic lateral sclerosis (ALS), Eaton Lambert syndrome) as these conditions may be exacerbated by the administration of BTX-A. BTX-A should also be avoided in patients with a history of Guillain Barre syndrome, hypersensitivity to BTX-A, and cow's milk allergy (specific to Dysport). If there is an active infection at any potential injection site, then the area should be allowed to heal prior to injection. A thorough understanding and familiarity of muscles of facial expression are essential to obtaining optimal results. Not only are the anatomic variations important to recognize, but also the functional anatomy as it may differ substantially from patient to patient. Each patient must be examined carefully to determine which muscle group(s) may contribute to any given furrow or wrinkle. As this is critical in the development of a treatment plan that will effectively reduce the activity of unaesthetic muscle effects.

Crow's Feet/Peri-Orbital Rhytids

The orbicularis oculi muscle encircles the orbit and acts in a sphincter-like fashion to close the eye and protect the globe. The lateral and inferior aspects of this muscle, when activated may create significant rhytids and furrows that can be easily treated with BTX-A. Careful examination of this region is necessary to identify asymmetries, laxity of the lower eyelid, and the presence of herniated fat in the lower eyelids. Some patients will not tolerate higher dosages of BTX-A and may result in untoward effects. Patients with laxity of the lower eyelid when injected, may result in ectropion and possibly exacerbation of any cheek/malar ptosis. The orbicularis oculi may also aid in elevation of malar elevation/projection. Over-injection can thus lead to loss of projection or ptosis. Injection into the lower eyelid region can also lead to increased scleral show or further herniation of the lower eyelid fat pads if the orbicularis tone is diminished.

Allergan has provided data in its studies that show the efficacy of using 12 units per side (24 units total) to the peri-orbital region. This treatment showed significant improvement in the lateral canthal lines of the test subjects versus placebo [7]. It is important to inject the most active segments of the orbicularis oculi and to have multiple sites of injection. This will help reduce any irregularities caused by active portions of the muscle that have not been treated.

Glabella

The glabellar region is one of the most common sites patient's request for injection and treatment. Careful examination of this area needs to be performed prior to injection. The procerus and corrugator supercilli muscles along with the medial aspect of the orbicularis oculi muscles contribute to furrows in this region. The contribution each muscle bundle makes to these furrows may vary significantly between patients. When asked to make an angry face, act as though they are smelling something (i.e., "wrinkle their nose") or frown, these glabellar muscles will move the brows inferomedially. In some patients, however, the brow may move superomedially. Consequently, when BTX-A is injected into this region, the outcome may vary from patient to patient.

Allergan recommends injecting the glabella with 20 units of Botox which is also the same dosage recommended for Xeomin [7, 9]. 50 units of Dysport is recommended to treat this same region [8]. Males may require higher dosages and there may be some preliminary evidence that using higher doses may result in a greater duration of effect. Care should be taken to inject above the supraorbital rim. When injecting, the non-injecting hand should be used to hold the tissue in a stable position. The patient may be asked to elevate their brow and then make a facial expression (as discussed above) to help identify the active portions of the muscles that need to be treated. Most of the BTX-A will be used to treat the corrugator muscles and a small amount will be used to treat the procerus muscle (see Photos 20.1 and 20.2).

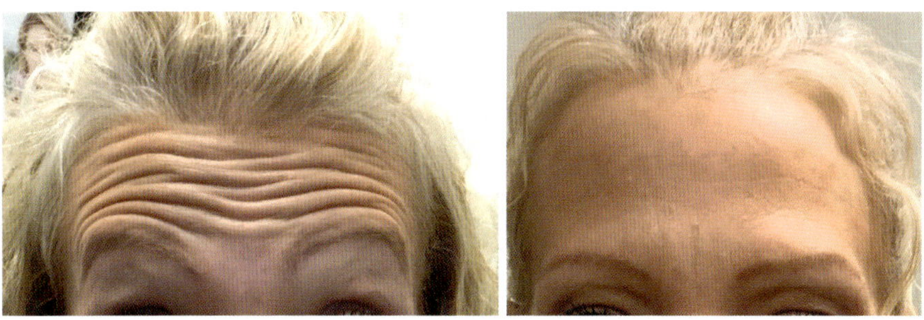

Photo 20.1 Forehead before and after treatment

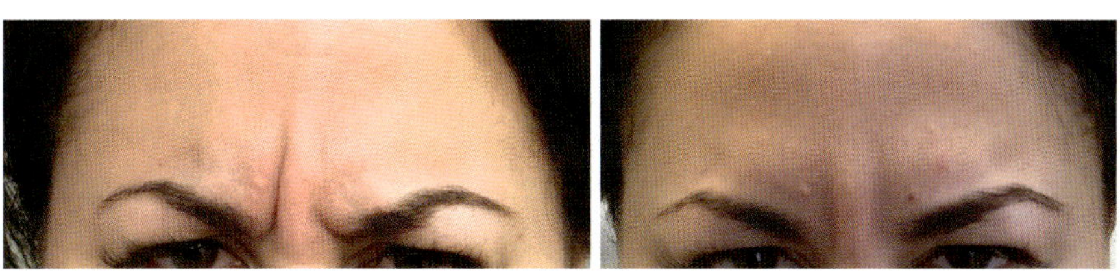

Photo 20.2 Glabella before and after treatment

Non-cosmetic Indications

Although the focus of this chapter is on cosmetic uses, BTX-A is FDA approved for a number of therapeutic indications, including bladder dysfunction, chronic migraine, spasticity, cervical dystonia, primary axillary hyperhidrosis, blepharospasm, and strabismus. It is also routinely used for treatment of patients with myofascial pain, although this use is considered "off-label." Although the pathophysiology of myofascial pain has not been fully elucidated, the role of muscle hyperactivity is thought to be central. It is thought that hyperactive skeletal muscle bands develop in response to trauma, strain, or overuse, and that these trigger points evoke a referred pain pattern [17]. Therefore, proposed treatment modalities aim to arrest, stabilize, or reverse this muscle overactivity. The ability of BTX-A to elicit a weakening or paralytic effect on the muscle may only account for part of the explanation for its analgesic effect. In addition to its effect on acetylcholine release, Botox also has an inhibitory effect on the release of substance P, which is a potent neurotransmitter in the activation of neurological inflammation [18].

The suggested injection pattern for chronic migraine headaches is described in the Botox Prescribing Information and includes a total of 155 Units into seven different muscle groups. In contrast, the injection technique for treatment of myofascial pain usually focuses on only the easily accessible muscles of mastication (masseter and temporalis), and because this indication is off-label, there is less clear guidance on a specific injection pattern. This author (JC) typically uses 100 units, with 35 units injected into the bilateral masseter, and 15 units injected into the bilateral temporalis. These muscles are much larger than the muscles of facial expression, and therefore larger quantities of neuromuscular blocker are needed to achieve a therapeutic effect. The injector should be aware that the target of masticatory musculature is expected to be deeper than the muscles of facial expression which are immediately subcutaneous. Especially for the masseter in a patient with more adipose tissue, there is occasionally the need for a longer needle than the standard ½" needle on a TB syringe.

Complications

A variety of complications have been reported, ranging from minor issues like bruising and asymmetry to major problems like anaphylaxis, dysphagia, and breathing difficulties. With the relatively smaller doses required for cosmetic indications, major complications are exceedingly rare and facial cosmetic use of Botox has a very well-established track record of safety [7, 19, 20]. Hypersensitivity to botulinum toxin has been reported, and usually manifests as soft tissue edema or urticaria. Bruising and bleeding at the injection site is not uncommon, and for this reason most practitioners suggest discontinuation of aspirin and other NSAIDs one week prior to injection [21].

Other preventative measures include icing immediately before injection (also has analgesic effect), injecting superficially, and avoiding vessels. Hematoma formation, caused by inadvertent vascular puncture, is less likely. Some authors advocate the use of vein illumination devices as helpful in identifying smaller vessels, especially in dark-skinned patients.

Most functional complications can be attributed to unintended spread of neurotoxin, or neuromuscular blockade of unintended muscles which can be due to improper injection technique or misidentification of facial muscular anatomy. Brow or eyelid ptosis are particularly undesirable complications both because of the ease of detection of even small asymmetries, and because of the potential for visual disturbance. When injecting the glabella, care should be taken to stay at least 1 cm above the superior orbital rim and inject perpendicular to the muscle. Diffusion of neurotoxin can cause weakness of the levator palpebrae superioris, causing upper eyelid ptosis. Further laterally, the "safe-zone" for injection of the forehead to avoid brow ptosis is generally considered to be at least 2–2.5 cm above the superior orbital rim. Similarly, injection of crow's feet is best performed no closer than 1–1.5 cm from the orbital rim to avoid diplopia caused by neurotoxin spread into the orbit, weakening the lateral rectus or inferior rectus.

Non-functional complications related to cosmetic asymmetry are easier to manage. These include peaked lateral brows ("Spock eyebrow"), uneven brow position, uneven smile, etc. It is recommended to wait 2 weeks after initial injection before doing a "touch-up" to allow for variations in timing of muscle response to neurotoxin [5].

Other complications may include:

- Oral incompetence
- Lower lid laxity/ectopion
- Speech impediment
- Dysphagia/neck weakness

Ptosis as a complication of neurotoxin injection too close to the upper lid, can be at least partially treated with apraclonidine (Iopidine; Alcon Labs Inc, Ft Worth, TX) 0.5% drops used 30 min before social situations. This α-adrenergic agonist stimulates Mueller's muscle, causing several hours of transient lid opening (see Photo 20.3)

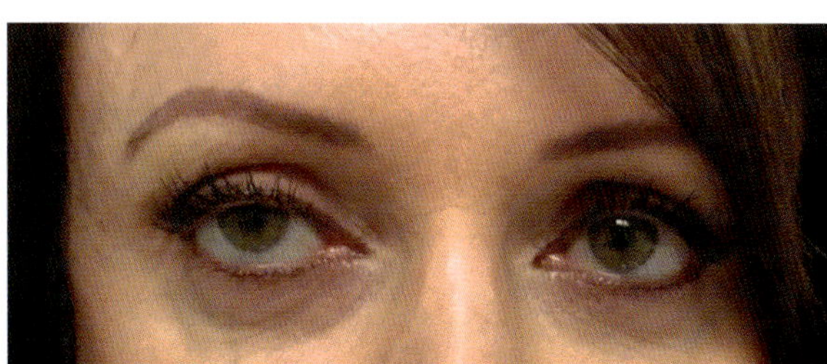

Photo 20.3 Right eyelid ptosis

Conclusion

In summary neuromuscular blockade injections as an adjunct for facial rejuvenation is a very viable and safe option. The treatment is easily administered in the outpatient setting and requires no additional equipment. One of the advantages of this technique is the temporary result.

References

1. Plastic Surgery Statistics Report https://www.plasticsurgery.org/documents/News/Statistics/2018/plastic-surgery-statistics-full-report-2018.pdf
2. Scott A, Rosenbaum A, Collins C. Pharmacologic weakening of extraocular muscles. Invest Ophthalmol Vis Sci. 1973;12(12):924–7.
3. Scott A. Botulinum toxin injection into extraocular muscles as an alternative to strabismus surgery. J Pediatr Ophthalmol Strabismus. 1980;17(10):21–5.
4. Scott A, Kennedy R, Stubbs H. Botulinum A toxin inection as a treatment for blepharospasm. Arch Ophyhlamol. 1985;103(3):347–50.
5. Carruthers J, Fagien S, Mattarasso SL, et al. Consensus recommendations on the use of botulinum toxin type A in facial aesthetics. Plast Reconstr Surg. 2004;114:1s–22s.
6. Carruthers J, Carruthers J. Treatment of glabellar frown lineswith Clostridium botulinum A exotoxin. Dermatol Surg. 1992;18:17–21.
7. Botox® (onabotulinumtoxin A) for injection. Prescribing Information. Irvine, CA: Allergan, Inc., 2017
8. Dysport™ (abotulinumtoxinA) for injection. Prescribing Information. Ipsen Pharmaceuticals and Galderma Laboratories, 2016
9. Xeomin™ (incobotulinumtoxinA) for injection. Prescribing Information, Franksville, WI: Merz Pharmaceuticals, LLC., 2010
10. David Crow, https://www.ft.com/content/49570b38-221f-11e8-9a70-08f715791301-,8 Mar 2018 (Financial Times Limited 2018)
11. Huang W, Foster J, Rogachefsky A. Pharmacology of botulinum toxin. J AmAcad Dermatol. 2000;43(2. Pt 1):249–59.
12. Kane MAC. Chapter 3 Botulinum toxin. In: Neligan PC, Warren RJ, editors. Vol 2 Aesthetic surgery of plastic surgery. Philadelphia, PA: Elsevier Health Scineces; 2012.
13. Prescribing Information. Solstice Neurosciences, San Francisco, CA May, 2010
14. Kim A, Jung J, Pak A, Cutis 2013;(Suppl):12–18
15. Seeley BM, et al. Effects of homeopathic arnica montana on bruising in face-lifts. Arch Facial Plast Surg. 2006;8:54–9.
16. Rowe DJ, Baker AC. Perioperative risks and benefits of herbal supplements in aesthetic surgery. Aesth Surg. 2009;29(2):150–7.
17. Smith HS, Audette J, Royal MA. Botulinum toxin in pain management of soft tissue syndromes. Clin J Pain. 2002;18:S147.
18. Guyer BM. Mechanism of botulinum toxin in the relief of pain. Curr Rev Pain. 1999;3:427.
19. Ney J, Joseph K. Neurologic uses of botulinum neurotoxin type A. Neuropshychiatr Did Treat. 2007;3(6):785–98.
20. Truong D, Duaane D, Jankovic J, et al. The efficacy and safety of botulinum type A toxin (Dysport) in cervical dystonia: results of the first US randomized, double blind, placebo controlled study. Mov Disord. 2005;20(7):783–91.
21. Qaqish C. Botulinum toxin use in the upper face. Atlas Oral Maxillofacial Surg Clin N AM. 2016;24:95–103.

Facial Fillers

21

Mina Boulos, Steven Halepas, and Elie M. Ferneini

Introduction

Minimally invasive procedures are becoming more popular as modality treatments for patients requesting cosmetic improvements. Facial fillers have become the main alternative to surgical facial rejuvenation. Facial fillers are being utilized in almost all regions of the face including the eyes, chin, cheeks, lips and nasolabial regions [1]. Most facial fillers are safe and predictable with very little risk of adverse events. Complications to facial fillers however can be detrimental, ranging from slight edema to infection to even blindness or stroke. It is therefore very critical that the practitioner is well versed in the procedural technique, the materials and the complex facial anatomy [2].

Materials

There are many different types of fillers that are better indicated for certain procedures.

M. Boulos
Thomas Jefferson University Hospital, Philadelphia, PA, USA
e-mail: mina.boulos@jefferson.edu

S. Halepas
Department of Oral and Maxillofacial Surgery, New York Presbyterian Hospital, Columbia University Medical Center, New York, NY, USA
e-mail: sh3808@cumc.columbia.edu

E. M. Ferneini (✉)
Beau Visage Med Spa, Greater Waterbury OMS, Cheshire, CT, USA

Division of Oral and Maxillofacial Surgery, University of Connecticut, Farmington, CT, USA

E. M. Ferneini, M. T. Goupil (eds.), *Office-Based Maxillofacial Surgical Procedures*, https://doi.org/10.1007/978-3-030-22371-7_21

Dermal Fillers

1. Absorbable dermal fillers (temporary)
   (a) Collagen
   (b) Hyaluronic acid
   (c) Calcium hydroxylapatite
   (d) Poly-L-lactic acid
2. Nonabsorbable dermal fillers (permanent)
   (a) Polymethylmethacrylate beads
   (b) Silicone

The dermal fillers are categorized based on duration of effect—temporary vs. permanent. The goal of any filler, beyond achieving esthetic results, is to be biocompatible as well as have limited potential for adverse effects. The temporary fillers are collagen (which is no longer available in the United States), Hyaluronic acid, Calcium hydroxylapatite, and Poly-L-lactic acid.

Hyaluronic acid (HA) is a naturally occurring molecule found in the extracellular matrix. It primarily holds its shape by binding and absorbing water molecules, therefore it's hydrophilic. HA functions mainly to hydrate, lubricate, and stabilize the connective tissue. The difference between naturally occurring HA and the dermal filler is that the latter contains more cross-linking structures, which makes the filler more resistant to degradation and giving HA a life of up to 18 months. The benefit to HA being a naturally occurring substance is that no allergy testing is needed. HA should be injected into the subcutaneous or deep dermal layers, which allows it to activate fibroblasts. The viscosity, also known as the G' value, of these fillers should be noted . The higher the viscosity, the longer the lasting effect of the filler. Adverse effects noted of HA fillers are increased incidence of bruising, pain, and swelling [3].

Types of HA

1. Restylane-L
2. Juvederm Ultra, Ultra Plus
3. Restylane Lyft
4. Juvederm Voluma
5. Volbella
6. Restylane Refyne & Defyne
7. Belotero
8. Revanesse

Calcium Hydroxylapatite (CaHA) is a naturally occurring mineral found in bone and teeth. This filler is composed of microspheres which are delivered in a suspension of glycerin and sodium methylcellulose. The suspension medium is absorbed in roughly 2–3 months, which supports the ingrowth of fibroblasts while allowing production new collagen. This dermal filler is biodegradable, nontoxic, nonmutagenic, nonantigenic, nonirritating, and ideal for deep creases and for areas where bone loss is the main etiology of facial volume loss. The benefits of one treatment can last 1–2 years. Adverse effects noted of CaHA fillers are pain, redness, swelling, bruising, and inflammation. It is very important to make sure that the product is not injected superficially because it will appear as nodules below the skin. If incorrectly injected, this can lead to even more pain, severe bruising, asymmetrical correction, firmness, textural changes, nodules as mentioned, and granulomas, which would further decrease the esthetic outcome and result in an unhappy patient [3].

Types of CaHA

1. Radiesse

   Poly-L-lactic acid is a biodegradable synthetic polymer, which, upon injection, stimulates collagen production. It does this through stimulation of fibroblasts which allows for the formation of a matrix of collagen and elastic fibers. This is the longest lasting of the temporary dermal fillers with a possible duration of 3 years. Results are noted at 4–6 weeks postoperatively as the edema subsides so intervals between injections should be no less than 4 weeks. This, like CaHA, can result in nodules if injected too superficially. It is important to massage the injected area aggressively while and immediately after to prevent from this happening. Adverse effects noted of PLLA fillers are bruising, edema, and inflammation.

Types of PLLA

1. Sculptra

   The permanent fillers are Polymethylmethacrylate (PMMA) and Silicone. These should be used in those patients that have completed multiple application of fillers or have had a trial run with a nonpermanent correction. The permanent nature of this treatment should be stressed to patients to assure understanding.

   Polymethylmethacrylate (PMMA) Beads is only offered in the Artefill preparation, which is a combination of bovine collagen and PMMA microspheres. The biodegradeable portion (collagen) is absorbed over the course of the first 3 months postoperatively leaving the beads to be encapsulated by fibrous tissue allowing for permanent correction [4]. If this method is chosen, it should be done so where the skin is thick enough so the material cannot be palpated. If the patient has proven allergies to bovine collagen or if they suffer from an autoimmune condition, this treatment should be avoided. Because of this potential complication, patients should undergo allergy testing prior to administration of this filler.

Types of PMMA

1. Bellafil

   Silicone has been around for many years and has been used for soft tissue augmentation. This is because it is inexpensive, does not promote bacterial growth, can be sterilized, and can be stored at room temperature. It has proven to be invaluable when treating facial rhytids (glabellar frown lines, nasolabial folds, labial commissures, etc.), lip augmentation, nasal irregularities post rhinoplasty, etc.

Anatomy

It is vital for the practitioner to understand the basic anatomic structures in order to avoid potentially irreversible consequences. Below is a brief overview of important anatomic landmarks to be familiar (Fig. 21.1).

The supratrochlear artery exits the superomedial orbit about 2 cm lateral to the midline. This vessel is often within 5 mm of the vertical plane just inferior to the transverse third of the forehead and medial to the medical canthal vertical line [5]. The artery becomes subcutaneous 15–25 mm above the supraorbital rim. The artery is just 1–2 mm deep to the muscle layer which makes it easily compromised in the injection of facial fillers. Glabellar frown lines demarcates the corrugator and the procerus muscles and the supratrochlear artery has been reported to be within 6 mm from this in most circumstances [6].

The superficial temporal artery is the terminal branch of the external carotid artery as it travels superiorly to the external acoustic meatus (Fig. 21.2). The superficial temporal artery normally divides into a parietal and a frontal branch. These arteries are of concern to the surgeon because of their superficial nature. In the temporal region, fillers should be injected either deeply or superficially. Deep injections should be in the periosteal plane.

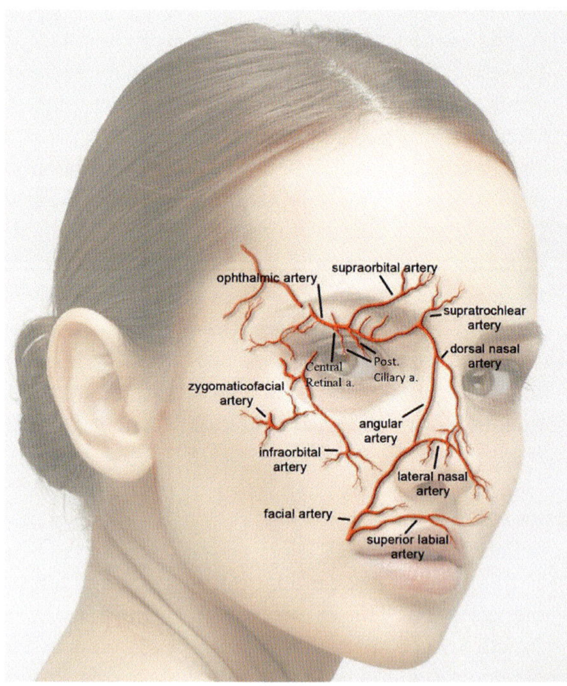

Fig. 21.1 Diagram of important regional vascularity

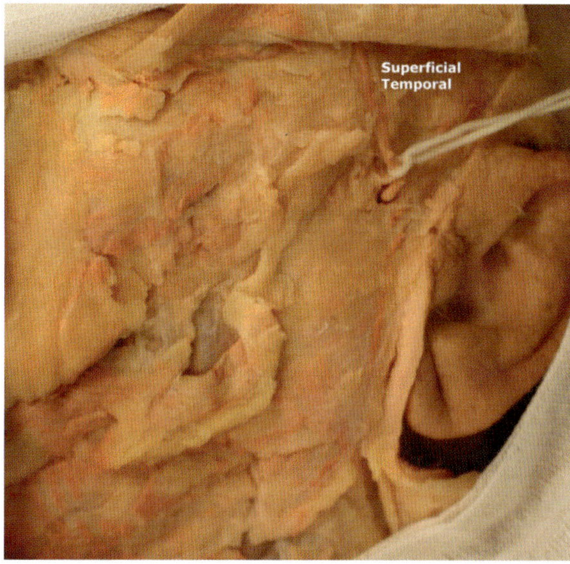

Fig. 21.2 Superficial temporal artery. Please note how superficial this artery is

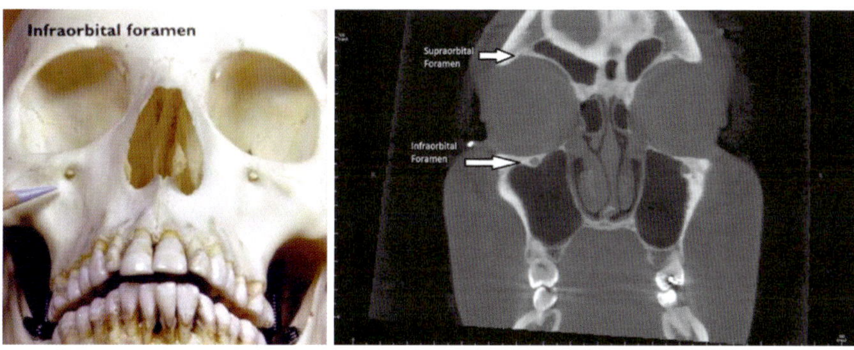

Fig. 21.3 Location of the infraorbital foramen

The infraorbital branch of the maxillary artery exits the infraorbital foramen and supplies the skin of the lower lid and middle face. The mean distance from the infraorbital rim to the infraorbital foramen has been reported to be 9.6 ± 1.7 mm [7] (Fig. 21.3). The surgeon must be mindful to avoid filler embolization in this areas as well as injury to the corresponding nerve. Midface injections should always be deep to avoid intravascular cannulation.

Lower lip injections need to be within the vermillion border no greater than 2 mm deep. The inferior labial artery is usually posterior at the mucosal-muscular interface and below the superior border of the lip. Intravascular injection in the location can lead to tissue/lip necrosis.

Anesthesia

Some patients will benefit from local anesthetics prior to the application of facial fillers while others will be able to tolerate the injections without anesthetics.

One option is the utilization of topical spray anesthetics such as dichlorotetrafluoroethane or ethyl chloride topical skin refrigerant spray. These topical sprays are marketed for application to the cheek and nasolabial folds only, not the oral mucosa Apply the spray for a duration of 30–60 s. After the appropriate time, the filler can be injected in a more comfortable way for the patient. It should be noted that the topical spray has only a superficial effect and that noxious stimuli will still elicit a response from the deeper dermal pain fibers. The patient should be informed that the spray will feel very cold [8].

In addition to the sprays, one can use the various topical local anesthetics such as lidocaine pastes. Another alternative would be using ice. Ice dampens the pain response and is extremely inexpensive, safe, and easy. The surgeon can have the patient hold the ice on the site of planned injection for 1–2 min. The advantage of this method is that the ice can then be used postoperatively, which will allow for a decrease in subsequent bruising and edema [8].

The final anesthetic option is one most commonly used for surgical procedures, which is a local anesthetic block. Injectable local anesthetics include Lidocaine, Carbocaine, Septocaine, Marcaine, etc. These anesthetics can come with or without epinephrine. The patient's medical history and allergies should be considered prior to choosing the appropriate local anesthetic. The downside to the use of these local anesthetics is the prolonged duration of action since these outpatient minimally invasive procedures are relatively short in procedural time. Transcutaneous injections are an option but should be avoided if possible as they can disrupt the surgical area and affect the surgeon's judgment on what the area needs as far as amount of filler. If direct injection is the preferred method, the provider should mark out the sites to be injected prior to the delivery of anesthesia. For example, infraorbital nerve blocks may be utilized for upper lip anesthesia, and mental nerve blocks can be utilized for lower lip anesthesia. Distraction techniques such as pressure adjacent to the injection site with a cotton tip applicator may further help reduce pain from the needle insertion [8].

Injection Techniques

Once the patient is probably anesthetized, the next step would be to proceed with the injection of the filler. The three main injection methods are:

1. Threading [3, 8]
   (a) Indication: Vermilion Border, Nasolabial Fold
   (b) Technique:
      - Place needle to the hub in the deepest portion of the wrinkle at the level of the dermis or subdermal tissue.
      - Deposit filler as the needle is removed.
        - NOTE: To confirm the needle is beyond the dermis, the provider should apply downward pressure. If the skin dimples, the needle must

be further advanced as the needle is still in the dermal layer. The needle must also not be visible through the skin. If there is minimal resistance upon injection, the needle is likely in the subcutaneous tissue.

2. Serial Droplet [3, 8]
   (a) Indication: Glabellar Creases, Periorbital Hollows, Philtral Columns, Fine Wrinkles
   (b) Technique:
      - Place needle in the deepest portion of the dermis.
      - Deposit a very small amount of filler. Multiple droplets must be placed throughout the stretch of the wrinkle/crease. These should be placed as closely as possible to allow for continuity. The areas should then be massaged to allow continuous and uniform correction.
         – NOTE: Multiple needles may be needed due to blunting.
3. Fanning [3, 8]
   (a) Indication: Folds, Deep Malar Injections
   (b) Technique:
      - Place the needle in the subdermis or subcutaneous tissue at a 30° angle.
      - Inject the filler slowly and steadily as the needle is passed back and forth. The needle should be retracted and redirected just prior to being withdrawn to achieve the appropriate coverage of the area to be corrected. If the area is a fold, the needle should be passed beneath the fold extending 2 mm bilaterally for a 4 mm wide band.
         – NOTE: Do NOT overcorrect as the product will take a few weeks before the final lasting result will be seen. The provider must give time for the inflammation to settle. Overcorrection will result in a less esthetic outcome.
4. Cross-hatching [1]
   (a) Indication: Oral commissure, Large areas of correction (i.e., peri-oral area)
   (b) Technique:
      - This technique is basically sequential applications of the threading technique. The sites of injection should be marked out prior to application, which will be in a cross-hatching pattern.

As with anything, it is crucial to understand the local anatomy of the area to be augmented. Things to identify include nerves and blood vessels. Below, the injection techniques are discussed based on the areas to be corrected (Fig. 21.4).

Tear Trough/Infraorbital Hollows

The tear trough and infraorbital hollows can be corrected using either PLLA or HA.

If the provider selects PLLA as the filler of choice, they should start the injection at the lateral canthus as this is the junction where the thin eyelid skin and thicker midface skin meet. The filler should be deposited in a linear and retrograde fashion along the inferior rim using a tunneling technique. The provider must only place the filler deep into the orbicularis muscle or just superficial to the periosteum while remembering to massage the site upwards towards the tarsal plate. This decreases

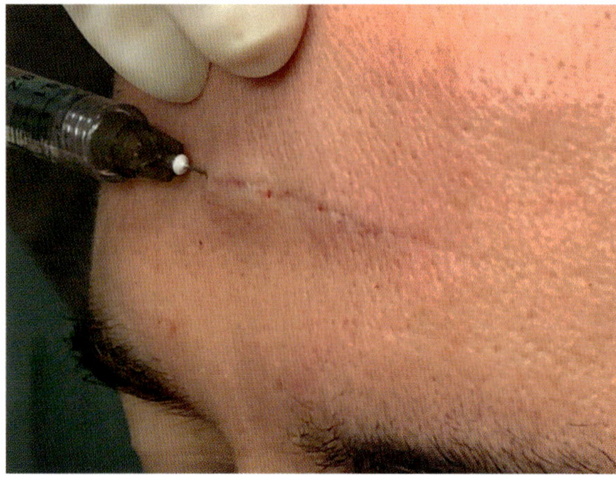

Fig. 21.4 Horizontal forehead lines corrected with Restylane-L

the likelihood of obtaining a nodular appearance of the augmented area. The same process can be performed on the medial aspect of the inferior rim. It is important to not overfill the sites. The recommended total of filler material is 3 mL on each side per session, which can be repeated two more times at subsequent sessions over a 4-month period [1].

Patient selection and operator experience must be seriously considered when using PLLA due to the potential adverse effects. The appropriate patient would be one who suffers from mild to moderate volume loss and minimal midface skeletal volume loss

An alternative to PLLA would be to use an HA product like Juvederm. The benefits are that the adverse effects are much more limited in comparison to PLLA. This technique is different however. It must be delivered using a threading technique and deposited anterograde as well as retrograde in the periosteal plane. The injections must being in the medial aspect of the area to be augmented and proceed laterally with constant massaging of the sites and application of ice to reduce postoperative swelling. Things to keep in mind while using HA include [1]:

1. Keep the needle moving while injecting to avoid cannulation of an artery
2. Avoid visible veins
3. Do not overcorrect

Supraorbital Hollow

HA is ideal for augmentation of the supraorbital region [9]. The injections should be anterograde with multiple small strokes along with rim. The provider should perform multiple injections that start laterally and move medially into the suborbicularis plane. Things to keep in mind while using HA include [1]:

1. Amount deposited at a time should be no more than 0.25 mL
2. Use a 30-gauge or 31-guage needle that is 0.5–1 inches in length or 30-guage microcannula
3. Inject slowly and avoid the supraorbital notch as to not damage the neurovascular bundle

Crow's Feet/Lateral Orbital Region

Botulinum neurotoxin type A is ideal for the crow's feet/lateral orbital region. Due to the potential toxicity, this is very technique sensitive. The injections should be superficial with the needle pointing away from the eye. The ideal angle of the needle to the skin should be kept between 20° and 30°, 1–2 cm from the orbital rim, and should go no deeper than the external aspect of the orbicularis oculi muscle. Serial small deposits of the material should be placed 1 cm apart and should follow a semicircle from the infra-lateral brow along the lateral orbital rim. Things to keep in mind while injecting [1]:

1. Needle should be 20°–30° to the skin
2. Stay 1–2 cm away from the orbital rim
3. Target only the superficial muscle fibers
4. Inject small amounts
5. Inject slowly with the bevel parallel to the skin

Temporal Hollow

HA is the ideal filler for augmentation of the temporal hollow. It is crucial to identify all the vasculature in this area prior to starting as there are many veins. If not identified, the provider risks puncturing them with the needle. The amount of filler needed depends solely on the amount of augmentation required. The technique should be an anterograde deposition of material. The depth and needle used depend on the amount of augmentation needed. The basic guidelines are [1]:

- Mild deficiency: 0.5 mL/side
  - Needle: 30-guage
  - Level of injection: Subcutaneous
- Moderate deficiency: 1–2 mL/side
  - Needle: 30-guage (superficial) or 27-guage (deep)
  - Level of injection: Subcutaneous or Supraperiosteal/Intramuscular
- Severe deficiency: 3+ mL/side
  - Needle: 27-guage
  - Level of injection: Supraperiosteal/Intramuscular

Cheek Augmentation

For cheek augmentation, the provider can use either calcium hydroxylapatite (CaHA), poly-L-lactic acid (PLLA), or hyaluronic acid (HA) (Fig. 21.5).

If the area requiring the filler is the malar or submalar regions, CaHA is particularly effective and should be used if possible. The preferred technique for ideal results is a multi-level and cross-hatching approach in an inverted triangular pattern. This provides structural support for enhancement of the cheek thereby providing a more esthetic result. The provider should inject the filler via multiple consecutive serial punctures using a 25-guage 1.5-inch or 27-guage 1-inch needle to inject 2–4 mL of filler. The injections should begin lateral to the nasolabial fold at the area superficial to the zygomatic bone and move towards the submalar soft tissue [1].

PLLA may also be used for augmentation of the midface. Again, this will be most effective when injected in a layered fashion as was CaHA to provide structural support and the most esthetic result. The injections should begin at the naso-facial sulcus, and small amounts (0.1 mL) should be injected directly above the periosteum. Serial injections should be done along the maxilla and zygomatic bone. As before, the injections should be being just inferior to the muscle and then subsequent layers of material should be placed as you move superficially. The layers of fillers should be placed just above the periosteum layer, at the subcutaneous/muscular junction, and, finally, in the deep subcutaneous tissue. Be sure to massage the area aggressively during and after the injections for 2–5 min to avoid nodule formation. The patient should also be instructed to do the same two times a day for the week following the procedure.

HA is another filler option for correction of a deficient cheek. Again, the layering fashion is key to obtain the best possible esthetic result. A cross-hatching technique should be utilized using 5–8 tunnels throughout the deficient area. The filler should be injected in a retrograde fashion. The use of a cool ultrasound gel to massage the area is recommended to adequately distribute the product. If the provider is using Voluma (a newer HA), a 23-guage needle should be used to deliver the filler in

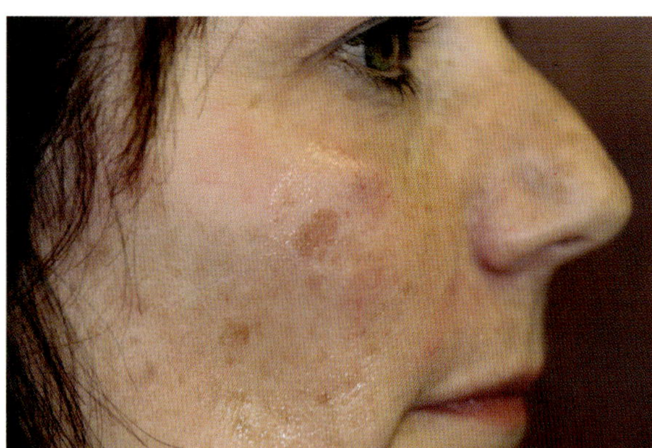

Fig. 21.5 Cheek augmentation with radiesse

retrograde or anterograde fashion. The delivery can be done via bolus, fanning, and/or cross-hatching technique in the supraperiosteal or subcutaneous tissue layer. It is advisable to use ice prior and immediately after administration for better patient comfort [1].

Chin Augmentation

For chin augmentation, the provider can use either calcium hydroxylapatite (CaHA), poly-L-lactic acid (PLLA), or hyaluronic acid (HA). The injection sites on the skin should be marked if anesthetic is to be delivered adjacent to the sites of augmentation as they will be distorted. The mental foramen should be identified and injections of filler should be at least 1 cm away [1].

If the provider is using CaHA or PLLA, the technique is similar. The injections begin at the prejowl sulcus in serial puncture fashion and should extend medially to mentalis muscle. The filler should be placed in the deep submuscular layer using a retrograde threading technique. This should be followed by massaging of the area to ensure distribution of the product and no nodular formation. CaHA works well if patient requests increased volume of the jawline or augmentation of the prejowl sulcus. If using it in the chin area, a linear threading or cross-hatching technique is ideal for best esthetic results. PLLA works well if the patient requests increased jawline definition, correction of their dimples or if they suffer from the peau d'orange appearance of the chin.

The technique is different if HA if the filler chosen. Such as was used in the cheek augmentation section of this chapter, this will be deliver via layering technique just above the periosteum if the goal is correction of volume loss. If the aim to correct wrinkles, it should be delivered subcutaneously. The filler can be delivered using anything from an 18-guage to a 23-guage needle and is based on provider preference. A midline (going from the lower lip to the inferior border of the mandible) and horizontal line (perpendicular to the midline) should be placed on the chin. If using Perlane, the provider should use an 18-guage and begin the injection from the midline and move laterally. The first layer should be placed just above the periosteum using a tunneling technique [1].

Complications

Complications from facial fillers can range from mild to quite severe. Examples of mild complications would be short-term ecchymosis, erythema, or edema. The use of small gauge needles, slow injection techniques, and blunt cannulas can reduce postoperative bruising [2].

More severe complications can include: (1) hypersensitivity reactions, (2) arterial compression/obstruction of blood flow, or (3) intravascular injection causing a TIA and/or blindness [3, 10–12]

Infections following soft tissue fillers is rare, estimated between 0.04% and 0.2% [13]. Infections from facial fillers generally occur early after the insertion but can present years later. These infections can sometimes be difficult to treat and can require debridement of the area and a long course of antibiotics.

One of the most devastating complications is risk of blindness following facial filler injections. The central retinal artery is a branch of the ophthalmic artery supplying blood to the optic nerve. Blockage of this artery would have devastating consequences to the patient's vision. Clinical signs of central retinal artery occlusion are a pale swollen retina with the patient reporting complete loss of vision in the effected eye [14].

Conclusion

Soft tissue facial fillers are excellent options to offer patients who are interested in facial cosmetic improvements. There are numerous different types of facial fillers available and it is important to be well versed with the different material in order to obtain the best clinical outcome. These procedures are very safe as long as the provider is familiar with the basic anatomical landmarks. Prevention is the key to avoiding the majority of severe complications. When complications occur it is important that the surgeon recognizes them and acts early.

References

1. Ferneini E, Jackson T, Ferneini C, Banki M. A review of new facial filler techniques for facial rejuvenation. Am J Cosmet Surg. 2014b;31:166–73.
2. Ferneini EM, Hapelas S, Watras J, Ferneini AM, Weyman D, Fewins J. Surgeon's guide to facial soft tissue filler injections: relevant anatomy and safety considerations. J Oral Maxillofac Surg. 2017b;75:2667.e1–5.
3. Ferneini E, Boynton T, Almunajed H, Dimitrov K, Banki M. Review of facial fillers and injectable neurotoxins. Am J Cosmet Surg. 2013b;30:53–60.
4. Kulichova D, Borovaya A, Ruzicka T, Thomas P, Gauglitz GG. Understanding the safety and tolerability of facial filling therapeutics. Expert Opin Drug Saf. 2014;13:1215–26.
5. Kleintjes WG. Forehead anatomy: arterial variations and venous link of the midline forehead flap. J Plast Reconstr Aesthet Surg. 2007;60:593–606.
6. Vural E, Batay F, Key JM. Glabellar frown lines as a reliable landmark for the supratrochlear artery. Otolaryngol Head Neck Surg. 2000;123:543–6.
7. Hwang SH, Kim SW, Park CS, Cho JH, Kang JM. Morphometric analysis of the infraorbital groove, canal, and foramen on three-dimensional reconstruction of computed tomography scans. Surg Radiol Anat. 2013;35:565–71.
8. Dayan SH, Bassichis BA. Facial dermal fillers: selection of appropriate products and techniques. Aesthet Surg J. 2008;28:335–47.
9. Muhn C, Rosen N, Solish N, Bertucci V, Lupin M, Dansereau A, Weksberg F, Remington BK, Swift A. The evolving role of hyaluronic acid fillers for facial volume restoration and contouring: a Canadian overview. Clin Cosmet Investig Dermatol. 2012;5:147–58.
10. Ferneini EM, Jacob Gady M, Erik Nuveen M. Complications associated with facial soft-tissue fillers. Am J Cosmet Surg. 2014a;31:238–42.

11. Ferneini EM, Ferneini AM. An overview of vascular adverse events associated with facial soft tissue fillers: recognition, prevention, and treatment. J Oral Maxillofac Surg. 2016;74:1630–6.
12. Scheuer JF, Sieber DA, Pezeshk RA, Campbell CF, Gassman AA, Rohrich RJ. Anatomy of the facial danger zones: maximizing safety during soft-tissue filler injections. Plast Reconstr Surg. 2017;139:50e–8e.
13. Ferneini EM, Beauvais D, Aronin SI. An overview of infections associated with soft tissue facial fillers: identification, prevention, and treatment. J Oral Maxillofac Surg. 2017a;75:160–6.
14. Beleznay K, Carruthers JD, Humphrey S, Jones D. Avoiding and treating blindness from fillers: a review of the world literature. Dermatol Surg. 2015;41:1097–117.

Neck Procedures

22

Erik J. Nuveen, Mohammad Banki, and Eric Ress

Introduction

One of the most frequent requests by patients seeking treatment from a maxillofacial cosmetic surgeon is to improve the neck and jawline [1]. Cervicoplasty, more commonly known as "neck lift" can be performed to address these patient requests especially in those patients between the ages of 40 and 75 years old [2]. In Ellenbogen and Karlin's seminal 1980 publication [2], the authors described some important criteria to consider when evaluating surgical success in cervical lifts. These criteria include the cervicomental angle, jawline definition, cervical banding, and submental adiposity.

Identification of the patient's chief complaint is of utmost importance with all patient interactions, but especially in elective cosmetic operations. Although different patients present with a variety of questions and concerns, it is important to address each individual's particular concerns when developing a treatment plan. Patient selection when performing cosmetic procedures requires a thorough preoperative evaluation in order to optimize the surgical care rendered and to achieve the best results. In addition to a comprehensive assessment, knowledge of the head and neck anatomy can improve surgical outcomes by addressing the specific tissues that will be manipulated. The four tissues that we surgically or nonsurgically modify in

E. J. Nuveen (✉)
Cosmetic Surgery Affiliates, Oklahoma City, OK, USA

Department of Oral and Maxillofacial Surgery, The University of Oklahoma, Oklahoma City, OK, USA

M. Banki
Artistic Contours, Warwick, RI, USA

E. Ress
UConn School of Dental Medicine, Farmington, CT, USA
e-mail: ress@uchc.edu

E. M. Ferneini, M. T. Goupil (eds.), *Office-Based Maxillofacial Surgical Procedures*, https://doi.org/10.1007/978-3-030-22371-7_22

maxillofacial cosmetic procedures are: skin, fat, muscle/fascia, and bone. It is best to evaluate each and recommend treatments for all four layers, followed by a summary of the comprehensive treatment recommendation.

Skin

Aging of the skin results in generalized loss of hydration, thinning of the epidermis and dermis, increased vascular fragility, and loss of subcutaneous fat, and accumulation of fat deep to the platysma. Surgical procedures that modify the underlying structures rely on the skin's ability to contract and redistribute in order to preclude a need for further removal of excess skin. When skin is significantly damaged due to exposure to pharmaceutical agents, oxidation, radiation, and the age the aging process, a planned excision of skin must be performed to limit the need for future revisions and to maximize patient satisfaction.

Fat

Fat lies in two separate planes within the neck, one being the subcutaneous plane and the second layer of fat resides in the deeper subplatysmal plane. These fatty layers are most commonly modified by either a closed or open liposuction technique or by direct removal of fat through its excision with surgical blade or electrocautery. Alternatively, adding more fat via fat grafting techniques may occasionally be indicated in order to restore a softer and a more youthful appearance to an aging neck with a significant loss of subcutaneous fat.

Muscle and Fascia

Banding or webbing of the neck especially in the neck midline is a common complaint expressed by patients seeking cosmetic modification. As we age, platysmal banding tends to occur due to the attenuation of the platysma's medial retaining ligaments [3]. These ligaments maintain the medial edges of this muscle approximated to the deep cervical fascia. These anatomical changes could also be the result of fat loss in the subcutaneous plane. This occurs mostly as a result of hormonal incompetence (seen in post-menopausal women) or simply as part of the normal aging process.

Bone

The anatomic shape of the mandible and its relationship with the hyoid bone and its position within the neck establish the cervicomental angle. Microgenia or an inferiorly positioned hyoid may hinder the surgeon's ability to achieve ideal results.

Diminutive chin projection can be modified with osseous advancement genioplasty or through prosthetic implant placement. Male patients often associate a strong jawline with masculinity, and therefore the patient may attempt to grow facial hair or develop a habitual chin posturing in order to mask this "deficiency." The lack of lateral neck definition or a poorly defined jaw line may be the result of inadequate bony support of the cervical soft tissues at the gonial angles.

Procedure

The procedure begins by recording preoperative vital signs as well as auscultation of the heart and lungs. It is critical that preoperative photos are obtained preoperatively for proper documentation and comparison purposes with the post-operative A written informed consent is verified. This is followed by a "time out" in order to verify patient's identity and confirm the proposed operation. Next, intravenous access is gained and a maintenance fluid such as a 0.45% solution of NaCl is started. Intravenous anxiolytics such as midazolam are administered to reduce patient's preoperative anxiety and to benefit from these agents' hypnotic and amnestic properties. The patient is then brought into the operating room where he or she is placed in the supine position on the operating room table. Blood pressure, electrocardiogram, pulse oximetry, and capnography monitors are utilized to closely observe and record all pertinent physiologic parameters intraoperatively.

Moderate sedation is initiated followed by administration of local anesthetic to the incision site as previously marked. A 22-gauge spinal needle on a 10 cc syringe is then utilized to inject approximately 350–500 cc of tumescent fluid into the subcutaneous plane. The tumescent solution contains lidocaine 2% with 1:100,000 epinephrine mixed in a 0.9% NaCl solution. This mix would allow for: (1) local anesthesia (to better manage pain and to lower the need for intraoperative opioids), (2) hemostasis (to prevent excess blood loss), and (3) lipoaspiration. The maximum safe allowable volume is dependent on the patient's weight and must be calculated preoperatively in order to avoid an accidental overdose. At this point, the patient's face and neck are prepared from hairline to below the clavicles in routine fashion using an antiseptic solution such as iodoprovidone.

A planned incision measuring approximately 3 cm is made inferior to the submental crease using a #15 blade. A dissection is made using facelift scissors in the subcutaneous plane, leaving roughly 5 mm of fat attached to the undersurface of the skin. This provides a layer of cushioning and prevents injury to the dermal plexus of the skin.

The dissection would continue to about 2 cm below the inferior border of the mandible and down to the cervical crease. Posteriorly, the dissection should continue in order to allow rotation and advancement of skin after removal of the excess fat and correction of muscle malposition. Particular attention should be made to the lateral aspect of the submental incision. Inadequate resection of adipose tissue is considered poor surgical technique resulting in a prominent "dog ear" deformity.

Open lipoaspiration is performed throughout the region, removing all adipose tissue from the platysmal surface. Attention is then focused on the midline decussation. If subplatysmal flat is evident, it is either resected with direct visualization or via Bovie electrocautery. Although "over-resection" has been shown to be associated with contour irregularities in some cases, [4, 5] we along with Feldman et al. [6] have not found this to occur with proper midline plication or anterior digastric resection. A Weider retractor is utilized to allow for direct visualization of the operative field.

Once the subplatysmal fat is removed, the medial borders of the platysma muscle are easily identifiable. The medial borders of the platysma muscle are dissected laterally from the underling tissue with either electrocautery or facelift scissors to a depth of 2 cm to assure medial mobilization and prevent bunching of the tissue. An inferior cut back of 8 cm or more from the midline is performed and carried down to the level of the cervical crease. Midline plication is then performed with 4-0 PDS suture. The bites of muscle should be at least 1 cm from the midline to ensure strength of re-approximation and to minimize pull through. The most caudal bite should include the deep fascia overlying the hyoid to provide for an ideal cervicomental angle of 105–120° [7]. As described by Feldman [7] in his corset platysmaplasty, a running interlocking suture is placed with a buried knot from inferior to superior and back.

In cases where the patient experiences massive weight loss or has poor hyoid position there are limitations in creating the ideal cervicomental angle. In this case, the entire platysma muscle can be resected at the level of the hyoid and one centimeter below the mandibular border. When this modification is performed care must be taken to avoid unmasking a ptotic submandibular gland or causing a prolonged recovery due to a more aggressive resection. The efficacy and safety of this procedure is well documented.

Liposuction is routinely performed above the platysma using either open or closed techniques. Access is made with a 4.0 mm stab incision centrally with an #11 blade as well as bilateral incisions at the lobular creases. Particular care must be taken when addressing the jowl region with both resection and lipoaspiration. In the event of compartment ptosis or septal dehiscence, fat must be removed by aspiration or chemical dissolution (Kybella) to maximize patient satisfaction [8]. Extreme caution should be used when chemical dissolution is administered due to close proximity to the marginal mandibular nerve.

Upon completion of resection and recontouring, redraping of the skin may result in excess that cannot be reliably predicted. This excess skin must be ressected and requires careful incision planning to utilize skin tension lines. The incision should extend from the preauricular crease, below the lobule, to the postauricular crease, and finally ending at the hairline. Greater laxity may require a longer incision to limit bunching of skin over the sternocleidomastoid muscle. Additionally, the incision should be beveled to assure ideal hair follicle regrowth.

To maximize longevity of cervicoplasty procedures, it is beneficial to perform a subplatysmal dissection and advancement with fixation to the mastoid fascia. Aging results in anterior advancement of the muscle and a woven mattress "tuckster" suture serves to improve the submandibular plane definition [9]. This is similar to a modified Giampapa suture suspension applied immediately inferior to the mandibular border rather than at the depth of the cervicomental angle. A platysmal window technique has been advocated by some as a method to avoid injury to the greater auricular nerve [10]. A simple submandibular dissection at any location immediately anterior to Erb's point will suffice to provide access. Although this technique provides a dissection from underlying fascia, it is perhaps the surgical denervation of the cervical plexus that may result in the greatest of improvement in longevity of neck modification.

The Z-Plasty Neck Lift

In patients with medical conditions that preclude intravenous sedation or extensive undermining procedures, the Z-plasty neck lift offers an alternative (Figs. 22.1 and 22.2). This procedure is often chosen by males due to concerns of the stigma of facelift or postauricular incision scars related to neck lift surgery. Surgeons are generally very familiar with a standard z-plasty procedure.

The Z-plasty is performed after evaluation of anterior neck laxity. If the patient has anterior banding or skin laxity, it is most commonly confined to the region of the medial border of the platysma muscle from the submental crease to the cervical crease. A standard z-plasty may be sufficient to enhance the region. More commonly, a double z-plasty with superior and caudal excision, often called a goblet z-plasty are needed to create the ideal neck form. This can routinely be performed with local anesthesia alone and allows access to the subcutaneous fat, platysma and subplatysmal fat. Closure is performed with 4-0 monocryl and 5-0 fast absorbing gut.

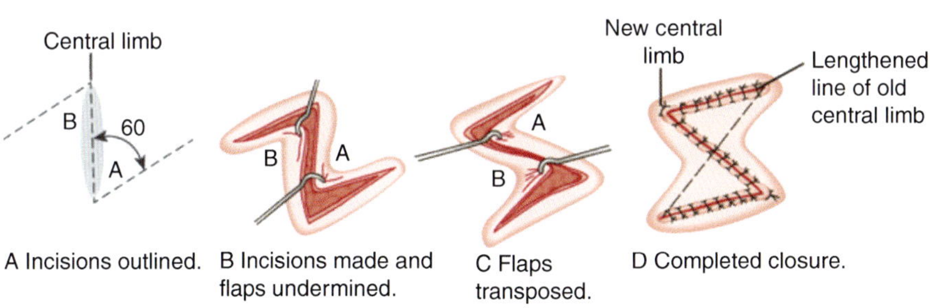

Source: Gerard M. Doherty: Current Diagnosis & Treatment: Surgery, 14th Edition
www.accessmedicine.com

Fig. 22.1 Schematic diagram of a z-plasty rotation of skin

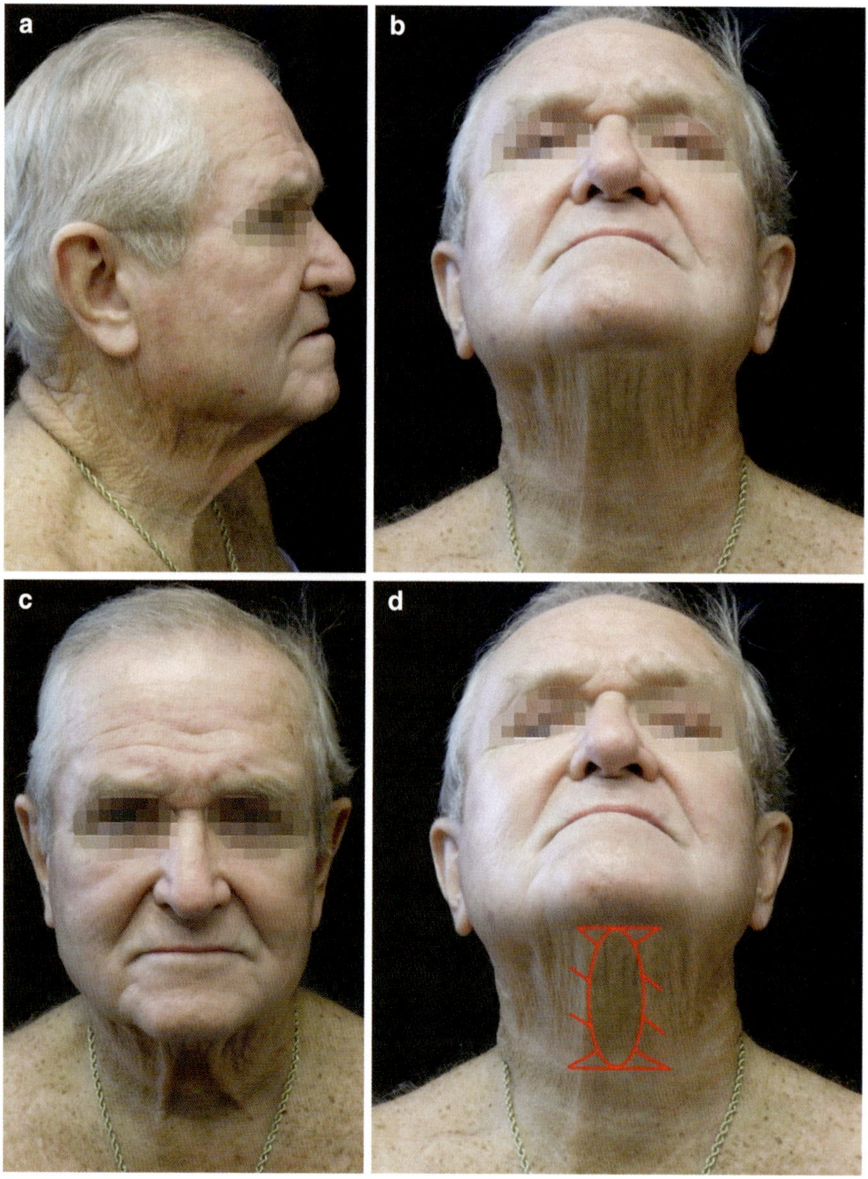

Fig. 22.2 (**a–d**) Preoperative images of a patient presenting for a neck lift. Please note the anterior neck laxity and anterior banding. (**e**) Immediate postoperative image of a patient who underwent a neck lift

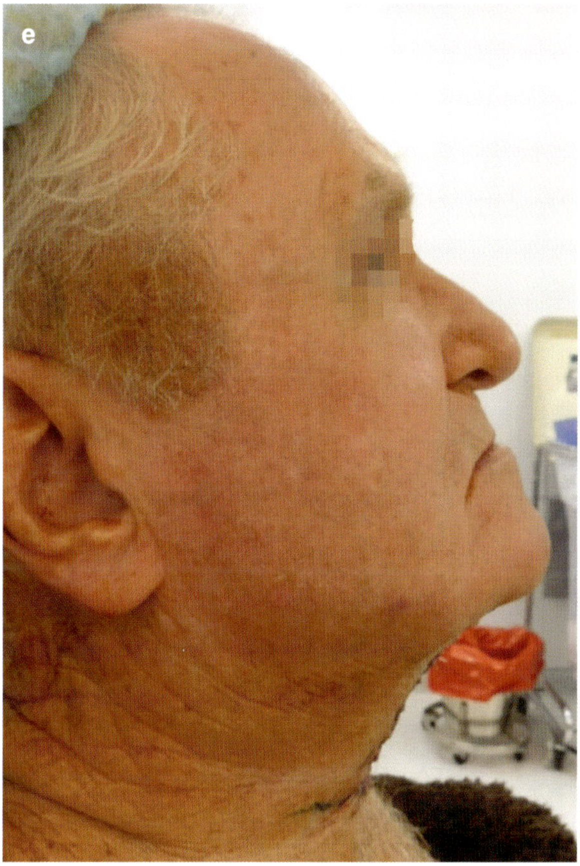

Fig. 22.2 (continued)

Complications

A wide range of complications, while rare, can and do occur following neck lift surgery including acute hematomas requiring emergent surgical evacuation to mild self-resolving contour irregularities. It is critical to understand the various etiologies of different neck rejuvenation complications in order to devise appropriate prophylactic strategies and timely interventions to minimize operative risks. Moreover, appropriate patient selection, mastery of head and neck anatomy, meticulous attention to surgical technique, and comprehensive postoperative care are all critical factors in minimizing and preventing neck lift surgery complications.

Hematoma

There is around a 3–8% rate of hematoma occurrence following neck lift, and the risk is unchanged with the use of a deep plane approach [11]. The rate is 3% in women and increases to 8% in men and those with hypertension, particularly with systolic blood pressures above 150. The risk also increases with the use of certain medications that increase bleeding risk, including aspirin, nonsteroidal anti-inflammatory medications, and melatonin [12]. Prophylactic measures to reduce the risk of postoperative hematoma include ensuring adequate blood pressure control perioperatively and appropriate cessation of medications that increase bleeding risk. Patients with a history of bruisability should have a coagulation workup. Those at high risk for hematoma formation may benefit from the use of tissue sealants during surgery [13]. Postoperative placement of a drain does not significantly minimize hematoma risk [14]. In the event of a postoperative expanding hematoma, urgent evacuation of the blood and surgical exploration for hemostasis is critical. Serious complications including airway compression and skin flap necrosis may occur if not addressed. By contrast, small stable hematomas or seromas may be treated by needle aspiration and a pressure dressing, and can be monitored for resolution. An organized hematoma may not be easily aspirated, and could be removed via a smaller opening through the original incision, suction evacuation, wound closure, and a pressure dressing.

Induration

Following the resolution of a hematoma or seroma, induration may occur. Initial management includes local massage, with or without the injection of a corticosteroid such as triamcinolone 10 mg/mL about one month postoperatively. The patient should be advised that subdermal atrophy and skin hyperpigmentation are potential adverse effects of triamcinolone. These unwanted results may be avoided by using a dilute injection and depositing it deep in the subcutaneous tissue. Often, induration resolves with the aforementioned conservative treatments. However, if skin contour irregularity does not resolve after several months to a year, the surgeon may counsel the patient on an additional procedure to undermine the affected area to enable skin contraction with healing.

Nerve Injury

The most commonly injured nerve in cervicofacial rhytidectomy is the great auricular nerve, and the most frequently injured motor nerve is the marginal mandibular nerve. Injury to the greater auricular nerve can result in temporary loss of sensation to the posterior and inferior outer ear, as well as neuroma. Injury can be prevented by careful dissection in the region inferior to McKinney point where the great auricular nerve runs most superficially. Alternative surgical approach utilizing the preauricular incision circumvents the potential risk of injuring the great auricular nerve. Treatment of any resulting neuroma, which often presents as a painful superficial mass, includes surgical removal [15]. Marginal mandibular nerve injury is the most common motor nerve injury in neck lift procedures, however is often a transient tractional injury which resolves with a few weeks to months. The marginal mandibular nerve innervates the depressor anguli oris, depressor labii inferioris, and mentalis muscles, and disruption can cause weakness of the ipsilateral lower lip. Injury to cervical branch of the facial nerve can also occur and can mimic paralysis of the marginal mandibular nerve, however patients with cervical branch injury are able to evert the lower lip given spared activity of the mentalis muscle [16].

Skin Contour Irregularities

There are many causes of irregularities in the skin contour following neck lift procedures. Removal of too much fat superficial to the platysma is a common cause. Excess fat removal may be prevented by using a small cannulas for liposuction, aiming the cannula opening away from the dermis, and ensuring a conservative approach to fat removal. Preoperatively, gently pinching the neck can help determine excess fat to be removed, with the aim to leave 3–5 mm of subcutaneous fat cushion on flap. If overzealous fat removal results in a single concavity, effective treatments include the injection of hyaluronic acid or other fillers, and focal fat grafting. However, if the dermis has adhered onto the platysma, then the skin may need to be undermined off of the muscle and redraped, with or without fat grafting. Insufficient undermining of skin may cause postauricular skin contour irregularities, and are relatively more common in short scar procedures. The surgeon can release the band with complete undermining of the affected skin and a small area surrounding it.

Infection

There is a miniscule chance of infection following cervicofacial rhytidectomy at around 0.6% [17]. Nonetheless, an increasing proportion of infections are attributed to methicillin-resistant staphylococcus aureus (MRSA). A careful preoperative evaluation with attention to risk factors for MRSA infection is essential. Increased risk is associated with history of prior hospitalizations, diabetes, obesity, smoking, work in healthcare, and/or perioperative antibiotic use. With the increase in MRSA infections, surgical centers have increasingly adopted the routine use of preoperative infection screenings, including cultures of the respiratory tract, groin, and wounds. One proposed practice includes treating asymptomatic MRSA colonized patients with mupirocin nasal ointment 3 times daily, 2% triclosan washes twice daily for 5 days, and chlorhexidine mouthwash 2–3 times daily for 5 days [18]. Other recommendations include initiating preoperative mupirocin nasal swab treatment to all patients, cleaning the surgical site with chlorhexidine gluconate, giving prophylactic antibiotics within an hour postoperatively, giving supplemental oxygen, and ensuring good blood sugar control. Abscesses noted postoperatively should be evaluated for treatment with incision and drainage, culture of the fluid, and initiation of broad-spectrum empiric antibiotics and adjustment based on culture sensitivities.

Platysmal Bands

The persistence of platysmal bands may represent inadequate skin tightening intraoperatively or loosening of sutures. Conservative treatment involves botulinum toxin injection [19]. A surgical option includes submentoplasty, which can effectively treat persistent platysmal bands, submental fat, and redundant submental skin [20]. The procedure uses a submental incision followed by wide local skin undermining, removal of excess submental tissue, and plication of the medial margins of the platysma muscle. A different revisional approach also using a submental incision includes using a corset platysmaplasty [21].

Prominent Submandibular Gland

A large submandibular salivary gland or a ptotic normal-sized gland may present after neck lift surgery as fullness in the submandibular triangle of the neck. Preoperatively, the surgeon can gauge the position and size of the submandibular gland by palpation of the neck during consultation. Intraoperatively, a ptotic submandibular gland can be addressed in a number of ways. To aid in repositioning the ptotic submandibular gland, a midline-to-mastoid submandibular sling suture may be performed [22]. A suture passed through the deep temporal fascia, the gland, and the medial surface of the mandible in a basket fashion has also been reported to yield long-term efficacy in treatment of submandibular fullness caused by normal-sized ptotic glands [23]. Placement of sling sutures can lead to complaint of neck fullness, however. Creation of a platysma muscle and hyoid bone fascia cradle has been described as an alternative [24]. Alternatively, partial gland resection has been recommended by some, with good aesthetic result [25]. Injury to nerves (hypoglossal nerve, lingual nerve, mylohyoid nerve, and marginal mandibular branch of the facial nerve), hemorrhage with potential need for reoperation, xerostomia, sialoma, and hollowness in the submandibular triangle secondary to over-resection of the gland are all potential complications of resection [26]. Postoperatively, less invasive options can also be considered. Injection of botulinum toxin to shrink the gland or injection of filler to soften the contour of the gland can address fullness caused by the submandibular gland after neck lift surgery [27].

Hairline Disruption

Hairline disruption can occur in neck surgery with extension of the postauricular incision through the postauricular sulcus or on the posterior surface of the concha to the occipital hairline. It is critical to approximate the hairline intraoperatively to minimize distortion upon healing. One strategy is to bevel the incision to preserve hair follicles through the incision site [28]. Alternatively, a w-plasty can be performed to minimize the appearance of a scar [29]. To minimize scarring, a tension-free skin closure is key. In cases of occipital hairline displacement, hair restoration can be considered postoperatively to achieve a more natural hairline [30].

Earlobe Deformity

Excess tension on the earlobe from the skin flap attachment may result in anterior migration of the earlobe attachment point, giving it a "pixie ear" appearance. This complication can be prevented by ensuring a normal tension closure of skin intraoperatively. Correction of a pixie ear deformity includes cutting the subcutaneous scar anchoring the earlobe in place, and superiorly shifting the infralobular and postauricular skin flap into the postauricular sulcus [31].

Conclusion

Neck rejuvenation procedures can dramatically improve the youthful appearance of the cervicomental angle. A thorough preoperative assessment, careful intraoperative technique, and appropriate postoperative care are vital to ensuring not only the success of the operation but more importantly patient safety and surgical outcome satisfaction. The most urgent complications include expanding hematomas, which demand immediate evacuation and close follow-up. Induration may result, and may require revisional surgery if skin contour irregularities persist. The great auricular nerve is the most frequently injured nerve, and the marginal mandibular branch of the facial nerve is the most commonly injured motor nerve. Infection as a result of surgery is uncommon; however, surgeons should be wary of increasing prevalence of methicillin-resistant Staphylococcus aureus in infectious complications. Finally, any nonresolving platysmal bands following the primary surgery may be addressed with botox injections, corset platysmaplasty, or submentoplasty. In general, neck rejuvenation is a relatively safe procedure with few complications and gratifying results.

References

1. Nuveen E, Zhu TR, Banki M. Neck procedures. In: Ferneini EM, Castiglione CL, Banki M, editors. Complications in maxillofacial cosmetic surgery. Cham, Switzerland: Springer; 2018. p. 209–19.
2. Ellenbogen R, Karlin JV. Visual criteria for success in restoring the youthful neck. Plast Reconstr Surg. 1980;66:826–37.
3. Nahai F. Neck lift. In: Nahai F, editor. The art of aesthetic surgery. St. Louis, MO: Quality Medical Publishing; 2005. p. 1239–83.
4. Lambros V. Models of facial aging and implications for treatment. Clin Plast Surg. 2008;35(3):319–27.; discussion 317. https://doi.org/10.1016/j.cps.2008.02.012.
5. Narasimhan K, Stuzin JM, Rohrich RJ. Five-step neck lift: Integrating anatomy with clinical practice to optimize results. Plast Reconstr Surg. 2013;132(2):339–50.
6. Feldman JJ. Neck lift my way: an update. Plast Reconstr Surg. 2014;134(6):1173–83. https://doi.org/10.1097/PRS.0000000000000712.
7. Feldman JJ. Corset platysmaplasty. Plast Reconstr Surg. 1990;85(3):333–43.
8. Ramírez OM. Advanced considerations determining procedure selection in cervicoplasty; part one: anatomy and aesthetics. Clin Plast Surg. 2008;35(4):679–90.
9. Reece EM, Rohrich RJ. The aesthetic jaw line: management of the aging jowl. Aesthetic surgery journal. 2008;28(6):668–74.
10. Cruz RS, O'reilly EB, Rohrich RJ. The platysma window: an anatomically safe, efficient, and easily reproducible approach to neck contour in the face lift. Plast Reconstr Surg. 2012;129(5):1169–72.
11. Nahai F, Bryce A. Deep plane procedures in the neck. In: Aston SJ, Steinbrech D, Walden J, editors. Aesthetic plastic surgery. New York: Elsevier; 2009. p. 231–42.
12. Wong WW, Gabriel A, Maxwell GP, et al. Bleeding risks of herbal, homeopathic, and dietary supplements: a hidden nightmare for plastic surgeons? Aesthet Surg J. 2012;32:332–46.
13. Farrior E, Ladner K. Platelet gels and hemostasis in facial plastic surgery. Facial Plast Surg. 2011;27(4):308–14.
14. Kosins AM, Scholz T, Cetinkaya M, Evans GR. Evidence-based value of subcutaneous surgical wound drainage: the largest systematic review and meta-analysis. Plast Reconstr Surg. 2013;132(2):443–50.
15. De Chalian T, Nahai F. Amputation neuromas of the great auricular nerve after rhytidectomy. Ann Plast Surg. 1995;35:297–9.
16. Daane SP, Owsley JQ. Incidence of cervical branch injury with "marginal mandibular nerve pseudo-paralysis" in patients undergoing face lift. Plast Reconstr Surg. 2003;111:2414–8.
17. Zoumalan RA, Rosenberg DB. Methicillin-resistant. Arch Facial Plast Surg. 2008;10:116–23.
18. Malde DJ, Abidia A, McCollum C, et al. The success of routine MRSA screening in vascular surgery: a nine year review. Int Angiol. 2006;25:204–20.
19. Kane MA. Nonsurgical treatment of platysma bands with injection of botulinum toxin a revisited. Plast Reconstr Surg. 2003;112:125S–6S.
20. Bitner JB, Friedman O, Farrior RT, Cook TA. Direct submentoplasty for neck rejuvenation. Arch Facial Plast Surg. 2007;9(3):194–200.
21. Feldman JJ. Correcting problems from a previous neck lift. In: Feldman JJ, editor. Neck lift. St. Louis, MO: Quality Medical Publishing, Inc.; 2006. p. 497–519.
22. Gamboa GM, Vasconez LO. Suture suspension technique for midface and neck rejuvenation. Ann Plast Surg. 2009;62(5):478–81.
23. Guyuron B, Jackowe D, Iamphongsai S. Basket submandibular gland suspension. Plast Reconstr Surg. 2008;122:938–43.
24. Lukavsky R, Linkov G, Fundakowski C. A novel approach to submandibular gland ptosis: creation of a platysma muscle and hyoid bone cradle. Arch Plast Surg. 2016;43(4):374–8.
25. Auersvald A, Auersvald LA. Innovative tactic in submandibular salivary gland partial resection. Plast Reconstr Surg Glob Open. 2015;2(12):e274.

26. Mendelson BC, Tutino R. Submandibular gland reduction in aesthetic surgery of the neck: review of 112 consecutive cases. Plast Reconstr Surg. 2015;136(3):463–71.
27. Connell BF. Male facelift. Aesthet Surg J. 2002;22:385–96.
28. Kridel RW, Liu ES. Techniques for creating inconspicuous face-lift scars: avoiding visible incisions and loss of temporal hair. Arch Facial Plast Surg. 2003;5:325–33.
29. Atiyeh BS, Dibo S, Papazian N, Zgheib E. Overcoming limitations of short scar minimal access cranial suspension facelift for enhanced rejuvenation. J Craniofac Surg. 2015;26(3):800–6.
30. Radwanski HN, Nunes D, Nazima F, Pitanguy I. Follicular transplantation for the correction of various stigmas after rhytidoplasty. Aesthetic Plast Surg. 2007;31(1):62–8.. discussion 69-70
31. Feldman JJ. Earlobe shaping. In: Feldman JJ, editor. Neck lift. St. Louis, MO: Quality Medical Publishing, Inc.; 2006. p. 473–95.

Blepharoplasty

23

Joy Xun Chen, Alia Koch, and Mohammad Banki

Introduction

The eye is an important component of facial esthetics and blepharoplasty can play a vital role in restoring facial harmony and correcting the signs of aging. Actinic and degenerative changes of the facial soft tissues can lead to loss of elasticity of the skin, fat atrophy or redistribution, downward descent of the facial units, and excessive rhytides. Changes in the eyelid appearance as a result of aging may convey an appearance of fatigue, sadness, and diminish the esthetic appearance of the face. In some cases, excessive eyelid skin (dermatochalasis) or pseudoherniation of orbital fat (steatoblepharon) is significant enough to cause a pseudoptosis and obscure the superior visual fields. Blepharoplasty may be performed as an isolated procedure or in combination with other facial rejuvenation procedures such as brow or midface lift as the aging process affects the position of the forehead, brows, and cheek complex which all contribute to the position and appearance of the eyelids. Surgeons must evaluate the periorbital functional and esthetic relationships before performing blepharoplasty surgery. Additionally, patient selection, thorough preoperative assessment, understanding of periorbital anatomy, meticulous surgical technique, and appropriate postoperative care are essential for optimizing surgical outcomes and prevention of surgical complications.

J. X. Chen · A. Koch
New York Presbyterian Hospital, Columbia University Medical Center, New York, NY, USA
e-mail: xc2308@cumc.columbia.edu; ak2045@cumc.columbia.edu

M. Banki (✉)
Artistic Contours, Warwick, RI, USA

E. M. Ferneini, M. T. Goupil (eds.), *Office-Based Maxillofacial Surgical Procedures*, https://doi.org/10.1007/978-3-030-22371-7_23

Anatomical Considerations

Thorough understanding of the anatomy of the periorbital complex is vital in achieving optimal surgical results and avoiding potential complications. To understand the anatomy, the lid complex may be arbitrarily divided into two distinct portions: the upper eyelid and the lower eyelid.

The upper eyelid can be further divided into two segments. The first segment spans the zone between the lid margin and the lid crease. From superficial to deep, the upper eyelid consists of skin, subcutaneous tissue, orbicularis muscle, levator aponeurosis, tarsus or Müller's muscle superiorly, and conjunctiva. These layers are held tightly together by fibers of the levator aponeurosis that cross the orbicularis and insert into the dermis. The second segment of the lid begins at the crease and extends to the superior orbital rim. Its layers consist of skin, subcutaneous tissue, orbicularis muscle, orbital septum, preaponeurotic fat pads, levator aponeurosis, Müller's muscle, and conjunctiva. The eyelid crease is formed by septal fibers from the aponeurosis inserting onto the orbicularis intermuscular septa and the skin. It marks the position where the septum inserts into the aponeurosis, which is also the lowest extent of the preaponeurotic fat pads. If the fat recedes, the crease appears more superior. When the levator aponeurosis becomes stretched or disinserted from the tarsus, it retracts upward, pulling up the septal insertion. In Asian eyelids, the crease, when present, is lower because of the low insertion of the septum into the aponeurosis and thus the lower extension of preaponeurotic fat. Please refer to Figs. 23.1 and 23.2 for details.

When the eyelid opens, the lid crease skin is pulled superior and posterior by the aponeurosis as it retracts under the fat pad. The fat pushes the skin forward, resulting in a slight bulge in the lid above the crease. During downgaze, there is laxity in the aponeurosis resulting in a diminished or absent lid crease. Integrity of the medial and lateral canthal tendons is very important to maintain a proper lid position with aging. These anatomical relations are also influenced by the size and position of the globe within the orbit.

The lower eyelid follows similar anatomy. The capsulopalpebral fascia, equivalent to the levator aponeurosis, fuses with the orbital septum at or a few millimeters below the lower border of the tarsus. Movement of the lower lid is of small amplitude. The crease, if present, is faint and lies close to the lid border [1–3]. Please refer to Fig. 23.3 for details.

Sex, race, and age also influence the relationships of the landmarks of periorbital anatomy. These unique anatomic relationships are an important to take into consideration during surgical alterations of the periorbital region. In females, the brow and lid crease are higher and more arched, and the lid fold is less prominent. In males, the brow protrudes more anteriorly, and the eyelid crease is closer to the eyelid margin. In Caucasian women, the crease is usually 8–11 mm above the lid margin. In Caucasian men, it is usually 6–9 mm above the eyelid margin [4]. In contrast to Caucasian anatomy, the Asian eyelid has more fullness of the upper eyelid and narrower palpebral fissures with presence of medial epicanthal folds and a lid crease closer to the eyelid margin. The lid crease in the Asian population can be absent,

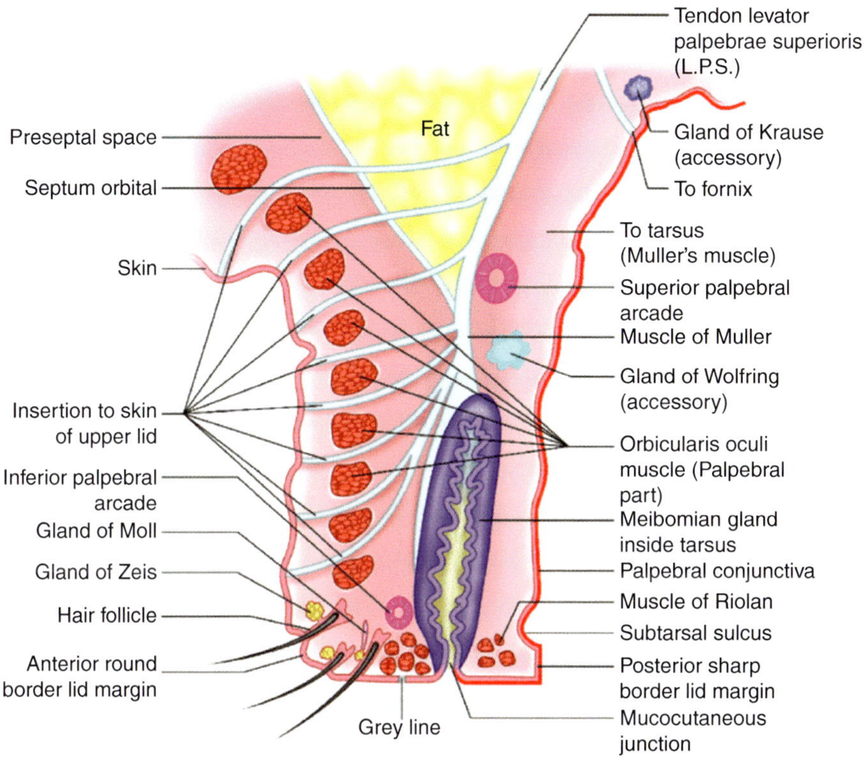

Fig. 23.1 Upper lid anatomy. Ansari M.W., Nadeem A. (2016) Anatomy of the Eyelids. In: Atlas of Ocular Anatomy. Springer, Cham

nasally tapered, and typically lies lower and flatter. This is because the orbital septum attaches to the levator aponeurosis at or slightly above the superior tarsal border or over the anterior surface of the tarsus, causing the lid fold to overlap and obscure the position of the eyelid crease [5].

Indications

Blepharoplasty is performed for various cosmetic and functionally indications. It can be used to enhance cosmetic appearance by creating or modifying eyelid crease or for achieving higher or symmetrical creases. Upper and lower eyelid blepharoplasties are often used to remove of excess skin and orbital fat and plays a vital role in facial rejuvenation.

Functionally, eyelids protect the globe, distribute tears on the surface of the eye, and facilitate the drainage of tears through the lacrimal apparatus. If any of these functions is impaired or significant ptosis of the upper eyelid blocks vision, surgical intervention may be indicated.

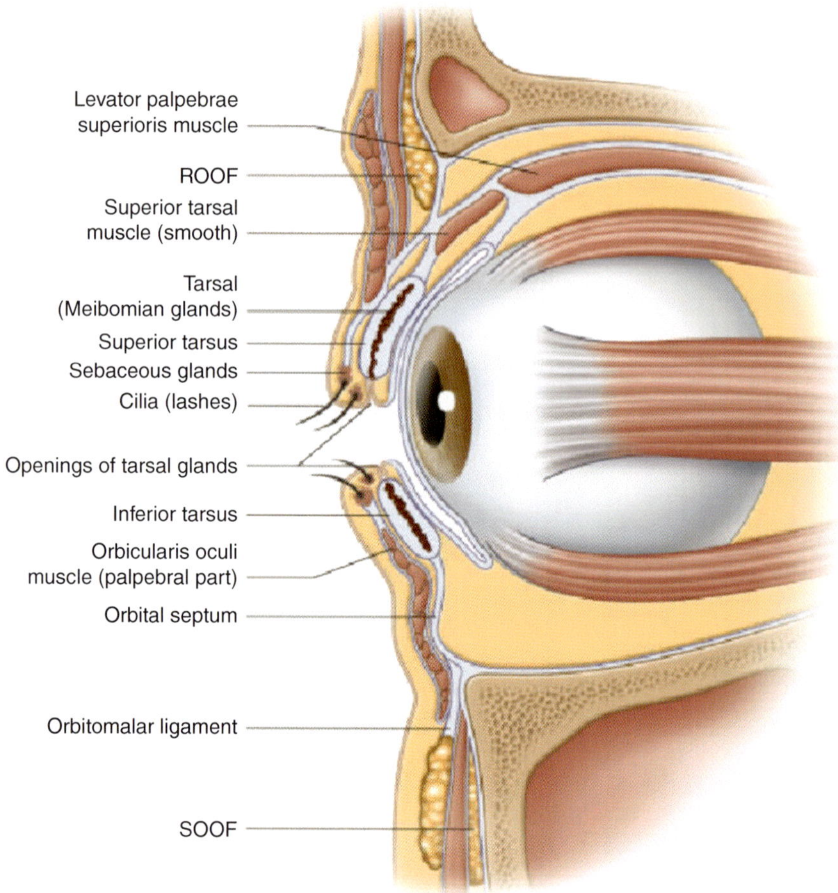

Fig. 23.2 Periorbital anatomy. Benyamini O.G., Hartstein M.E. (2013) Anatomy of the Eyelid. In: Shiffman M., Di Giuseppe A. (eds) Cosmetic Surgery. Springer, Berlin, Heidelberg

Dermatochalasis or sagging eyelids is a common condition with skin redundancy and lid atrophy of the upper eyelids mostly caused by aging. It is typically a bilateral condition and mostly seen in the elderly leading to both functional and cosmetic issues. The overall prevalence of dermatochalasis among individuals 45 years or older is reported to be 16% and is more frequent in males [6]. Dermatochalasis usually results from the normal physiological changes occurring in the periocular soft tissues with aging. Repeated contraction of the orbicularis muscle over time, along with gravity, leads to decreased elasticity of the skin and weakening of the connective tissues in the forehead. These factors result in lowering of the lateral third of the eyebrow and an appearance of excess skin in the lateral corner of the upper eyelid [7].

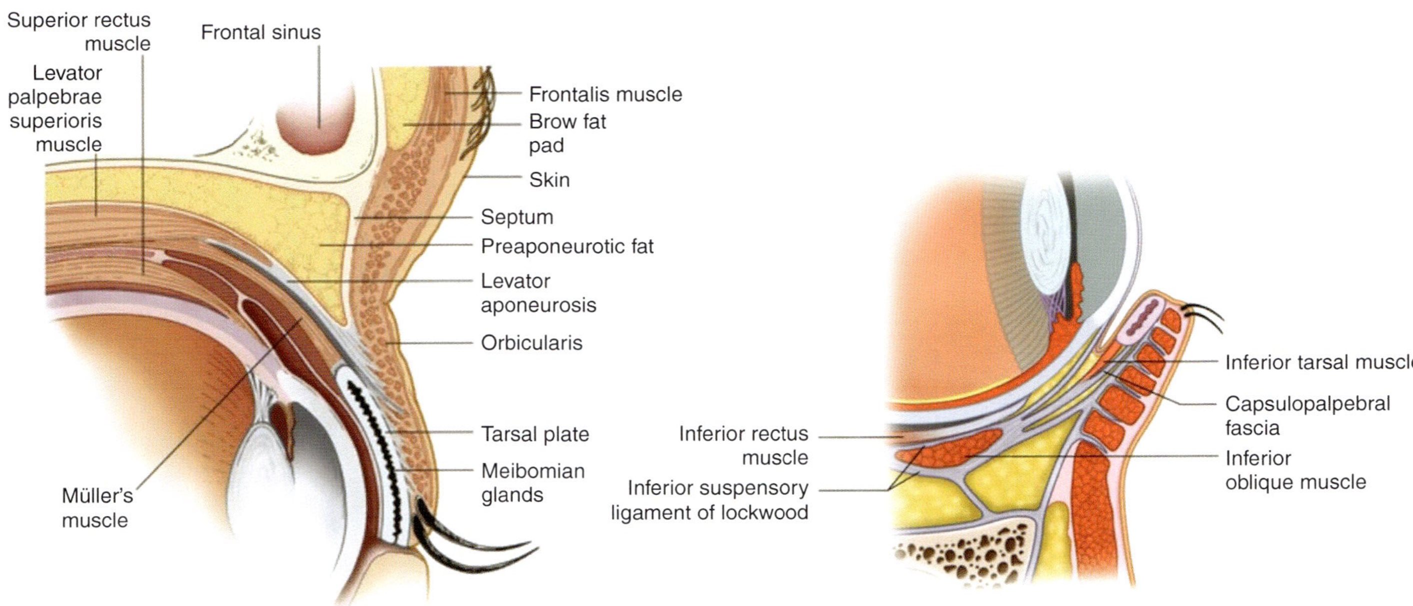

Fig. 23.3 Surgical anatomy of the upper and lower eyelid. Javier Servat J., Baylin E.B. (2018) Surgical Anatomy of the Eyelid. In: Gladstone G., Nesi F., Black E. (eds) Oculoplastic Surgery Atlas. Springer, Cham

The usual presentation is with cosmetic concerns of "droopy eyelids" which leads to a dull and aged appearance. Other complaints include ocular irritation secondary to chronic blepharitis, dry eye, and misdirected lashes associated with lateral lash ptosis and lateral hooding. Apart from the usual complaints, a significant number of patients report obstruction of the peripheral temporal visual field or reduction in the quality of vision, eventually leading to an impairment of daily activities. Restriction in the visual fields due to dermatochalasis is caused by the mechanical obstruction of the visual fields due to overabundance in the redundant eyelid tissue. In addition, the redundant eyelid tissue may cause the eyelashes to deviate and obscure patient's line of vision.

Steatoblepharon, or pseudoherniation of orbital fat, is another indication for blepharoplasty. It is often cosmetically unpleasing and can be associated with lash ptosis. Patients often complain of chronic "puffy" eyes and corneal irritation. Constant microtrauma caused by the ptotic lashes result in damage to the surface epithelium leading to dry eyes and irritation of the ocular surface [8].

Preoperative Evaluation and Diagnostic Approach

History and Evaluation

Prior to any surgical procedure, surgeons must perform a focused medical and comprehensive history and evaluation. Whether performed for cosmetic or functional indications, blepharoplasty is an elective procedure, and underlying medical conditions must be evaluated and treated prior to elective surgery. Specific questions should be asked about thyroid abnormalities, autoimmune and inflammatory diseases, dry eye syndromes, chronic blepharitis, and previous refractive surgery such as laser in situ keratomileusis (LASIK) or photorefractive keratectomy (PRK). Blepharoplasty is relatively contraindicated in patients with active or severe dry eye symptoms or recent corneal refractive surgery such as laser assisted in situ keratomileusis within the past 6 months. These patients are at increased risk for exacerbation of dry eye and development of keratopathy. Patients with thyroid eye disease should exhibit twelve months of stability in their orbitopathy before undergoing elective cosmetic surgery.

Current medications, including vitamins, herbal supplements, and nonsteroidal anti-inflammatory medications, need to be documented. To avoid a postoperative hemorrhage, preoperative clearance must be obtained to stop all medications that cause increased bleeding and platelet dysfunction.

The evaluation should include a thorough ophthalmologic evaluation that includes visual acuity, ocular motility, visual field testing, and basic tear secretion testing such as the Schirmer test. The Schirmer test is performed by placing a strip of test paper over the temporal palpebral conjunctiva and measuring the wetting on the strip after 5 min. If the measurement is less than 10 mm, the patient may have insufficient tear production, which may be a contraindication to blepharoplasty [9].

When evaluating patients who seek cosmetic improvement of the periorbital area, the surgeon should understand the patients' motives for undergoing surgery. Asking patients their expected outcomes for surgery can sometimes reveal unexpected motives or unrealistic expectations. In assessing expectations, the surgeon can help by carefully discussing the surgery and explaining the improvements to be expected. It is important to detail the cosmetic defects that cannot be changed by surgery and establish a realistic plan.

Physical Examination

The position and appearance of the different periorbital structures are evaluated along with the quality of the skin. In the forehead area, the level and shape of the hairline and the position of the brows are evaluated with specific attention to detecting brow asymmetry. The surgeon assesses the relationship of the brow position to the upper lid and makes an early decision as to whether isolated upper lid blepharoplasty is sufficient or whether brow position adjustment is necessary to achieve the desired results. It should be noted that the tail of the brow may be further pulled inferiorly following isolated upper eyelid blepharoplasty. Manual elevation of the brow to the desired position allows the patient and surgeon to assess the role the brows play in the appearance of the upper eyelid. This is done with the patient in an upright position and with the patient looking straight ahead. In males, the brow is positioned along the supraorbital rim. In females, the brow is elevated to a position at or up to 10 mm above the supraorbital rim.

Once brow position has been determined, the surgeon assesses the presence of excess skin, skin laxity, and fat herniation in the upper lid. Upper eyelid aging changes are typically a combination of excess skin or skin laxity, causing redundancy of the tissues. Excess or herniated fat causes the upper eyelid to have a protrusive appearance. The nasal fat pad, the middle fat pad, and the lacrimal gland in the upper eyelid influence the overhang of the upper lid fold. Precise measurements of the eyelid aperture should be recorded, noting the high point of the upper lid and the shape of the palpebral fissure. The position of the lid crease and fold should be documented. The amount of fat to be removed in all fat pad areas is estimated and position of the lacrimal glands is noted. The amount of excess skin should be evaluated after the surrounding structures have been corrected mentally. If a brow lift is also planned, the excess of lid skin will be less. Laxity of the canthal tendons is also noted and manually tightened with the finger before considering removal of any skin.

The inferior periorbital area is evaluated in a similar fashion. The quality of the skin is important, and cicatricial changes from certain dermatologic conditions can make the lower lid more susceptible to ectropion or entropion after surgery. The lower lid fat pads are also carefully assessed and the amount of fat to be removed is carefully calculated. The nasojugal area should be examined to detect tear trough deformities, which may need correction instead of fat pad removal [10].

Skin Marking

Preoperatively, surgical landmarks and planned skin excisions are marked on the patient. Many techniques are used for marking the upper eyelid incisions, but some basic principles should be followed to minimize complications and to achieve reproducible results. Markings should be made with the patient sitting upright in neutral gaze with brows properly positioned. The lid crease incision is marked first, generally following the eyelid crease in the upper lid. The natural eyelid crease is situated above the ciliary margin at approximately 8–9 mm in women and 7–8 mm in men. The lower limit of excision should be along the eyelid crease. Nasally, the incision should be limited by a line drawn upward from the medial commissure, avoiding the deep concavity of the medial canthal region. The lateral extent of the marking should be limited by an imaginary line joining the lateral end of the brow to the lateral canthus. Carrying the incision too far medially may result in scar band formation or medial webbing. Lateral extension of the incision beyond the orbital rim also results in a more prominent and visible scar.

For a clear margin of safety, the superior border of the incision should be at least 10 mm from the inferior border of the brow. This prevents excess skin removal that may cause lagophthalmos and also prevents the blepharoplasty excision from causing downward traction on the brow position. To assess the amount of skin to be removed, the surgeon may use the pinch technique. The patient is asked to gently close the eyelids and smooth forceps is used to grasp the excess skin above the eyelid crease incision just until the eyelashes begin to rotate upward. This is marked as the maximum amount of skin that may be safely removed. A minimum of 20 mm of vertical lid height from the inferior border of the brow to the ciliary margin should be preserved for normal eye closure. Please see Fig. 23.4 for surgical marking details.

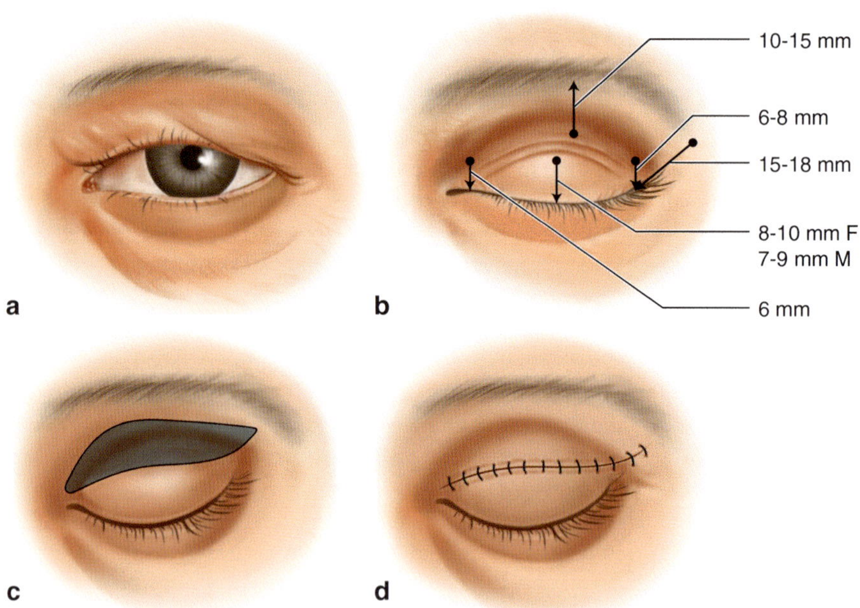

Fig. 23.4 (**a**) Dermatochalasia and lateral hooding of the upper eyelid. (**b**) It is critical to preserve approximately 10 mm of eye skin from the ciliary margin inferiorly and 10 mm from the inferior-most aspect of the eyebrow superiorly to avoid lagopthalmos. (**c**) Area of skin and muscle removal. (**d**) skin closure

Once the skin has been marked with the patient in an upright position, the surgeon gently presses on the globe to observe protrusion of the fat pockets. The location and amount of protrusive fat is assessed and considered for surgical contouring [11].

Anesthesia

Both topical and local anesthesia are used during blepharoplasty surgery. A topical anesthetic such as tetracaine may be used for conjunctival anesthesia if a protective corneal shield is used. Local infiltration provides sufficient surgical anesthesia for blepharoplasties and lidocaine is the most frequently used agent for infiltrative anesthesia. When used without epinephrine, the effects last approximately 30 min. Lidocaine with epinephrine is the anesthetic of choice for most blepharoplasty patients. The epinephrine causes vasoconstriction and therefore prolongs the duration of anesthesia up to 90 min and is beneficial for intraoperative hemostasis.

For local infiltration in upper lid blepharoplasty, 1–2 mL of anesthetic is placed subcutaneously at the surgical site with a 30 gauge needle. The surgeon should use enough agent for adequate anesthesia and hemostasis but no more than necessary because the volume of the local anesthetic disrupts the surgeon's ability to assess the contours of the tissues. When fat pads are to be contoured during the procedure, additional local anesthetic is injected into the fat pads intraoperatively after planes are surgically exposed as the initial subcutaneous injections do not adequately diffuse through the orbital septum to anesthetize the fat.

Systemic sedation can be used in conjunction with local anesthesia to increase patient comfort and decrease patient anxiety. Oral premedication with diazepam at a dose of 5–10 mg may be used to reduce the patient's anxiety. Intravenous sedation may also be administered for induction and maintenance of anesthesia during the surgery. The most frequently used agents include midazolam, ketamine, fentanyl, and propofol. Standard protocol for monitoring of sedation anesthesia should be strictly followed [12].

General Techniques

The patient should avoid using makeup on the day of surgery. Draping should be done carefully to avoid distortion of the brow and lateral canthi and to allow the patient to sit up, if necessary, during the operation. The amount of skin to be removed is marked before infiltration with local anesthesia.

Upper Lid Blepharoplasty

The lid is placed under traction and a Bard-Parker No. 15 blade or monopolar cautery is used to incise the skin to the level of the dermis. The skin flap is then removed with a blade or Wescott scissors, leaving the orbicularis intact. Gentle pressure is then placed on the globe to prolapse the orbital fat and help identify the orbital septum. The fat is exposed by making a small buttonhole centrally through the orbicularis and the septum above its insertion on the aponeurosis. The septum is opened laterally and medially from this buttonhole with Wescott scissors. The fat capsule is then opened and the fat is gently prolapsed with pressure and sectioned. Care must be taken to avoid pulling too much fat from the orbit. The paler nasal fat pad should be specifically exposed and resected to ensure a clean medial canthal area.

The aponeurosis is carefully separated from the orbicularis just above the tarsal border to encourage the formation of a good adherence between the aponeurosis and the skin where the lid crease is to be formed. The orbicularis can be tacked down to the aponeurosis immediately under the upper skin edge using three 6-0 plain gut sutures. Theses eyelid suspension sutures defines the position of the eyelid crease and controls the position of the fat pad in the lid. These techniques minimize the risks of ptosis and allow better attenuation of the lid crease in downgaze than firmer skin fixation.

The lid skin is closed with 6-0 nylon or prolene in a simple non-locking running suture. The area beyond the lateral canthal angle is closed with interrupted sutures to obtain an edge-to-edge closure without folds [13].

Lower Lid Blepharoplasty

Two specific techniques are used for lower lid blepharoplasty. The transcutaneous approach allows modification of the interaction between the muscle and the skin planes and makes lid tightening or canthal repositioning easier. When only fat prolapse is present with no excess skin, the transconjunctival approach allows surgical access without visible scar and avoids the risk of lid malposition.

Transcutaneous Approach

In the transcutaneous approach, the skin is marked 3 mm below the lash line from the inferior punctum to the lateral canthal angle. If excess skin is to be removed or if the orbicularis muscle is to be tightened, the incision is extended laterally and downward toward the earlobe for a short distance. Local anesthetic can be injected through the conjunctiva.

The skin is incised with a no. 15 blade and scissor dissection exposes the suborbicularis plane and the anterior surface of the orbital septum. The septum is easily identified by pushing gently on the globe to prolapse the fat and opened with scissors. The capsule of each of the fat pads is opened. The temporal and central fat pads are one continuous pad separated by a vertical band of fascial connections between the capsulopalpebral fascia and the orbital septum [1]. Care is taken to tease the fat out of the respective pockets without excessive traction in order to avoid deep bleeding in the orbit. In the medial lid the fat capsule is opened separately, and care must be taken to protect the inferior oblique at the time of excision. The fat is carefully examined and hemostasis achieved before it is allowed to retract into the orbit.

A canthopexy can be used to lift a sagging lateral angle by placing a suture through the lateral canthus and attaching it to periosteum. If horizontal lid laxity is present, a tarsal strip procedure can be performed and a small triangle of skin and orbicularis muscle may be excised laterally. Hemostasis is attained carefully before the skin is closed with a continuous suture of 6-0 nylon.

Transconjunctival Approach

With the transconjunctival approach, the lid is everted over a medium-size Desmarres retractor. The lateral fat pad is exposed via a buttonhole through the conjunctiva laterally about 4 mm from the inferior tarsal border. The fat is cauterized at the base and carefully cut with fine scissors. This approach allows early identification of the lateral fat pad before any bleeding occurs. The incision can then be extended medially to expose the central and medial pads, which are removed in the same way. Closure of the conjunctiva is completed with a few 6-0 plain catgut sutures [13, 14].

Postoperative Care

For postoperative care, antibiotic ointment is applied on cutaneous incisions followed by a medium-pressure bandage applied to the lids. The patient can start applying cold packs to the surgical site for 10 min each hour during the first evening and then four or five times the next day. Patients should only require light analgesia following surgery. Severe pain is not expected with blepharoplasties and warrants immediate examination to rule out orbital hemorrhage or corneal abrasion. The sutures on the skin can be removed 5–7 days postoperatively if non-resorbable sutures are used [12].

Complications

Retrobulbar Hemorrhage

Retrobulbar hemorrhage is a rare but serious complication following blepharoplasty. Bleeding in the retrobulbar space may cause an acute compartment syndrome that can lead to ischemic injury to the optic nerve and permanent vision loss. Retrobulbar hemorrhage is most common after lower eyelid blepharoplasty. To avoid this devastating complication, the use of careful and diligent hemostasis at the time of the surgery is of the utmost importance. Hypertension control and discontinuing the use of antiplatelets and medications that predispose to bleeding prior to and after surgery should also be strongly considered. Retrobulbar hemorrhage is a medical emergency and require immediate surgical intervention to prevent vision loss. Severe pain, elevated ocular pressure, and vision changes should raise suspicion for retrobulbar hemorrhage. If retrobulbar hemorrhage is suspected, the wound is opened and re-explored to evacuate the hematoma and find the source of the hemorrhage. Lateral canthotomy and cantholysis may be performed if the intraorbital pressure remains elevated or if the hematoma cannot be completely evacuated. In extreme circumstances, orbital decompression may be required to decrease the orbital pressure [15].

Infection

Infections following blepharoplasty are rare because of the rich vascularity of periorbital area. Perioperative prophylactic antibiotics are often unnecessary. Mild erythema, swelling, drainage, and pain, is often indicative of preseptal cellulitis which is amenable to outpatient treatment by oral fluoroquinolones or third-generation cephalosporins. If orbital cellulitis is suspected, urgent computed tomography is indicated to assess for postseptal abscess and cavernous sinus thrombosis. Patients with orbital cellulitis often present with severe pain, erythema, swelling, changes in vision, extraocular muscle dysfunction, and abnormal pupillary reflexes. Treatment of orbital cellulitis requires hospitalization for intravenous broad-spectrum antibiotics and possible surgical drainage [9].

Excessive Skin Removal

Excess skin removal or inappropriately placed skin incisions can cause cosmetic and functional issues. Excessive skin removal from the upper lid may result in lagophthalmos, ectropion of the upper lid, or exacerbation of brow ptosis. This complication can be avoided with meticulous preoperative measurement of the amount of skin to be removed. Mild lagophthalmos may occur in the immediate postoperative period secondary to edema or myotoxicity of the orbicularis muscle from local anesthetic. Severe lagophthalmos may result from excess skin resection, scar contraction, or adherence of the orbital septum to the skin. Prolonged lagophthalmos may result in serious complications such as exposure keratopathy, stromal scarring, and vision loss. A second operation may be required to release the adherent scar tissue or to place a skin graft to repair the shortening in the upper eyelid [15].

Blepharoptosis

Blepharoptosis is an uncommon complication that may occur secondary to inadvertent levator injury during the procedure. To prevent injury to the levator aponeurosis, conservative dissection beyond the preaponeurotic fat compartments is recommended. Transient postsurgical ptosis is sometimes observed secondary to eyelid edema or hematoma. Corrective surgery should be delayed for at least 3 months in case of spontaneous improvement. Surgical repair of the levator aponeurosis is usually required if the ptosis persists longer than 6 months [9].

Lid Malposition

Lid malposition is a relatively common complication following blepharoplasty. Malposition includes lid retraction, entropion, and ectropion. Retraction and ectropion are caused by excessive skin resection, edema, or scar contraction. Complications from retraction and ectropion include dryness, conjunctival irritation, and exposure keratopathy. Entropion is usually caused by posterior lamellar deficiency. Management of lid malposition is a surgical challenge and is best handled by an experienced oculoplastic surgeon [15].

Conclusion

Blepharoplasty is an elegant surgical procedure for periorbital rejuvenation and restoring facial harmony that can be performed safely in an office setting. However, it is a technically challenging procedure with the potential to cause serious complications. Attaining successful outcomes relies on a solid understanding of periorbital anatomy, thorough preoperative assessment and planning, meticulous surgical technique, and the ability to recognize potential complications. In the hands of a skilled surgeon, blepharoplasty can be used to provide profound cosmetic and functional results for the patient.

References

1. Siegel RJ. Essential anatomy for contemporary upper lid blepharoplasty. Clin Plast Surg. 1993;20:209–12.
2. Doxanas MT, Anderson RL. Eyebrows, eyelids and anterior orbit, Ch 4. In: Doxanas MT, Anderson RL, editors. Clinical orbital anatomy. Baltimore: Williams & Wilkins; 1984. p. 57–88.
3. Jindal K, Sarcia M, Codner MA. Functional considerations in aesthetic eyelid surgery. Plast Reconstr Surg. 2014;134:1154–70.
4. Morrison CM, Langevin CJ. Eyelid and periorbital aesthetic surgery, Ch 22. In: Siemionow MZ, Klein E, editors. Plastic and reconstructive surgery. London: Springer-Verlag; 2010. p. 297–310.
5. Chen WPD. Asian blepharoplasty and the eyelid crease. 2nd ed. New York, NY: Elsevier; 2006.
6. Flowers RS, Flowers SS. Precision planning in blepharoplasty. Clin Plast Surg. 1993;20:303–10.
7. Bosniak SL. Cosmetic blepharoplasty. New York: Raven Press; 1990. p. 37–58.
8. Cahill KV, Bradley EA, Meyer DR, Custer PL, Holck DE, Marcet MM, et al. Functional indications for upper eyelid ptosis and blepharoplasty surgery: a report by the American Academy of Ophthalmology. Ophthalmology. 2011;118:2510–7.
9. Wu C, Wu A, Banki M. Complications of blepharoplasty, Ch 15. In: Ferneini, et al., editors. Complications in maxillofacial cosmetic surgery. Cham: Springer; 2018. p. 183–97.
10. Jelks GW, Jelks EL. Preoperative evaluation of the blepharoplasty patient. Bypassing the pitfalls. Clin Plast Surg. 1993;20:213–24.
11. DeMartelaere SL, Shepler TR, Blaydon SM, Neuhaus RW, Shore JW. Incisional guidelines when marking the skin in upper eyelid blepharoplasty. In: Hartstein ME, Holds JB, Massry GG, editors. Pearls and pitfalls in cosmetic oculoplastic surgery. New York, NY: Springer; 2008.
12. Castro E, Foster JA. Upper lid blepharoplasty. Facial Plast Surg. 1999;15:173–81.
13. Naik MN, Honavar SG, Das S, Desai S, Dhepe N. Blepharoplasty: an overview. J Cutan Aesthet Surg. 2009;2:6–11.
14. Jacono AA, Moskowitz B. Transconjunctival versus transcutaneous approach in upper and lower blepharoplasty. Facial Plast Surg. 2001;17:21–8.
15. Klapper SR, Patrinely JR. Management of cosmetic eyelid surgery complications. Semin Plast Surg. 2007;21:80–93.

Genioplasty

24

Joy Xun Chen and Alia Koch

Introduction

The chin is the inferior topographic limit of the face and thus play a pivotal role in the perception of facial proportions. Proper chin positioning and morphology is an essential component of overall facial harmony. Vertical deficiency or excess of the chin disrupts the balance of facial thirds. Horizontal deficiency or excess of the chin can result in a cosmetically displeasing facial profile. Genioplasty is a versatile procedure that can address functional and cosmetic concerns of the patient. In younger patients, this procedure is typically performed during rhinoplasty or orthognathic surgery to give harmonious balance to the face. In older patients, it is usually performed simultaneously with facial and neck rhytidectomy to give definition to the jaw line and to improve the pre-jowl sulcus. Osseous genioplasty can also increase the upper airway space by repositioning the genioglossus and geniohyoid muscles anteriorly and therefore may be a useful component in obstructive sleep apnea. Osseous genioplasty was first described by Trauner and Obwegesser in 1957 and has continued to be a vital component in the oral and maxillofacial surgeon's arsenal [1].

Anatomy

The chin encompasses a region of the face below the labial mental fold that includes both soft tissue and bone. The soft tissue portion includes the labial mental fold superiorly, the oral commissures laterally, and the submental cervical crease inferiorly. The bony portion of the chin includes the mandibular symphyseal and

J. X. Chen (✉) · A. Koch
New York Presbyterian Hospital, Columbia University Medical Center, New York, NY, USA
e-mail: xc2308@cumc.columbia.edu; ak2045@cumc.columbia.edu

E. M. Ferneini, M. T. Goupil (eds.), *Office-Based Maxillofacial Surgical Procedures*, https://doi.org/10.1007/978-3-030-22371-7_24

parasymphyseal region inferior to the root apices of the anterior teeth. The depressor angularis, depressor labi inferioris and mentalis attach to the anterior surface of the bony chin. Attached to the genial tubercle of the lingual surface of the chin are the tendinous attachments of the geniohyoid and genioglossus muscles. The anterior bellies of the digastric muscles are attached to the posterior portion of the inferior border of the symphysis.

The sensory innervation to the cutaneous chin, the lower lip, and the vestibular mucosa is derived from the mental nerve. It is a continuation of the inferior alveolar nerve and exits the mandible via the mental foramen located between the first and second mandibular premolars. As the nerve travels to the foramen, it takes on an upward trajectory that must be taken into consideration when planning the location and angle of a horizontal osteotomy. To avoid nerve injury, the osteotomy should be placed at least 5–7 mm caudal to the foramen and be executed at a caudal-oblique angle. The motor innervation to the muscles within the soft tissues of the chin occurs through the marginal mandibular and cervical branches of the facial nerve. Care must be taken to protect the soft tissue when making osteotomies to avoid direct facial nerve injury [2].

Preoperative Assessment

Evaluation of the chin in three dimensions is necessary for proper diagnosis and genioplasty treatment planning. From the frontal view, the chin and inferior border of the mandible should be well defined and provide separation of the lower third of the face from the neck. The midline of the chin should also be coincident with the facial midline with no significant deviation or asymmetry. The chin width should be in harmony with the bizygomatic and bigonial facial widths.

The chin's vertical dimension plays an important role in balancing vertical facial thirds. The middle third from glabella to subnasale and the lower third from subnasale to soft tissue menton should be approximately equal in males and females. The lower third can be further subdivided into the upper and lower lip, as seen in Fig. 24.1. The upper lip length should be approximately half the lower lip length, which is 40 mm (±2) in females and 44 mm (±2) in males. Excessive lower facial height may warrant a reduction osseous genioplasty. Deficiencies in vertical chin height may be improved with osseous genioplasty and an interpostional bone graft. Midline asymmetries and chin deviations may require a combination of ostectomy and grafting [2, 4].

Chin projection is an important aspect of the facial profile. A lateral cephalometric radiograph provides accurate image of the facial skeleton and the overlying soft tissues from which to judge profile esthetics when taken with the patient in their natural head position with the condyles seated in the fossa and with a normal freeway space between the teeth. For anteroposterior soft tissue analysis, a vertical line perpendicular to the floor can be drawn through subnasale to assess the relative prominence of the nose, lips, and chin. Ideally, soft tissue pogonion should be 3 mm

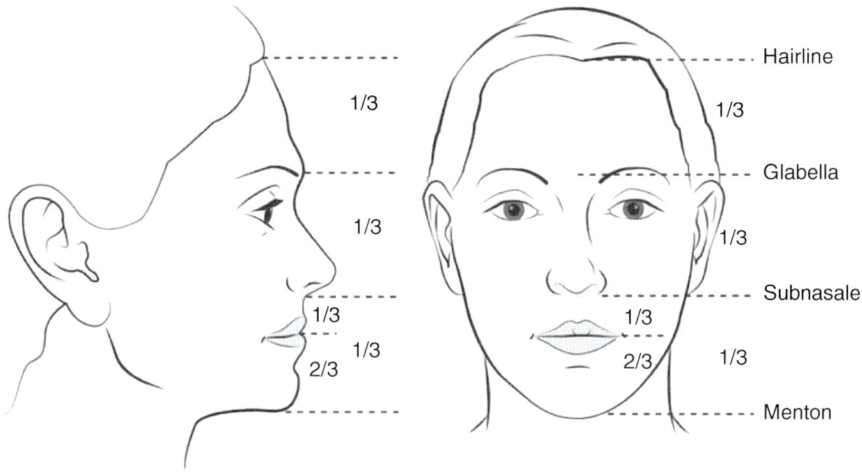

Fig. 24.1 Division of facial thirds [3]

(±3) behind this line, with the lips slightly anterior. Generally, a stronger chin is considered masculine, and a more retrusive chin is considered feminine. The bony chin position can be assessed with NB–pogonion and A–pogonion relationships to the lower incisor. The lower incisor tip and pogonion relationship to the NB line should be 2:1 to 1:1. These analyses assume that the maxilla and mandible are in the proper anterior-posterior relationship to one another and that the lower incisor inclination is normal [4].

It is important to assess other factors such as chin shape, depth of the labiomental fold, lower lip position, and mandibular position. Cultural differences should also be taken into consideration as a weak chin is generally considered more esthetic in Asian cultures whereas a stronger projection is generally desired in Western cultures.

With the advent of technology, virtual surgical planning is increasingly utilized for genioplasties. With virtual surgical planning, cutting guides, positioning guides, custom plates, and custom implants can be fabricated to ensure esthetic outcome and decrease surgical time [5]. This is especially helpful in genioplasties where there is significant asymmetry to be corrected.

Osseous Genioplasty

Osseous genioplasty is more versatile than alloplastic implants in correcting three-dimensional chin position. It can be used to manage vertical and anteroposterior excess or deficiency and correct midline asymmetries. Osseous genioplasty is often performed in combination with orthognathic surgery, though careful assessment is needed as chin projection is influenced by rotation of the maxillomandibular complex.

Anesthesia

Local anesthetic with a vasoconstrictor is recommended for anesthesia and hemostasis. Intravenous sedation can be administered in conjunction with local anesthesia for induction and maintenance of anesthesia during the surgery to increase patient comfort. The most frequently used agents include midazolam, ketamine, fentanyl, and propofol. Standard protocol for monitoring of sedation anesthesia should be strictly followed.

Surgical Technique

Local anesthesia is administered in mandibular blocks as well as infiltration into the submucosal tissue of the chin. The patient is then placed into maxillomandibular fixation with arch bars or maxillomandibular fixation screws to help stabilize the mandible during surgery.

An incision is made through the lip mucosa with 15 blade or electrocautery 3–10 mm below the mucogingival junction extending from canine to canine. Care should be taken not to extend the incision far laterally in either direction as this can damage the mental nerve as it exits the foramen. The mentalis muscle is then divided in an oblique angle so that an adequate cuff is left attached to periosteum for muscle resuspension on closure. The incision is then carried down to bone and subperiosteal dissection is performed with a #9 periosteal to fully expose the symphysis down to the inferior border. Subperiosteal dissection is then carried posteriorly into the premolar region, keeping the elevator along the inferior border. Excessive dissection along the inferior border should be avoided to preserve vascular supply to the advanced segment. A well vascularized pedicled segment is vital in postoperative healing and preventing long-term bone resorption. Dissection is then finally carried superiorly to identify and expose the mental nerve where it exits the foramen.

Using a thin fissure bur, the symphyseal midline is marked in a straight line across the intended osteotomy. To avoid injury to the mandibular teeth and mental nerve, the horizontal osteotomy should be at least 5 mm below the apices of the mandibular canines and 6 mm below the mental foramen. In advancement genioplasty, the osteotomy should extend posteriorly to the molar region in order to avoid excessive notching of the mandibular border.

The osteotomy is initiated posteriorly through both cortices of the inferior border. As the saw is advanced anteriorly, it should be gradually uprighted, reaching 90° at the midline. A finger on the operator's nondominant hand should be used to palpate the tip of the saw extraorally to ensure that both cortices are cut and to avoid over-insertion of the blade that can result in trauma to the mylohyoid and genioglossus muscles and excessive bleeding. The same osteotomy is carried out on the opposite side, with both osteotomies connecting at the midline. If the genial segment is not easily mobilized, the osteotomy should be rerun with the saw to ensure that both cortices have been fully cut. Forcing the segment to mobilize may result in irregular fracturing and sharp bony edges.

Bony fixation is then carried out with plates or positional screws depending on the surgeon's preference and the type of movement desired. Any osteotomy gaps should be grafted with autogenous or allogeneic bone. Please refer to Fig. 24.2 for surgical steps.

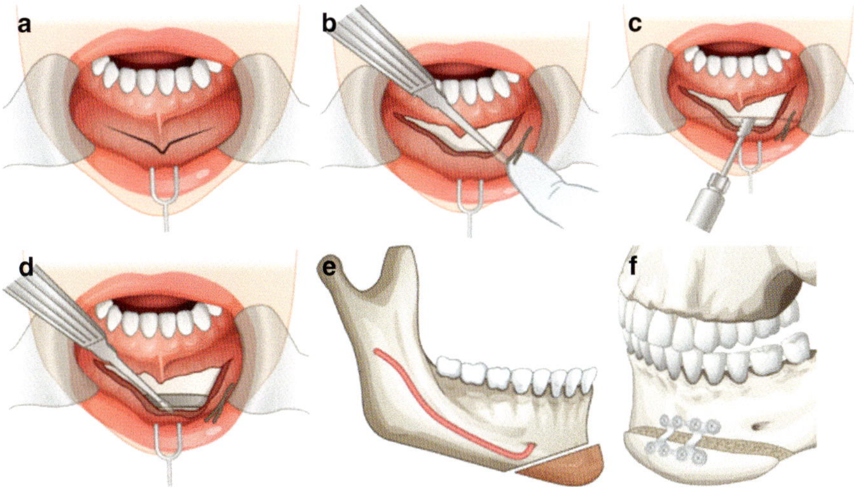

Fig. 24.2 Surgical technique as viewed caudad to cephalad. (**a**) Surgical incision extending from canine to canine. (**b**) Subperiosteal dissection carried to the inferior border. (**c**) Osteotomy with a sagittal saw. (**d**) Mobilizing the genial segment. (**e**) Oblique osteotomy 6 mm below the mental foramen. (**f**) Rigid fixation [6]

The wound is then thoroughly irrigated and closed in two layers. The mentalis muscle is resuspended using vicryl sutures to maintain soft tissue contour and prevent chin ptosis. The mucosa is then closed in a continuous running fashion with chromic gut. A surface pressure dressing is placed to support the soft tissue envelope, minimize edema, and prevent hematoma formation [2, 7].

Alloplastic Augmentation

Synthetic high-density porous polyethylene implants are common in facial augmentation and can be used in several anatomical areas such as the nose, cheek, or chin. Numerous companies manufacture products such as Medpor® and Gore-Tex® implants that can be used for alloplastic augmentation of the chin. Alloplast implants are limited to the correction of a vertical or transverse chin deficiency. A narrow chin or disruption of the jaw line with jowling may benefit from augmentation with an alloplastic implant to enhance chin projection and lateral jaw line contour. Implants offer several advantages, including ease of placement, shorter surgical time, and structural stability. They can be placed via a submental incision and are often placed in conjunction with other cosmetic procedures such as rhytidectomy, platysma plication, or neck liposuction [2]. One potential downside to alloplastic implants is an increase in infection rate, although the infection rates quoted in recent literature seem to be about equal to that of osseous genioplasty. This may be attributed to the development of better implant material. A recent study by Ferneini et al. shows that MedPor implants with larger pores of 100–300 μm allows for a lower infection risk long term due to the ability for macrophages to infiltrate [8].

Complications

One potential complication of genioplasty is hematoma formation which can be devastating depending on the location. Anterior hematomas are often benign and can be treated with pressure dressing or needle evacuation. Expanding hematomas in the floor of the mouth can cause airway obstruction and result in an airway emergency. To prevent this complication, judicious hemostasis is warranted during surgery. A thorough preoperative history should also be taken to check for any coagulopathies and medications that can disrupt platelet function and hemostasis [9].

Inferior alveolar nerve injury is another potential intraoperative complication. This can occur if the nerve runs low in relation to the inferior border of the mandible and the situation is not appreciated preoperatively and adjusted for during surgery. Up to 50% of patients complain of temporary postoperative paresthesia or anesthesia due to edema or stretching from the retractors. Only about 3.5% of patients experience permanent neurosensory disturbances secondary to nerve injury. To minimize the risk of nerve transection, careful presurgical imaging should be done and the osteotomy should be at least 7 mm below the mental foramen. If the nerve is transected, a neurorrhaphy procedure can be attempted [9, 10].

To avoid chin ptosis or a "witch's chin" deformity, the surgeon should avoid excessive stripping of the mentalis muscle. Care should be taken to ensure adequate resuspension of the mentalis muscle when closing. In addition, appropriate chin dressing should be placed to provide additional support to the chin and to prevent hematoma formation [11].

Conclusion

Genioplasty, whether performed via osteotomy or allograft augmentation, can play a pivotal role in altering the profile esthetics of the face. When performed with diligent preoperative assessment, meticulous planning, and precise surgical execution, genioplasty can restore esthetic balance between the skeletal and soft tissue components of the lower face. Both allograft implant augmentation and osseous genioplasty can be performed in the office setting and should be an integral component in the armamentarium of an oral and maxillofacial surgeon.

References

1. Trauner R, Obwegeser H. The surgical correction of mandibular prognathism and retrognathia with consideration of genioplasty. I. Surgical procedures to correct mandibular prognathism and reshaping of the chin. Oral Surg Oral Med Oral Pathol. 1957;10:677–89.. contd
2. Guyuron B, Kinney BM. Aesthetic plastic surgery video atlas e book. New York, NY: Elsevier Health; 2011. p. 179–97.
3. Johnson M. Genioplasty. In: Wong BF, Arnold M, Boeckmann J, editors. Facial plastic and reconstructive surgery. Cham: Springer; 2016.
4. Posnick JC. Orthognathic surgery: principles and practice. New York, NY: Elsevier; 2014. p. 1564–678.

5. Costa PJC, Demétrio MS, Nogueira PTBC, Rodrigues LR, Júnior PDR. A new proposal for three-dimensional positioning of the chin using a single computer-aided design/computer-aided manufacturing surgical guide. J Craniofac Surg. 2018;29:1963–4.
6. Park S. The osseous genioplasty. In: Park S, editor. Facial bone contouring surgery. Singapore: Springer; 2018.
7. Kademani D, Tiwana P. Atlas of oral and maxillofacial surgery: Elsevier Health Sciences; 2015. p. 282–97.
8. Ferneini E, Halepas S. Antibiotic prophylaxis in facial implant surgery: review of the current literature. Conn Med. 2018;82:693–597.
9. Sood A, Caldemeyer C, Ferneini E. Complications of genioplasty. In: Ferneini E, Castiglion C, Banki M, editors. Complication in maxillofacial cosmetic surgery. Cham: Springer; 2017.
10. Ousterhout DK. Sliding genioplasty, avoiding mental nerve injuries. J Craniofac Surg. 1996;7:297–8.
11. Richard O, Ferrara JJ, Cheynet F, Guyot L, Thiery G, Blanc JL. Complications of genioplasty. Rev Stomatol Chir Maxillofac. 2001;102:34–9.

Printed by Printforce, the Netherlands